Immune Hematology

Jenny M. Despotovic

Editor

Immune Hematology

Diagnosis and Management of Autoimmune
Cytopenias

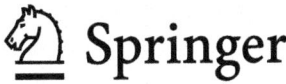 Springer

Editor
Jenny M. Despotovic
Baylor College of Medicine
Texas Children's Hospital
Houston, TX
USA

ISBN 978-3-030-10344-6   ISBN 978-3-319-73269-5   (eBook)
https://doi.org/10.1007/978-3-319-73269-5

Printed on acid-free paper

This Springer imprint is published by the registered company Springer International Publishing AG part of Springer Nature.
The registered company address is: Gewerbestrasse 11, 6330 Cham, Switzerland

Preface

The autoimmune cytopenias are a fascinating and clinically challenging group of disorders characterized by the development of autoantibodies against self-antigens on the surface of hematopoietic cells. The pathophysiology of these disorders is complex and incompletely understood but is generally related to loss of self-tolerance due to immune dysregulation. These disorders can be primary or secondary to underlying systemic autoimmunity or immune deficiency. The diagnosis of these disorders can be challenging and varies significantly according to disease and underlying pathology. While antibody testing is a cornerstone of diagnosis in some autoimmune cytopenias, it offers low sensitivity and specificity for others.

This book offers an extensive overview of immune thrombocytopenia (ITP), autoimmune hemolytic anemia (AIHA), Evans syndrome, thrombotic thrombocytopenic purpura (TTP), and autoimmune neutropenia (AIN). Each section contains chapters covering historical background, pathophysiology, differential diagnosis, diagnostic workup, and management, offering a much more in-depth review of these disorders than is available in most hematology or immunology textbooks. Readers will find many useful figures, tables, and diagnostic algorithms to complement the text.

The first part covers ITP, a condition in which autoantibodies are generated against platelet antigens resulting in peripheral destruction of circulating platelets and often profound thrombocytopenia. The trigger of the development of platelet antibodies is often not identified but is typically thought to result from an environmental stimulus such as infection. The pathophysiology of this disorder is complex and involves the generation of antiplatelet antibodies, T-cell imbalance with a shift in the T-cell profile favoring decreased self-tolerance, and abnormal production of platelets. There are a variety of treatments available for both acute control of bleeding symptoms and long-term management and each will be comprehensively reviewed in Part I.

Part II covers AIHA and Evans syndrome. Autoimmune hemolytic anemia is a rare but potentially life-threatening disorder resulting from antibodies against endogenous erythrocytes and often severe hemolytic anemia. The complications of hemolytic anemia can be devastating and this part highlights the importance of early diagnosis and prompt treatment of the various forms of AIHA. As each type of AIHA has a different pathophysiology, each requires a different management strategy. Evans syndrome is historically defined as the combination of AIHA and ITP but currently encompasses any two (or more) autoimmune cytopenias occurring simultaneously or separately. The antibodies which cause the cytopenias are not cross-reacting but discrete antibodies, and therefore highlight a more generalized immune dysregulation which typically becomes a chronic disease with a number of important complications often requiring immunomodulatory therapy.

Thrombotic thrombocytopenic purpura (TTP) is the focus of Part III. This is a fascinating autoimmune cytopenia caused by autoantibodies against a disintegrin and metalloproteinase with a thrombospondin type 1 motif, member 13 (ADAMTS13), resulting in microangiopathic hemolytic anemia and often severe thrombocytopenia due to consumptive coagulopathy. Prior to the use of plasma exchange, this disorder was almost universally fatal. Experts in this field provide the latest information available on the pathophysiology and treatment of TTP in this part.

Finally, Part IV covers autoimmune neutropenia (AIN), a common cause of severe neutropenia in childhood with a typically benign clinical course. Given the extensive differential diagnosis of severe neutropenia, the authors of this part provide critical information on the typical presentation and biology driving AIN, as well as approach to workup and treatment, if needed.

Within this book, readers are offered an in-depth and comprehensive review of the autoimmune cytopenias. Any hematologist, immunologist, general practitioner, or trainee wanting better understanding of these entities from a historical and pathological perspective, or requiring relevant and up-to-date information regarding diagnosis and management of the immune hematologic disorders, will benefit from these expert contents.

Houston, TX   Jenny M. Despotovic

Contents

Contributors

Vicky R. Breakey, MD, MEd, FRCPC (Peds) Department of Pediatrics, McMaster University, Hamilton, ON, Canada

Alicia K. Chang, MD Section of Hematology-Oncology, Department of Pediatrics, Baylor College of Medicine, Texas Children's Hospital, Houston, TX, USA

Satheesh Chonat, MD Pediatric Hematology, Department of Pediatrics, Emory University School of Medicine and Aflac Cancer and Blood Disorders Center, Children's Healthcare of Atlanta, Atlanta, GA, USA

Clay Cohen, MD Department of Pediatric Hematology and Oncology, Baylor College of Medicine, Houston, TX, USA

Kandace L. Gollomp, MD Division of Hematology, The Children's Hospital of Philadelphia, Philadelphia, PA, USA

Amanda B. Grimes, MD Baylor College of Medicine, Texas Children's Hospital, Houston, TX, USA

Kristina M. Haley, DO, MCR Pediatric Hematology/Oncology, Department of Pediatrics, Oregon Health and Science University, Portland, OR, USA

Michele P. Lambert, MD Division of Hematology, The Children's Hospital of Philadelphia, Philadelphia, PA, USA

Omar Niss, MD Division of Hematology, Department of Pediatrics, Cincinnati Children's Hospital Medical Center and University of Cincinnati College of Medicine, Cincinnati, OH, USA

Taylor Olmsted Kim, MD Section of Hematology/Oncology, Department of Pediatrics, Texas Children's Cancer and Hematology Centers, Baylor College of Medicine, Houston, TX, USA

Jacquelyn M. Powers, MD, MS Pediatric Hematology/Oncology, Baylor College of Medicine, Texas Children's Cancer and Hematology Center, Houston, TX, USA

Shawki Qasim, MD Baylor College of Medicine, Texas Children's Hospital, Houston, TX, USA

Sarah E. Sartain, MD Baylor College of Medicine, Texas Children's Hospital, Houston, TX, USA

Russell E. Ware, MD, PhD Division of Hematology, Department of Pediatrics, Cincinnati Children's Hospital Medical Center and University of Cincinnati College of Medicine, Cincinnati, OH, USA

Part I
Immune Thrombocytopenia (ITP)

Chapter 1
Background of Immune Thrombocytopenia

Kristina M. Haley

Introduction

Immune thrombocytopenia (ITP, formerly idiopathic thrombocytopenic purpura) is an acquired disease characterized by immune-mediated destruction of normal platelets and suppression of platelet production that is associated with variable bleeding symptoms [1]. Primary ITP is characterized by isolated thrombocytopenia in the absence of any clear underlying cause or initiating factor [2]. Secondary ITP is defined as ITP that is associated with an underlying cause or precipitating factor [3]. The variable disease definitions and the heterogeneity of symptoms suggest that the actual incidence is not clear [1]. However, a 2009 study of published ITP literature estimated the incidence of ITP in adults to be 3.3 per 100,000 adults/year, while the incidence of ITP in children was estimated to be 1.9–6.4 per 100,000 children/year [4]. There is a female preponderance in young adults, but in older adults, ITP affects males and females equally [1]. In pediatric patients, ITP affects males more often in the younger years and females more often in the older years [5].

Patients with ITP present with isolated thrombocytopenia (though anemia secondary to blood loss may be present) and variable bleeding symptoms which range from asymptomatic to severe, life-threatening bleeding. The diagnosis of ITP is one of exclusion [6]. The natural history in the majority of pediatric patients with ITP is spontaneous resolution, and treatment is aimed at ameliorating symptoms while awaiting spontaneous resolution. The majority of adult patients receive some upfront treatment, but majority of many will not require ongoing therapy. The likelihood of remission decreases as the duration of ITP increases [1].

The underlying etiology of ITP is immune dysregulation resulting in a combination of increased platelet destruction and impaired platelet production [5, 7]. Antiplatelet

K. M. Haley, DO, MCR
Pediatric Hematology/Oncology, Department of Pediatrics, Oregon Health and Science
University, Portland, OR, USA
e-mail: haley@ohsu.edu

© Springer International Publishing AG, part of Springer Nature 2018
J. M. Despotovic (ed.), *Immune Hematology*,
https://doi.org/10.1007/978-3-319-73269-5_1

antibodies, directed at platelet and megakaryocyte surface glycoproteins, develop secondary to a loss of tolerance of these self-antigens [5]. Antiplatelet antibodies bind to circulating platelets and result in their phagocytosis by splenic macrophages. In addition, antiplatelet antibodies bind to megakaryocytes and result in impaired megakaryocyte maturation and/or apoptosis [5, 7]. Dysregulation or dysfunction of T cells likely also plays a role in impaired self-tolerance and in development of autoimmunity [5, 8]. The understanding of the mechanisms at play in ITP is evolving and shaping the understanding of the disease and the recommendations for treatments. The pathophysiology of ITP will be comprehensively reviewed in Chap. 2.

In this chapter, the historical understanding of ITP, the evolution of the terminology around ITP, and the clinical presentation including distinction between primary and secondary ITP as well as the development of a differential diagnosis will be discussed.

Historical Perspective

Long before platelets were identified, clinical symptoms associated with thrombocytopenia were noted and recorded. Early descriptions of otherwise healthy individuals with purpura likely fit our current definition of ITP and are recorded as early as 1025 [9]. The classical clinical description of ITP was first noted by Paul Gottlieb Werlhof in 1735, as he described a 16-year-old female with mucosal bleeding which developed following an infection [9, 10]. The link to thrombocytopenia was not made until years later, as platelets were not described until the 1800s, with the advent of improved microscopy techniques [11]. The first drawing of platelets occurred in 1841, but it was not until 1882 that the term "platelets" was used to describe an independent blood cell line with hemostatic function [11, 12]. The first report connecting thrombocytopenia and petechiae or purpura was published in 1883 [9]. Just a few years later, it was observed that the appearance of petechiae correlated with thrombocytopenia and the disappearance correlated with resolution of thrombocytopenia [9]. Despite these observations, the underlying pathophysiology of the thrombocytopenia remained unknown.

Two theories emerged in the early twentieth century regarding the etiology of thrombocytopenia: decreased platelet production vs. increased platelet destruction [10, 13]. In support of impaired production, Ernest Frank posited that a toxic substance produced by the spleen resulted in impaired platelet production by megakaryocytes [9, 10]. And, in opposition, Paul Kaznelson proposed that there was increased platelet destruction in the spleen [9, 10]. Though still a student, Kaznelson convinced his mentor to perform a splenectomy on one of his patients with chronic ITP, and the patient's thrombocytopenia improved [9]. This debate over decreased production vs. increased destruction continued over the next few decades. In 1942, Troland and Lee suggested that a substance produced by the spleen, what they called "thrombocytopen," caused ITP. Observations by Dameshek and Miller, published in 1946, ultimately led to the conclusion that ITP was due to an abnormality of the spleen which led to impaired megakaryocyte production of platelets [10, 14].

A series of experiments conducted by William Harrington and James Hollingsworth in 1951 provided evidence in support of peripheral destruction as the etiology of ITP. Dr. Harrington infused whole blood from a patient with known ITP into himself and others in order to determine the effect on circulating platelets. He became severely thrombocytopenic and developed bleeding symptoms soon after the infusion. Bone marrow examination done before and after the infusion demonstrated increased megakaryocytes at the time of thrombocytopenia. His platelet count recovered within 1 week. Of note, he had a generalized seizure soon after the infusion and was hospitalized due to his bleeding symptoms and thrombocytopenia. He performed this experiment again on volunteers from his lab and non-ITP patients and found similar findings in a subset of those infused. This was the first study to demonstrate the importance of host factors in the development of ITP. He later demonstrated that the factor resulting in thrombocytopenia was in the gamma-globulin fraction of plasma [9, 10, 12]. While these series of experiments would never be approved in today's research milieu, they led to a significant improvement in our understanding of the pathophysiology of ITP, specifically highlighting the role of decreased platelet survival secondary to a humoral factor [9]. In the same year as the Harrington and Hollingsworth experiments, Evans and colleagues attributed the syndrome to an antiplatelet antibody [10]. Several years later, additional work demonstrated that the antiplatelet antibody was associated with immunoglobulin G (IgG) [9] and directed against platelet glycoproteins [13].

Interestingly, the debate of increased destruction vs. decreased production continued even once antiplatelet antibodies were identified. Studies with radiolabeled platelets demonstrated significant heterogeneity in platelet turnover, with many patients producing less platelets than expected for the degree of thrombocytopenia [15]. These experiments revitalized the idea that decreased platelet production contributed to the thrombocytopenia seen in ITP. Experiments performed evaluating the effect of antiplatelet antibodies on megakaryocytopoiesis confirmed impaired platelet production in ITP [16, 17]. Evaluation of megakaryocyte ultrastructure using electron microscopy has added additional data in support of impaired platelet production in ITP [18]. However, the absence of antiplatelet antibodies in a proportion of patients spurred an additional hypothesis to explain the thrombocytopenia in ITP: cytotoxic T-lymphocyte (CTL)-mediated platelet lysis. Early experiments demonstrated increased CTL expression of cytotoxic genes as well as increased platelet lysis by CTLs in patients with active ITP and no platelet lysis in patients with ITP in remission [19]. Further, improved understanding of the immune system as well as further study of chronic ITP resulted in appreciation for the importance of immune dysregulation in the development of ITP.

Terminology

The abbreviation ITP has been defined in a number of ways over the years, including idiopathic thrombocytopenic purpura, immune thrombocytopenic purpura, and immune thrombocytopenia. In addition, other aspects of ITP, such as response criteria or bleeding symptoms, have been variably defined. These inconsistencies have resulted in difficulty in standardization of research, in applicability of research results to different clinical populations, and in communications regarding ITP. An International Working Group (IWG) was formed and convened in 2007 to address the inconsistencies and develop standardization in terminology.

In 2009, the culmination of the collaborative efforts of the International Working Group (IWG) was published and provided a reference for terminology [3]. The 2011 American Society of Hematology (ASH) guidelines on ITP call for the utilization of the IWG standard terminology as well as refinement of the terminology in areas of continued debate [20].

The IWG proposed that the acronym ITP stands for immune thrombocytopenia [3]. The term "idiopathic" was removed from the definition, while the term "immune" was kept in order to highlight the known pathophysiologic mechanisms. Purpura was removed due to the variability of this clinical finding. Immune thrombocytopenia is defined as isolated thrombocytopenia in the absence of any underlying cause [2]. The threshold for diagnosis was set at a platelet count of $100 \times 10^9/L$ [3, 19, 20]. The IWG also proposed that secondary immune thrombocytopenia be broadly defined as all immune-mediated thrombocytopenia that is not primary ITP

Table 1.1 Examples of conditions associated with secondary ITP

Autoimmune and immune dysregulation disorders	Evans syndrome Autoimmune lymphoproliferative syndrome (ALPS) Systemic lupus erythematosus (SLE) Antiphospholipid antibody syndrome (APS) Autoimmune thyroid disease Combined variable immunodeficiency (CVID)
Malignant lymphoproliferative disorders	Chronic lymphocytic leukemia (CLL) Large granular T-lymphocytic leukemia Hodgkin lymphoma
Infections	*Helicobacter pylori* Human immunodeficiency virus (HIV) Hepatitis C Cytomegalovirus (CMV) Varicella zoster virus (VZV)
Drug effects	Strong evidence for quinine, quinidine, trimethoprim/sulfamethoxazole, vancomycin, penicillin, rifampin, carbamazepine, ceftriaxone, ibuprofen, mirtazapine, oxaliplatin, suramin, glycoprotein IIb/IIIa inhibitors (abciximab, tirofiban, eptifibatide), heparin
Others	Vaccine side effect (MMR) Post bone marrow or solid organ transplantation

[3]. Further, the IWG recommended that secondary ITP should be designated by the terminology "secondary ITP" followed by the associated disease or drug in parentheses [3]. Secondary causes of ITP include medications, viral infections such as hepatitis C or human immunodeficiency virus, and autoimmune disorders such as systemic lupus erythematosus or antiphospholipid antibody syndrome (Table 1.1—causes of secondary ITP).

ITP was previously split into two groups: acute ITP and chronic ITP. Acute ITP was described as a self-limited disease lasting less than 6 months, and persistent thrombocytopenia beyond 6 months was termed chronic ITP. A challenge to these definitions was that acute ITP could only truly be defined retrospectively. The IWG proposed three phases of ITP which can be used both prospectively and retrospectively: newly diagnosed (0–3 months), persistent (3–12 months), and chronic ITP (>12 months) [3]. These distinctions have been widely implemented and are important as they may help guide therapy or prognostication. For example, there is still a significant chance of remission in those with persistent ITP, which may help guide decisions regarding aggressiveness of therapy [22]. Definitions of disease severity are less well-defined. Historically, disease severity (mild, moderate, severe) has been correlated solely with degree of thrombocytopenia. The IWG recommended that the designation of severe ITP should be reserved for clinically significant bleeding that necessitates intervention [3]. This definition may result in decreased intervention in a patient with significant thrombocytopenia but no clinical bleeding [21].

Response criteria were a major focus of the IWG to facilitate comparison of clinical studies and to guide therapy. While they acknowledged that clinically relevant endpoints would be ideal, surrogate endpoints like platelet count are objective and more easily compared [3]. The IWG proposed the following definitions [3]:

- Complete response (CR): any platelet count of at least 100×10^9/L
- Response (R): any platelet count between 30 and 100×10^9/L PLUS resolution of bleeding symptoms
- No response (NR): any platelet count less than 30×10^9/L or less than doubling of the baseline count
- Corticosteroid dependence: ongoing need for continuous corticosteroid or frequent courses of corticosteroids beyond 2 months to maintain a platelet count at or above 30×10^9/L and to avoid bleeding

Notably, patients with corticosteroid dependence are considered nonresponders. Duration of response is measured from the achievement of CR or R to loss of CR or R. Patients with refractory ITP are defined as those who fulfill two criteria: (1) nonresponder to splenectomy or relapse after splenectomy and (2) severe ITP or high risk for bleeding [3]. The various types of therapy were also more clearly defined by the IWG. On-demand therapy was defined as any therapy used to temporarily increase the platelet count to safely perform invasive procedures or to treat major bleeding or in the event of trauma. Adjunctive therapy includes any therapy that is not ITP specific. For example, antifibrinolytics, hormonal therapy, and DDAVP are considered adjunctive therapies [3].

The standardized terminology developed by the IWG has been incorporated into treatment guidelines [2, 20], facilitating communications between treating providers. In addition, the establishment of clear definitions and terms for ITP has helped to classify patients into subgroups, to design clinical trials, and to interpret and apply results [6]. The adaptability of the IWG consensus terminology was evaluated in a clinical population of pediatric patients in 2012 [23]. In this study, the majority of patients with ITP could be easily classified using the new criteria. However, the investigators noted a few limitations. Specifically, the authors found the exclusion of secondary ITP by the IWG in the application of the standardized terminology to result in exclusion of several patients with Evans syndrome. This population of patients often has symptomatic ITP that is challenging to treat and would benefit from inclusion in clinical studies as well as from comparison using standardized terminology. Further, the authors found that the duration of response criteria was difficult to apply retrospectively. Finally, the authors note that the IWG terminology is limited in its definition of refractory ITP in a pediatric patient [23].

Presentation

ITP should be suspected in a patient presenting with an isolated thrombocytopenia, an otherwise unremarkable peripheral smear, and exam findings significant for expected bleeding for platelet count [8]. Bleeding is the most common presenting symptom in ITP [7] and is typically mucocutaneous, resulting in petechiae, purpura, and bruising. Examples of more significant bleeding include epistaxis, oral bleeding, urinary bleeding, gastrointestinal bleeding, and/or heavy menstrual bleeding [7]. Intracranial hemorrhage is a rare but life-threatening complication. Pediatric patients typically have an acute onset of bleeding symptoms and are otherwise clinically well. A preceding viral infection is seen in approximately two-thirds of pediatric patients [25]. In contrast, ITP can be insidious in adults and more frequently becomes a chronic disease [26].

Severe hemorrhage is rare in patients with platelet counts $>30 \times 10^9$/L [5, 22]. A recent systematic review analyzed the incidence of severe hemorrhage across several prospective ITP studies [21]. Intracranial hemorrhage (ICH) occurred in 0.4% of newly diagnosed pediatric patients with ITP and 0.6% of adult patients with ITP [21]. There is a higher incidence of ICH in chronic ITP, occurring in 1.3% and 1.8% of pediatric and adult patients, respectively [21]. Other severe bleeding occurred in 20.2% of pediatric patients and 9.6% of adult patients with ITP [21]. In the systematic review, no predictors of severe bleeding were identified, but association of severe bleeding with lower platelet counts (below $10–20 \times 10^9$/L) and minor bleeding was observed [21]. The heterogeneous nature of ITP and the lack of prediction tools make application of treatment algorithms difficult.

Primary ITP and Secondary ITP

As stated previously, primary ITP is defined as immune-mediated thrombocytopenia in the absence of any identified causative factors [7]. It is a diagnosis of exclusion. However, distinguishing primary ITP from secondary ITP can be difficult, as patients with primary ITP are sometimes found to have a positive direct antiglobulin test or other autoantibodies [1]. There is likely significant heterogeneity among patients with primary ITP, particularly between patients with self-resolving ITP and patients who develop chronic ITP. Further, some patients develop ITP following an infectious illness, while most people with the same infectious illness do not develop ITP. Differences in development of cross-reactive antibodies and in immune response likely influence the risk of ITP development [25].

Secondary ITP is defined as immune-mediated thrombocytopenia with an associated underlying cause (Table 1.1). Approximately 20% of ITP is secondary [8]. Frequently, the focus in treatment of secondary ITP is on the underlying disease, as optimal disease control typically results in improved thrombocytopenia. A review of adult patients with primary and secondary ITP noted that patients with secondary ITP were older and had higher platelet counts at diagnosis, suggesting a more insidious onset [26]. A variety of underlying disorders and medications have been associated with ITP, with the most common underlying disorder being an autoimmune disease [25].

It has been proposed that each underlying cause of secondary ITP mediates thrombocytopenia through different mechanisms [8]. In systemic lupus erythematosus (SLE), up to 25% of patients develop thrombocytopenia. The etiology of the thrombocytopenia is multifactorial and has been attributed to a combination of anti-platelet antibodies, immune complexes, antiphospholipid antibodies, vasculitis, thrombotic microangiopathy, hemophagocytosis, bone marrow abnormalities, and megakaryocyte antibodies [25]. Antiphospholipid antibodies (APLA) are found in a wide range of patients with ITP, though it is not clear what the clinical significance of these antibodies are and if they are involved in clearance of platelets [8]. Evans syndrome is the combination of immune cytopenias, including most commonly ITP and autoimmune hemolytic anemia but can also include immune neutropenia. ITP in Evans syndrome can be difficult to treat, and refractory disease is not uncommon [8, 25]. Similarly, ITP in autoimmune lymphoproliferative syndrome (ALPS) is less responsive to standard initial ITP therapy [8, 25] (see Section "Clinical Presentation" Chap. 3 and Part II Chap. 7 for more information on Evans syndrome and secondary causes of immune cytopenias).

Infection-related ITP is most commonly associated with *Helicobacter pylori*, hepatitis C virus (HCV), cytomegalovirus (CMV), human immunodeficiency virus, and varicella zoster virus (VZV). While *H. pylori* is not an uncommon infection, *H. pylori*-associated ITP is rare. The pathogenesis is related to molecular mimicry with the bacteria inducing antibodies that cross-react with platelets [8]. Current American Society of Hematology (ASH) guidelines do not recommend testing for *H. pylori* in pediatric patients with ITP and recommend testing in only those adult patients in whom treatment would be recommended if testing were positive [20]. Thrombocytopenia in HCV is likely multifactorial, a combination of immune-mediated platelet destruction, impaired thrombopoietin production, and marrow suppression [8]. ASH guidelines recommend testing adult patients with ITP for HCV [20] ITP in HIV is also likely multifactorial, owing to immune-mediated platelet destruction and viral suppression of megakaryocyte activity. Prior to the introduction of highly active antiretroviral therapy, ITP was common in patients with HIV [8]. ITP associated with HIV is generally responsive to typical ITP therapy [8].

The variable association of different underlying diseases with the development of ITP lends insight into the pathophysiology of ITP and underlying immune mechanisms. In general, secondary ITP treatment is aimed at treating the underlying disease. However, depending on symptoms, ITP-directed therapy may be needed while awaiting improvement of the associated diagnosis.

Differential Diagnosis

The differential diagnosis for isolated thrombocytopenia is broad and can be classified in a few different ways: (1) inherited vs. acquired, (2) consumption/destruction vs. production, or (3) platelet size. Historical clues, physical exam findings, and laboratory investigations can help narrow down the differential diagnosis. In addition, combining the classification methods can be helpful to guide historical questions, physical exam, and additional laboratory investigations. A prior normal platelet count can help rule out an inherited thrombocytopenia. However, a previous complete blood count is not always available. In the event of isolated thrombocytopenia without clinical bleeding, pseudothrombocytopenia must be ruled out by evaluation of the peripheral blood smear.

Further classifying the inherited thrombocytopenias according to platelet size can be a useful way to organize the differential diagnosis [27, 28] (Fig. 1.1) (Table 1.2). Large platelets are found in Bernard-Soulier syndrome, MYH9 disorders, and gray platelet syndrome, among others. Large platelets can also be seen in ITP, though they are variable in size and not typically uniformly large. Small platelets are seen in Wiskott-Aldrich syndrome (WAS) and X-linked thrombocytopenia, both X-linked disorders. WAS is also associated with immune deficiency and eczema, which can be helpful clinical clues in a male child presenting with thrombocytopenia. Normal-sized platelets are seen in congenital amegakaryocytic thrombocytopenia (CAMT), thrombocytopenia absent radii (TAR) syndrome, and familial platelet disorder with predisposition to acute myelogenous leukemia.

The list of acquired causes of thrombocytopenia is long [29] (Table 1.3). Further classifying the acquired thrombocytopenias into the categories of disor-

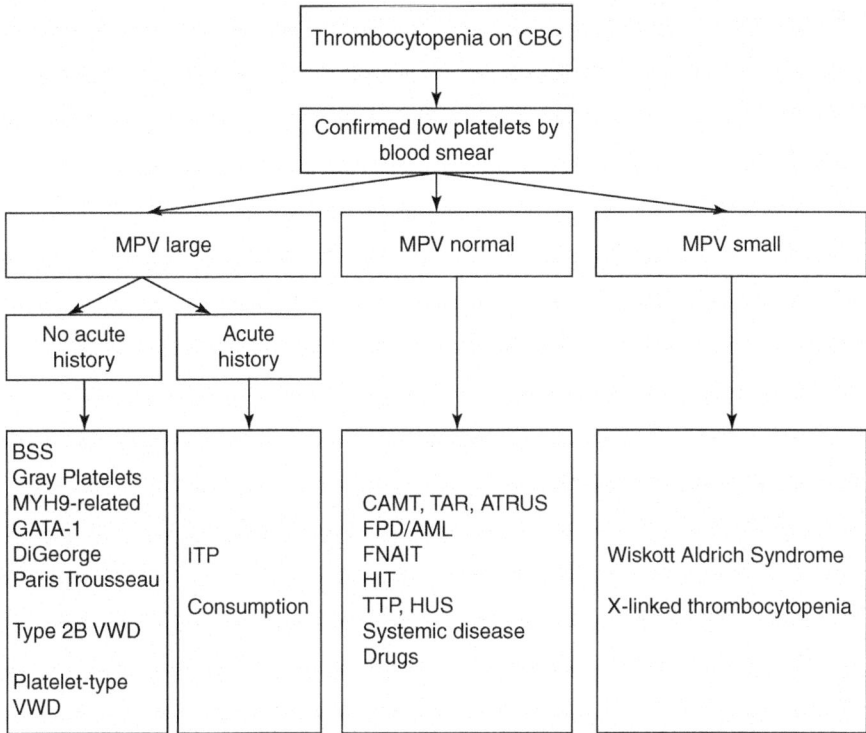

Fig. 1.1 Algorithm to diagnose thrombocytopenia by platelet size (adapted from *SickKids Handbook of Pediatric Thrombosis and Hemostasis* 2nd, revised and extended edition, with permission). *CBC* complete blood count, *MPV* mean platelet volume, *ITP* immune thrombocytopenia, *HIT* heparin-induced thrombocytopenia, *NAIT* neonatal alloimmune thrombocytopenia, *TTP* thrombotic thrombocytopenic purpura, *HUS* hemolytic uremic syndrome, *CAMT* congenital amegakaryocytic thrombocytopenia, *ATRUS* amegakaryocytic thrombocytopenia with radioulnar synostosis, *FPD/AML* familial platelet disorder and predisposition to acute myelogenous leukemia, *GPS* gray platelet syndrome, *TAR* thrombocytopenia absent radii, *THC2* autosomal dominant thrombocytopenia, *WAS* Wiskott-Aldrich syndrome, *XLT* X-linked thrombocytopenia

ders of production, destruction, and consumption can be helpful [30]. With regard to decreased platelet production, disorders of the bone marrow such as myelodysplastic syndromes and aplastic anemia as well as marrow infiltrative processes such as leukemia, lymphoma, or solid metastatic malignancies must be considered. Each of these would likely be associated with other blood cell line abnormalities, but depending upon the presentation, physical findings, and other lab findings, they should be considered. Increased platelet destruction is seen in ITP. As above, secondary causes of ITP such as infections and autoimmune disorders should be considered. Further, the patient's medication list should be reviewed for drugs known to be associated with thrombocytopenia by immune

Table 1.2 Inherited thrombocytopenia syndromes grouped by platelet size

Condition	Inheritance pattern	Gene implicated	Unique clinical/lab findings (in addition to bleeding symptoms)
Small platelets			
Wiskott-Aldrich syndrome	X-linked	*WAS*	Infections secondary to combined immunodeficiency, autoimmune conditions, eczema, cancer predisposition
X-linked thrombocytopenia	X-linked	*WAS*	None
Normal size platelets			
Congenital amegakaryocytic thrombocytopenia (CAMT)	Autosomal recessive	*MPL*	Pancytopenia/bone marrow failure in childhood
Amegakaryocytic thrombocytopenia with radioulnar synostosis	Autosomal dominant	*HOXA11*	Proximal radioulnar synostosis ± other skeletal anomalies, some with sensorineural deafness
Thrombocytopenia absent radii (TAR)	Autosomal recessive	Unknown	Shortened/absent radii bilaterally
Familial platelet disorder/ AML		*AML1*	Early onset myelodysplasia, acute myelogenous leukemia
Large platelets			
MYH9-related disorders	Autosomal dominant	*MYH9*	Sensorineural hearing loss, glomerulonephritis, cataracts
Gray platelet syndrome	Autosomal dominant and recessive types	*NBEAL2*	Alpha-granules absent, making platelets appear gray in blood smear, some develop myelofibrosis
X-linked thrombocytopenia with dyserythropoiesis	X-linked	*GATA-1*	Variable anemia ± evidence of hemolysis, hypercellular marrow with erythro- and myelodysplasia
Bernard-Soulier syndrome	Autosomal recessive	*GP1BA, GPIBB, GP9*	Bleeding due to platelet dysfunction
Velocardiofacial syndrome (DiGeorge)	Autosomal dominant	*22q deletion*	Dysmorphism, developmental and growth delay, cardiac anomalies, cleft lip/palate, hypoparathyroidism, immunodeficiencies
Paris-Trousseau/Jacobsen syndrome	Autosomal dominant	*11q23 (FLI1)*	Congenital impairment, dysmorphic features, cardiac anomalies, growth issues

Table 1.3 Acquired thrombocytopenias to include in the differential diagnosis of ITP

Production	Destruction	Consumption
Aplastic anemia	Primary ITP	Disseminated intravascular coagulation (DIC)
Myelodysplastic syndrome	Secondary ITP	Thrombotic thrombocytopenic purpura (TTP)
Bone marrow failure syndromes	Drug-induced (including heparin)	Hemolytic uremic syndrome (HUS)
Bone marrow infiltration (i.e., leukemia or lymphoma or in pediatrics, neuroblastoma)	Infection (e.g., EBV, CMV, HIV)	Hypersplenism
Infection (e.g., EBV, CMV, HIV)	Mechanical (e.g., mechanical valve)	HELLP syndrome
Nutritional deficiencies		Kasabach-Merritt syndrome
Bone marrow suppression		

mechanisms or by marrow suppression. Increased consumption associated with microangiopathic conditions should be considered, particularly in an ill patient with laboratory evidence of hemolysis or schistocytosis. If the patient has evidence of autoimmune hemolytic anemia, Evans syndrome should remain high on the differential.

Conclusion

The clinical syndrome of immune thrombocytopenia has been well documented for hundreds of years. However, until the discovery of the platelet, the connection between mucocutaneous bleeding and thrombocytopenia was unknown. Initial debates surrounding the etiology of ITP centered upon theories of increased platelet destruction vs. theories of decreased platelet production. However, with additional understanding of the immune system and autoimmunity, the two sides of the debate are now united and combined with an appreciation of a dysregulated immune system to give us our current understanding of the pathophysiology of ITP. Over the years, the terminology used to describe and study ITP has been variable. The current accepted terminology has been agreed upon and published and is now being widely applied and integrated into clinical guidelines and research studies. ITP does remain a diagnosis of exclusion, and it is important to consider other causes of thrombocytopenia when ITP is suspected; however, there are many clues which can quickly help lead to an accurate diagnosis. Improved understanding of the pathophysiology and the development of a common language to describe the clinical course and treatment response is allowing for significant continued progress in the field of ITP.

References

1. Cuker A, Cines DB. Immune thrombocytopenia. Hematol Am Soc Hematol Educ Prog. 2010;2010:377–84.
2. Provan D, Stasi R, Newland AC, Blanchette VS, Bolton-Maggs P, Bussel JB, et al. International consensus report on the investigation and management of primary immune thrombocytopenia. Blood. 2010;115:168–86.
3. Rodeghiero F, Stasi R, Gernsheimer T, Michel M, Provan D, Arnold DM, et al. Standardization of terminology, definitions and outcome criteria in immune thrombocytopenic purpura of adults and children: report from an international working group. Blood. 2009;113:2386–93.
4. Terrell DR, Beebe LA, Vesely SK, Neas BR, Segal JB, George JN. The incidence of immune thrombocytopenic purpura in children and adults: a critical review of published reports. Am J Hematol. 2010;85:174–80.
5. Neunert CE. Current management of immune thrombocytopenia. Hematol Am Soc Hematol Educ Prog. 2013;2013:276–82.
6. Cooper N. State of the art—how I manage immune thrombocytopenia. Br J Haematol. 2017;177:39–54.
7. Kistangari G, Mccrae KR. Immune thrombocytopenia. Hematol Oncol Clin North Am. 2013;27:495–520.
8. Cines DB, Bussel JB, Liebman HA, Luning Prak ET. The ITP syndrome: pathogenic and clinical diversity. Blood. 2009;113:6511–21.
9. Stasi R, Newland AC. ITP: a historical perspective. Br J Haematol. 2011;153:437–50.
10. Blanchette M, Freedman J. The history of idiopathic thrombocytopenic purpura (ITP). Transfus Sci. 1998;19:231–6.
11. Brewer DB. Max Schultze (1865), G. Bizzozero (1882) and the discovery of the platelet. Br J Haematol. 2006;133:251–8.
12. Anoop P. Immune thrombocytopenic purpura: historical perspective, current status, recent advances and future directions. Indian Pediatr. 2012;49:811–8.
13. Liebman HA. Immune thrombocytopenia (ITP): an historical perspective. Hematol Am Soc Hematol Educ Prog. 2008;2008:205.
14. Dameshek W, Miller EB. The megakaryocytes in idiopathic thrombocytopenic purpura, a form of hypersplenism. Blood. 1946;1:27–50.
15. Stoll D, Cines DB, Aster RH, Murphy S. Platelet kinetics in patients with idiopathic thrombocytopenic purpura and moderate thrombocytopenia. Blood. 1985;65:584–8.
16. Mcmillan R, Wang L, Tomer A, Nichol J, Pistillo J. Suppression of in vitro megakaryocyte production by antiplatelet autoantibodies from adult patients with chronic ITP. Blood. 2004;103:1364–9.
17. Chang M, Nakagawa PA, Williams SA, Schwartz MR, Imfeld KL, Buzby JS, et al. Immune thrombocytopenic purpura (ITP) plasma and purified ITP monoclonal autoantibodies inhibit megakaryocytopoiesis in vitro. Blood. 2003;102:887–95.
18. Houwerzijl EJ, Blom NR, Van Der Want JJ, Esselink MT, Koornstra JJ, Smit JW, et al. Ultrastructural study shows morphologic features of apoptosis and para-apoptosis in megakaryocytes from patients with idiopathic thrombocytopenic purpura. Blood. 2004;103:500–6.
19. Olsson B, et al. T-cell-mediated cytotoxicity toward platelets in chronic idiopathic thrombocytopenic purpura. Nature Medicine. 2003;9(9):1123–24.
20. Neunert C, Lim W, Crowther M, Cohen A, Solberg L Jr, Crowther MA, American Society of Hematology. The American Society of Hematology 2011 evidence-based practice guideline for immune thrombocytopenia. Blood. 2011;117:4190–207.
21. Neunert C, Noroozi N, Norman G, Buchanan GR, Goy J, Nazi I, et al. Severe bleeding events in adults and children with primary immune thrombocytopenia: a systematic review. J Thromb Haemost. 2015;13:457–64.
22. Imbach P, et al. Childhood ITP: 12 months follow-up data from the prospective registry of the Intercontinental Childhood ITP Study Group (ICIS). 2006;46:351–56.

23. Grace RF, Long M, Kalish LA, Neufeld EJ. Applicability of 2009 international consensus terminology and criteria for immune thrombocytopenia to a clinical pediatric population. Pediatr Blood Cancer. 2012;58:216–20.
24. Cines DB, Bussel JB. How I treat idiopathic thrombocytopenic purpura (ITP). Blood. 2005;106:2244–51.
25. Nugent DJ. Immune thrombocytopenic purpura of childhood. Hematol Am Soc Hematol Educ Prog. 2006;2006:97–103.
26. Lo E, Deane S. Diagnosis and classification of immune-mediated thrombocytopenia. Autoimmun Rev. 2014;13:577–83.
27. Cines DB, Liebman H, Stasi R. Pathobiology of secondary immune thrombocytopenia. Semin Hematol. 2009;46:S2–14.
28. Ayesh MH, Alawneh K, Khassawneh B, Khader Y, Kasasbeh A. Adult primary and secondary immune thrombocytopenic purpura: a comparative analysis of characteristics and clinical course. Clin Appl Thromb Hemost. 2013;19:327–30.
29. Balduini CL, Cattaneo M, Fabris F, Gresele P, Iolascon A, Pulcinelli FM, et al. Inherited thrombocytopenias: a proposed diagnostic algorithm from the Italian Gruppo di Studio delle Piastrine. Haematologica. 2003;88:582–92.
30. Lambert MP. What to do when you suspect an inherited platelet disorder. Hematol Am Soc Hematol Educ Prog. 2011;2011:377–83.
31. Stasi R. How to approach thrombocytopenia. Hematol Am Soc Hematol Educ Prog. 2012;2012:191–7.
32. Gauer RL, Braun MM. Thrombocytopenia. Am Fam Physician. 2012;85:612–22.

Chapter 2
Pathophysiology of Immune Thrombocytopenia

Taylor Olmsted Kim

Platelet Autoantibodies

ITP is caused, at least in part, by the development of platelet autoantibodies that lead to platelet destruction. This mechanism was first identified by Dr. William Harrington through his classic experiment published in 1951 [1]. As described in Chap. 1, Harrington infused blood from active chronic ITP patients into himself as well as a set of healthy volunteers [1]. Sixty-one percent of these patients then developed transient thrombocytopenia [1], highlighting not only the presence of an antiplatelet substance leading to the development of the ITP syndrome but also the apparent contribution of host factors, as not everyone who received the affected blood developed thrombocytopenia or clinical symptoms. In the 1960s, Shulman [2] infused plasma from ITP patients into healthy recipients. Shulman et al. discovered that resulting thrombocytopenia was proportional to the plasma dose. The causative plasma factor was absorbed by platelets and appeared in the immunoglobulin G fraction on ion-exchange chromatography [2]. Harrington and Shulman both concluded that thrombocytopenia in ITP was caused by platelet autoantibodies [1–3].

Subsequent studies sought to identify the causative platelet autoantibody with the goal of being able to diagnose ITP on the basis of positive antibody testing. Platelet-associated IgG assays were developed and found to be positive in the majority of chronic ITP patients. However, these tests lacked specificity and were positive in a portion of healthy patients as well, thereby limiting their utility [4]. In the 1980s, van Leeuwen [5] used antibody eluates from chronic ITP patients and found they could bind normal platelets, but not platelets from Glanzmann's thrombasthenia patients, who lack the GP IIb/IIIa surface receptor [5]. This finding suggested that in ITP, antibodies directed against platelets are specific for GP IIb/IIIa.

T. Olmsted Kim, MD
Section of Hematology/Oncology, Department of Pediatrics, Texas Children's Cancer
and Hematology Centers, Baylor College of Medicine, Houston, TX, USA
e-mail: teolmste@txch.org

© Springer International Publishing AG, part of Springer Nature 2018
J. M. Despotovic (ed.), *Immune Hematology*,
https://doi.org/10.1007/978-3-319-73269-5_2

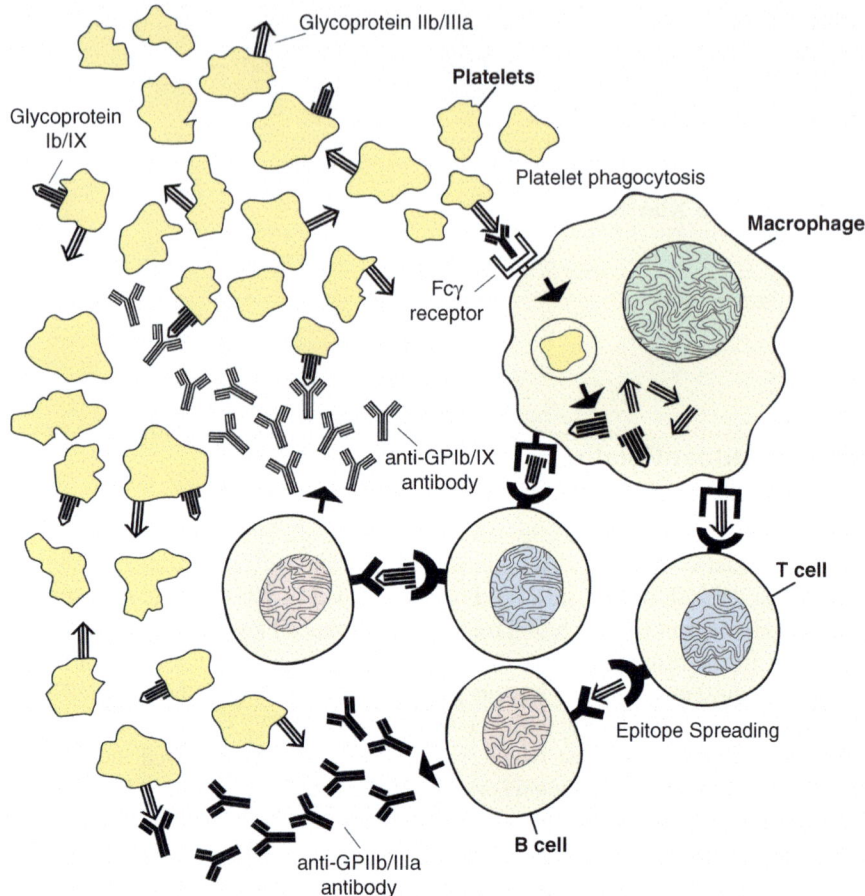

Fig. 2.1 Propagation of antibodies against platelet glycoproteins. Autoantibodies targeting platelet antigens, primarily glycoprotein IIb/IIIa. Opsonized platelets are bound by Fcγ receptors on macrophages and phagocytized. Platelet glycoproteins are presented by antigen-presenting cells. As additional platelet glycoproteins are expressed by activated antigen-presenting cells, they are recognized by T cells. T cells interact with B cell clones resulting in continued anti-glycoprotein IIb/IIIa antibody production in addition to new glycoprotein antibodies

Antigen-specific assays were later developed that identified autoantibodies against platelet surface proteins, primarily glycoprotein IIb/IIIa, but also glycoprotein Ib/IX [4]. Glycoprotein IIb/IIIa and glycoprotein Ib/IX are the most common targets of platelet antibodies in the setting of ITP (Fig. 2.1) [4]. Some patients have antibodies against multiple platelet surface antigens [4, 6]. However, even with more specific antigen-specific assays, only an estimated 50–60% of ITP patients have detectable antibodies [6, 7]. Platelet autoantibodies are derived from B cell clones, evidenced by highly conserved fragment antigen-binding (Fab) gene rearrangements within a single Ig heavy-chain variable region gene (Fig. 2.2) [8, 9].

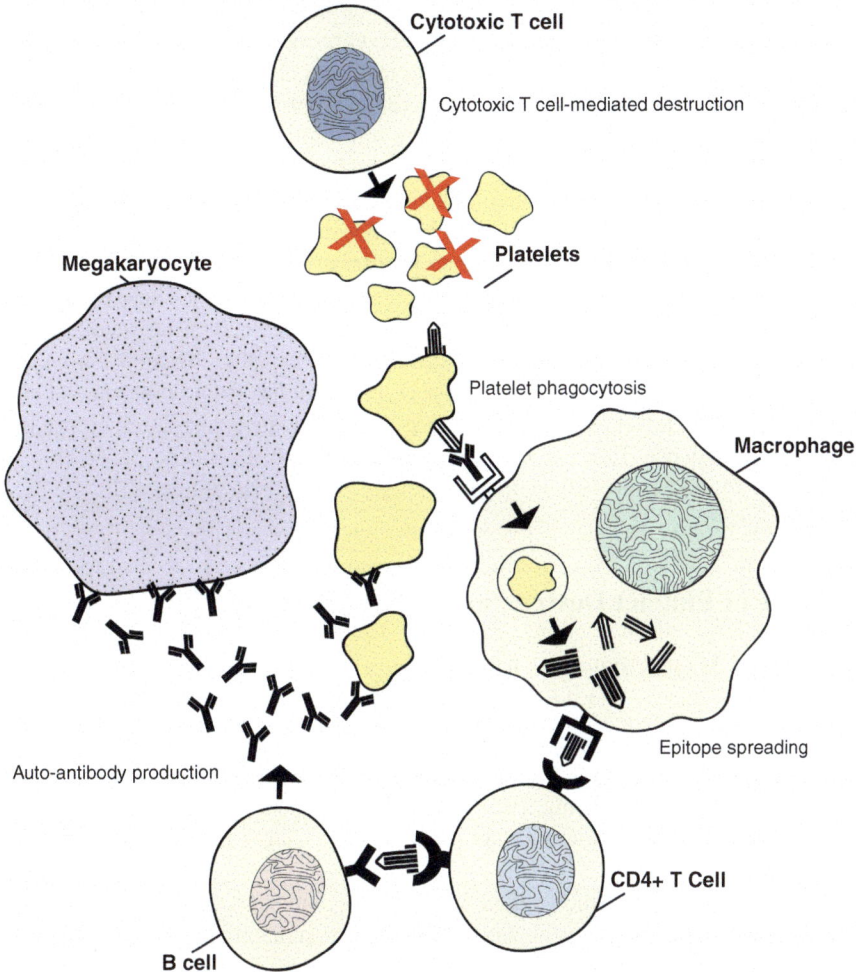

Fig. 2.2 Summary of ITP pathogenesis. Autoantibodies against platelet glycoproteins lead to platelet opsonization, phagocytosis, and destruction by the reticuloendothelial system. Cryptic epitopes from other platelet glycoproteins are then presented by antigen-presenting cells. CD4+ cells interact with B cells, leading to propagation of new antiplatelet autoantibodies. Antibodies are also produced against megakaryocytes, leading to impaired maturation and function. Cytotoxic CD8+ cells cause direct platelet destruction

Senescent platelets at the end of their 8–11 day life span are removed from circulation by the reticuloendothelial system in normal patients [10]. A fixed portion of platelets are also consumed daily in a supportive function at the endothelium [11]. In ITP, antibody-tagged platelets are destroyed by the reticuloendothelial tissues of the liver and spleen [12]. This has been demonstrated morphologically as well as in in vitro models assessing the uptake of ^{51}Cr-labeled platelets [12, 13]. Opsonized platelets are cleared via Fcγ receptors expressed on splenic macrophages and peripheral blood neutrophils. When surface FcγRIIIA expressed on macrophages engages anti-GPIIb/IIIa bound to a platelet, the complex is engulfed. Data suggest that low-affinity receptors FcγRIIA and FcγRIIIA remove antibody-bound platelets from circulation, while high-affinity receptors are not implicated in the same way [14, 15]. In addition to phagocytosis in the reticuloendothelial system, antibody-tagged platelets may also be a trigger for complement-mediated destruction [16].

This process of antibody-mediated phagocytosis is propagated when antigen-presenting cells interact with and induce proliferation of CD4+ T cells. Antigen-presenting cells engulf platelets bound by GPIIb/IIIa antibodies. These complexes are degraded and processed within the antigen-presenting cells. Activated antigen-presenting cells then go on to express GPIIb/IIIa antigens, thereby contributing to a positive feedback loop. They also express cryptic epitopes from other platelet glycoproteins. These novel peptides are expressed and recognized by T cell clones [9]. Interactions between T cell clones and B cell clones result in the production of GPIIb/IIIa antibodies as well as new platelet glycoprotein antibodies [9].

Balance of Platelet Destruction and Production

Abnormal Megakaryocyte Morphology

As early as the 1940s, light microscopy showed an increased number of large, young megakaryocytes in ITP patients. This finding would appear consistent with response to thrombocytopenia, except that these megakaryocytes showed no evidence of platelet production and had degenerative changes in both the nuclei and cytoplasm [11, 17, 18].

Electron microscopy studies done in the 1980s demonstrated evidence of apoptotic changes in the megakaryocytes of ITP patients, remaining consistent with earlier light microscopy findings [19]. In 2004, Houwerzijl et al. [19] studied the ultrastructure of bone marrow in ITP patients. Seventy-eight percent of patients had morphologic abnormalities which were increasingly prevalent in more mature megakaryocytes [19]. Seen most commonly in stage III megakaryocytes, cells had evidence of para-apoptosis with cytoplasmic vacuolization, mitochondrial swelling, condensed nuclei, and distention of the demarcation membranes. Megakaryocytes were also seen being phagocytized by neutrophils and macrophages [19].

Antibody Destruction of Megakaryocytes

Shortly after antibody-mediated platelet destruction was identified in ITP, evidence that megakaryocytes are also targeted expanded. Plasma from ITP patients infused into healthy donors resulted in para-apoptotic changes in megakaryocyte morphology [20]. In the 1970s, Rolovic et al. [21] used a rat model to show that infusion of antiplatelet antibody-rich serum resulted in thrombocytopenia, but also decreased maturation of megakaryocytes as well as the absolute number of stage III, mature megakaryocytes [21]. After assays for specific antibodies against GPIIB/IIIa and GPIIb/IX were created, these antibodies were discovered to target megakaryocytes directly. Cultured CD34+ cells from healthy human donors with serum from ITP patients [22]. Megakaryocyte production in culture was decreased, ranging from 26 to 90% reduction as compared to cells cultured in control plasma [22]. As with the prior rat studies carried out by Rolovic et al., in this model, megakaryocytes showed impaired maturation [11, 21, 22].

Inadequate Thrombopoietin Levels

Megakaryocyte progenitor growth and maturation is impacted by multiple cytokines, but most significantly by thrombopoietin (TPO). In ITP, the capacity of the megakaryocytes to produce new platelets is inadequate for the rate of platelet destruction [10, 23], and insufficient TPO levels may contribute to this inability to adequately respond to the thrombocytopenia.

TPO is constitutively expressed by the liver; however, it is produced to a lesser degree in other organs such as the bone marrow and spleen [23]. Intuitively, endogenous TPO levels should have a compensatory increase in the setting of thrombocytopenia. However, in the setting of ITP, TPO levels are not appropriately elevated. In 1998 Nichol et al. [23] measured TPO levels in healthy controls, aplastic anemia, and ITP patients [23]. Though the patients with aplastic anemia had appropriately high TPO levels in the setting of severe thrombocytopenia, the ITP patient population did not [23]. Studies in mice monitoring radiolabeled TPO showed a twofold increase in clearance for platelet-bound TPO in ITP as opposed to mice who were thrombocytopenic due to sublethal radiation [23]. It is theorized that in the setting of ITP, platelets may have more thrombopoietin receptors (Mpl receptor), thereby allowing for increased TPO binding and subsequent clearance [23]. Therefore, it appears that in ITP, there is not inadequate production of TPO, but rather inadequate levels due to excessive clearance by platelets prior to their destruction.

T Cell-Mediated ITP

T Cell-Propagated Autoantibody Production

The production of autoantibodies against platelet surface glycoproteins requires interaction with CD4+ T cells. Following exposure to GPIIb/IIIa fragments by antigen-presenting cells, CD4+ T cells stimulate antibody synthesis through interaction with B cells. CD4+ cells do not react in the same way to native platelet glycoproteins. The reason for this is not well understood; however, it is hypothesized that epitopes which are not normally exposed in a self-antigen are uncovered and then recognized by the immune system in the setting of circumstances such as an infection [24]. There is evidence that autoreactive T cells directed against GPIIb/IIIa are present in healthy individuals without thrombocytopenia. This suggests that in ITP, there are additional defects in immune tolerance which play a role in pathogenesis [25].

Helper T Cell Responses

Similar to other autoimmune diseases, there are increased pro-inflammatory T cell responses in ITP with increased CD4+ Th0/Th1 activation in association with decreased Th2 responses [6]. Showed that IL-2, IFN-γ, and IL-10 are increased in the sera of chronic ITP patients, consistent with the theory that ITP is mediated by Th1 cell activation [26]. This finding of a predominance of Th1 cytokines in ITP patients has been reproduced by other groups [27–30]. Mouzaki et al. [31] consistent with other works, found Th0 cytokine response in acute ITP patients and Th1 activation in chronic patients [31]. More interesting, Mouzaki et al. [31] discovered that ITP patients in remission or those treated with IVIG showed Th2 polarization [31]. These findings suggest an imbalance between Th0/Th1 and Th2 signaling as causative in active ITP [31, 32].

In contrast, other studies do not as clearly support the idea that Th0/Th1 responses are implicated in ITP. Crossly et al. studied peripheral blood mononuclear cells in chronic ITP. At baseline, these cells secreted low levels of IL-2 and IFN-γ (both Th1-type cytokines), and only when stimulated by interferon-α, did these secreted cytokine levels increase [33]. Other groups showed IL-4, secreted by Th2 cells, to be elevated in chronic ITP with no appreciable increase in IFN-γ levels over controls [34]. Talaat et al. [35] found IFN-γ and TNF-α, both Th1-type cytokines, as well as IL-4, IL-6, and IL-10, Th2 cytokines, to be elevated in ITP patients as compared to healthy controls [35]. Another group has reported in pediatric ITP, cytokines including IL-3, IL-4, IL-6, and IFN-γ may be actually affected by age as opposed to disease status [36].

Collectively, these studies suggest that T-helper cell responses play some role in ITP pathogenesis. The consensus remains that chronic ITP is associated with Th0 profiles, severe disease with Th1 responses, and quiescence with Th2 cytokines [32].

Role of Th17 Cells

A distinct subset of CD4+ Th cells, Th17 cells, characterized by IL-17 secretion, have previously been implicated in the development of inflammatory and autoimmune diseases such as systemic lupus erythematosus, allergic encephalomyelitis, multiple sclerosis, and collagen-induced arthritis [35, 37, 38]. Though contradictory data on their role exists, the current consensus is that Th17 cells contribute to the development of ITP [38, 39]. IL-17 is elevated in serum and plasma levels in pediatric patients with active disease and has increased expression from CD4+ cells in ITP patients [7]. Additionally, a Th17 transcription factor, retinoic acid-related orphan receptor gamma-t (RORγt), when overexpressed in mice was linked to the production of antiplatelet antibodies [37, 40]. Genetic studies have shown associations with an interleukin-17F gene polymorphism in chronic ITP as well [41].

Th17 cells may also contribute to ITP pathogenesis via production of IL-22. IL-22 is a pro-inflammatory cytokine in the IL-10 superfamily. Elevated IL-22 levels have been demonstrated in the plasma of active ITP patients as compared to controls [42]. Cao et al. [43] assessed IL-22 levels as well as the number of Th1, Th17, and Th22 cells in ITP patient samples before and after treatment with dexamethasone [43]. Steroid treatment resulted in a decrease in plasma IL-22 as well as a decrease in the number of Th1 cells [43]. These findings suggest regulation of Th1 responses as a mechanism for Th17 in ITP pathogenesis [43].

In vitro studies show positive correlation between Th1 and Th17 cytokines and the presence of cytotoxic $CD3^+CD8^+IFN-\gamma^+$ T cells [44, 45]. Direct cytotoxic destruction of platelets offers an alternative process for platelet destruction independent of autoantibody production described previously.

Regulatory T cells

There is evidence that Th17 cells work in balance with regulatory T cells (Tregs). Tregs are a subset of cells that constitute approximately 5–10% of the CD4+ T cell population [46, 47]. Tregs promote self-tolerance via suppression of effector T cell and B cell function via direct cell contact or cytokine-mediated mechanisms [38, 46, 48]. Tregs also interact with antigen-presenting cells [49–51].

There are substantial amounts of data to demonstrate decreased levels of circulating Tregs in all phases of ITP [38]. With decreased numbers of Tregs, a regulatory mechanism on antigen-presenting cells is removed, thereby resulting in decreased self-tolerance and subsequent platelet destruction [38]. Tregs from ITP patients have demonstrated decreased ability to inhibit T cell proliferation, as compared to inhibition by Tregs from healthy controls. This suggests an intrinsic defect in Tregs in ITP patients may contribute to disease pathogenesis [48]. Murine models of ITP also support theories regarding Tregs. Nishimoto et al. [52] showed in a cohort of Treg-deficient mice that 36% developed thrombocytopenia [52]. These thrombocytopenic mice went on to develop IgG platelet antibodies [52]. Transfer of Tregs from healthy mice prevented the development of thrombocytopenia [52].

B Cell-Mediated ITP

The role of B cells in ITP pathophysiology was initially believed to be due exclusively to the production of GPIIb/IIIa and GPIb/IX autoantibodies. However, studies suggest that the role for B cells in ITP is actually more complex than inappropriate production of autoantibodies alone.

TNFSF13B, a B cell-activating factor (BAFF), has been implicated in ITP development. BAFF levels are found at increased levels in those with active ITP as compared to controls [53]. Higher levels of BAFF, present in chronic ITP patients, correlate inversely with platelet count [54, 55].

The number of B cells present in the red pulp of the spleen is increased over controls [56]. Proliferating Ki67[+] B cells have also been identified in proliferative lymphoid nodules (PLN) in the spleen. Unlike cells in the germinal center, these cells do not express Bcl6, a transcriptional regulator of germinal center reactions, and do not demonstrate normal polarization. T follicular and regulatory T cells are also reduced in the PLN. Collectively, these findings reflect aberrancies in normal tolerance mechanisms and lack of appropriate T cell regulation in ITP patients [57].

B-Regulatory Cells

B-regulatory cells (Bregs), characterized by $CD19^+CD24^{hi}CD38^{hi}$ profile, inhibit T cell and monocyte activation. Bregs promote self-tolerance in the periphery through IL-10 secretion. Though their interaction is not fully understood, there is evidence that Bregs interact with Tregs [5]. In ITP patients, Bregs appear to have a decreased response to IL-10 stimulation, reduced number of Bregs, and lowered IL-10 in all B cell populations [38, 48].

A subset of $CD19^+CD24^+FOXP3^+$ Bregs are present at increased numbers in the spleens of ITP patients requiring splenectomy as opposed to those splenectomized due to trauma [58]. Conversely, this cell population is present at lower levels in the peripheral blood in other autoimmune diseases [59]. These findings preliminarily suggest this population of Bregs is sequestered in the setting of ITP, though their role in the disease remains incompletely understood.

Myeloid-Derived Suppressor Cells

Myeloid-derived suppressor cells (MDSCs) have been proposed to play a role in ITP pathogenesis. Myeloid-derived suppressor cells are a heterogeneous population of immature myeloid cells which suppress adaptive immunity [60]. These cells have been studied as a potential therapeutic target for cancer due to the role of MDSCs in tumor-mediated immune escape [60, 61]. MDSCs, characterized by $CD11b^+CD33^+HLA-Dr^{low}$, are present in decreased numbers and also function abnormally in both the peripheral blood and spleens of ITP patients [62]. In the absence of MDSCs, there is immune dysregulation through decreased number of Tregs and through altered function of Bregs [48, 62, 63].

Recent studies have demonstrated an MDSC-mediated mechanism for high-dose dexamethasone (HD-DXM) and intravenous immunoglobulin (IVIG) response in the treatment of ITP [62, 63]. MDSC function and numbers are restored by exposure to HD-DXM. In vitro, cells cultured with HD-DXM demonstrate expansion of the C11b+CD33+HLA-Dr^{low} population, increased expression of MDSC-produced cytokines IL-10 and TGF-ß, as well as attenuated CD4+ T cell proliferation and cytotoxic T cell-mediated platelet lysis [62]. Aslam et al. [63] took spleen cells from refractory chronic ITP patients and those derived from trauma patients and cultured them in the presence of intravenous immunoglobulin [63]. A significant increase in the C11b+CD33+HLA-Dr^{low} population in the ITP group correlated directly with rising IVIG concentration applied to culture media [63].

Initial studies propose MDSCs as the lynchpin regulating both T and B cells in the pathogenesis of ITP. Therapies which restore MDSC functioning may alleviate immune dysregulation in ITP. Further research is needed, but the discovery of this novel cell population holds promise.

Genetic Studies

Though our understanding of the complexities of immune derangements in ITP has grown, the underlying factors which predispose certain individuals to the development of these abnormalities and factors that drive the development of chronic ITP remain elusive. Gene expression differences in acute and chronic ITP have been proposed in small studies. Different gene expression profiles have been identified by DNA microarray analysis on T cells from newly diagnosed ITP patients and those with chronic ITP. Genome-wide expression profiles clustered without any overlap between the two cohorts in a dendrogram plot [64]. Differently expressed transcripts clustered by Gene Ontology (GO) annotations highlighted T cell activation, lymphocyte proliferation, and chemotaxis in newly diagnosed ITP patients. Chronic ITP patients showed increased transcript expression in B cell differentiation and CD8+ α:β T cell differentiation [64]. Another group showed elevated mRNA levels of vanin-1, an oxidative stress sensor in epithelial cells, in whole blood from chronic ITP patients as compared to acute patients [65]. These studies are all severely limited by sample size and the results have not been validated.

A number of studies have attempted to demonstrate the importance of specific genetic variants in ITP; however, all have been candidate gene approaches limited to relatively small numbers of patients, and none have held up to validation [66]. A few examples of these findings follow. The FCGR gene, encoding the Fcγ receptor, has been of interest based on the antibody-mediated component of ITP pathogenesis. Associations are weak and data mixed on which polymorphism within this gene carries any predictive value in ITP [67]. A single study has identified variants in HLA-DRB1 in ITP patients [68]. More recently, an IL-17F 7488TT polymorphism was found to be associated with severe thrombocytopenia at diagnosis of ITP [41].

Secondary ITP

Helicobacter pylori-*Related ITP*

Helicobacter pylori (*H. pylori*) infection is associated with the development of ITP. At the molecular level, it is hypothesized that this process is driven by molecular mimicry [69]. CagA, a *H. pylori* virulence gene, has been linked to the incidence of ITP and the presence of anti-GPIIb/IIIa antibody-producing B cells [69]. ITP related to *H. pylori* infection resolves with eradication of the bacterium in 0–7% of US cases, with up to 100% resolution in a Japanese review [70].

CMV-Related ITP

CMV has been linked to ITP [71, 72], causes delayed platelet recovery after bone marrow transplant, and causes thrombocytopenia in the setting of congenital infection [7, 71, 72]. Murine studies suggest that CMV virus has a direct cytotoxic effect on megakaryocytes and their progenitors [73].

Varicella Zoster-Related ITP

VZV-related thrombocytopenia develops in the case of neonates born to infected mothers, during viral reactivation, after vaccination, and may develop prior to the onset of viral dissemination and purpura fulminans [74, 75]. Similar to CMV, it is hypothesized that varicella zoster virus (VZV) infection damages megakaryocytes [74]. VZV may also lead to the development of antibodies which bind to platelets; however, the antiplatelet antibodies generated in VZV infection are not cross-reactive anti-varicella antibodies [74]. VZV specifically was reported to cause the development of anti-GPIb-IX antibodies [7, 74, 75].

Hepatitis C-Related ITP

The etiology of ITP secondary to hepatitis C is multifactorial. Thrombopoietin may be reduced in advanced hepatitis infection. Megakaryocytes may be infected, impairing platelet production [7]. Additionally, there is evidence of cross-reactive antibodies targeting platelet GPIIIa [76]. The hepatitis C virus structural protein E2 activates B cells via a B cell co-receptor [77, 78]. This leads to clonal expansion of B cell populations which may drive antiplatelet antibody production.

HIV-Related ITP

Thrombocytopenia appears to follow disease status and viral load in HIV [79, 80]. Treatment with HAART results in improvement in ITP [80]. Megakaryocytes express CD4 and co-receptors for HIV [81, 82]. Megakaryocytes are able to bind HIV, internalize the virus, and become infected [83]. In addition to the mechanism involving the megakaryocytes, the sera of HIV patients contains antiviral antibodies which are also cross-reactive with portions of GPIIIa, resulting in thrombocytopenia [82].

Malignancy-Related ITP

Hematologic malignancies are the most common neoplasms to be associated with ITP [7]. The mechanism for ITP in the case of chronic lymphocytic leukemia (CLL) is not entirely understood. The malignant clone does not appear to directly produce antiplatelet antibodies. Studies have shown an association with unmutated IgV_H, and ITP related to CLL appears to be the result of generalized immune dysregulation. Other autoimmune cytopenias develop commonly in CLL, with the most common being autoimmune hemolytic anemia [7, 84]. CLL cells may act as antigen-presenting cells, processing antigen and revealing cryptic epitopes to Th cells [85]. CLL-related ITP is also seen specifically following treatment with fludarabine and other purine analogues. These drugs specifically result in loss of CD4+, CD45RA+ cells, a population of autoregulatory T cells [85, 86]. ITP also develops in the setting of large granular T-lymphocytic leukemia (LGL). In LGL, a clonal population of CD8+ T cells may lead to cytotoxic effects on megakaryocytes; however, it is not known if this population is constitutively or transiently activated [87, 88]. ITP secondary to Hodgkin disease is rare, with an estimated prevalence of less than 1% of patients, and the mechanism by which this occurs is not known [7].

Other Autoimmune Disorders

Two to five percent of patients with ITP go on to develop systemic lupus erythematosus (SLE) [7]. In this condition there are multiple antibodies which could play a role in the development of ITP: antibodies against CD40L (expressed on Th cells, when bound by activated APCs), thrombopoietin and its receptor, and platelet glycoproteins [89, 90]. Systemic inflammation resulting in vasculitis, thrombotic microangiopathy, and hemophagocytosis leads to increased platelet consumption. Marrow damage and amegakaryocytosis in SLE could further impair platelet production [90]. SLE patients may develop antiphospholipid antibodies [91], also independently associated with development of ITP. Antiphospholipid antibodies (APLAs) bind epitopes on GPIIIa and some recognize markers which become expressed during platelet activation. Activation of coagulation may lead to further thrombocytopenia as platelets are consumed in thrombus formation [7].

Evans Syndrome

Evans syndrome is a rare disorder defined by either concurrent or sequential development of two autoimmune cytopenias [7, 92]. Most commonly, Evans syndrome involves ITP and warm autoimmune hemolytic anemia (AIHA), although autoimmune neutropenia can also be present [7, 93]. Evans syndrome is the result of immune dysregulation leading to autoantibody production [7]. In Evans syndrome, red cell antibodies are commonly directed against the Rh-locus and are distinct from those generated against platelets [7]. Limited studies of Evans patients have shown an imbalance in CD4/CD8 ratios, with a shift toward CD8 cells [7]. Evans syndrome is most often chronic and poorly responsive to therapy (see Section "Clinical Presentation" in Chap. 3 and Part II Chap. 2 for comprehensive review of Evans syndrome).

Autoimmune Lymphoproliferative Syndrome (ALPS)

ALPS is an inherited disorder, most commonly autosomal dominant, which is characterized by defective apoptosis of B and T cells [7]. The majority of ALPS patients carry a mutation in APT1, which encodes Fas (CD95/Apo-1) [7]. Active T and B lymphocytes highly express Fas. When Fas binds Fas ligand on activated T cells, a caspase cascade is triggered, ultimately resulting in apoptosis [92]. Some patients may have defects in the Fas ligand, caspase-8, or caspase-10 [7]. For approximately 24% of cases, no disease causing mutation could be identified [7, 92]. The result of these mutational defects is aberrant apoptosis of activated T and B lymphocytes. Without the ability to downregulate the immune response, ALPS patients develop autoimmune cytopenias, including immune thrombocytopenia, lymphadenopathy, hepatosplenomegaly, as well as cancer predisposition [92]. In addition to the aberrant Fas-mediated apoptosis and aforementioned clinical criteria, ALPS patients have greater than 1% double negative T cells (TCR α/β^+, $CD3^+$, $CD4^-$, $CD8^-$ T cells) [7].

ITP is a heterogeneous disorder with complex underlying pathophysiology. Research continues to identify immune pathways which do not function normally in ITP. However, further work is needed to tease out the breakpoints that initiate immune dysregulation leading to destruction of platelet populations and to understand what drives the host factors that lead to these changes.

References

1. Harrington WJ, Minnich V, Hollingsworth JW, Moore CV. Demonstration of a thrombocytopenic factor in the blood of patients with thrombocytopenic purpura. J Lab Clin Med. 1951;38:1–10.
2. Shulman NR, Marder VJ, Weinrach RS. Similarities between known antiplatelet antibodies and the factor responsible for thrombocytopenia in idiopathic purpura. Physiologic, serologic and isotopic studies. Ann N Y Acad Sci. 1965;124:499–542.
3. Harrington WJ, Sprague CC, Minnich V, Moore CV, Aulvin RC, Dubach R. Immunologic mechanisms in idiopathic and neonatal thrombocytopenic purpura. Ann Intern Med. 1953;38:433–69.
4. McMillan R, Wang L, Tani P. Prospective evaluation of the immunobead assay for the diagnosis of adult chronic immune thrombocytopenia purpura (ITP). J Thromb Haemost. 2003;1:485–91.
5. van Leeuwen EF, van der Ven JT, Engelfriet CP. von dem Borne AE. Specificity of autoantibodies in autoimmune thrombocytopenia. Blood. 1982;59:23–6.
6. Stasi R, Evangelista ML, Stipa E, Buccisano F, Venditti A, Amadori S. Idiopathic thrombocytopenia purpura: current concepts in pathophysiology and management. Thromb Haemost. 2008;99:4–13.
7. Cines DB, Bussel JB, Liebman HA, Luning Prak ET. The ITP syndrome: pathogenic and clinical diversity. Blood. 2009;113(26):6511–21.
8. Roark JH, Bussel JB, Cines DB, Siegel DL. Genetic analysis of autoantibodies in idiopathic thrombocytopenic purpura reveals evidence of clonal expansion and somatic mutation. Blood. 2002;100(4):1388–98.
9. Cines DB, Blanchette VS. Immune thrombocytopenic purpura. N Engl J Med. 2002;346(13):995–1008.
10. Aster RH, Jandl JH. Platelet sequestration in man. I. Methods. J Clin Invest. 1964;43:843–55.
11. Nugent D, McMillan R, Nichol JL, Slichter SJ. Pathogenesis of chronic immune thrombocytopenia: increase platelet destruction and/or decreased platelet production. Br J Haematol. 2009;146:585–96.
12. Handin R, Stossel T. Phagocytosis of antibody-coated platelets by human granulocytes. N Engl J Med. 1974;290(18):989–93.
13. Tsubakio T, Kurata Y, Kenayama Y, Yonezawa T, Tarui S, Kitani T. In vitro platelet phagocytosis in idiopathic thrombocytopenic purpura. Acta Haematol. 1983;70:250–6.
14. Ericson SG, Coleman KD, Wardwell K, Baker S, Fanger MW, Guyre PM, Ely P. Monoclonal antibody 197 (anti-Fc gamma RI) infusion in a patient with immune thrombocytopenia purpura (ITP) results in down-modulation of Fc gamma RI on circulating monocytes. Br J Haematol. 1996;92:718–24.
15. Crow AR, Lazarus AH. Role of Fcgamma receptors in the pathogenesis and treatment of idiopathic thrombocytopenic purpura. J Pediatr Hematol Oncol. 2003;25(Suppl 1):S14–8.
16. Tsubakio T, Tani P, Curd JG, McMillan R. Complement activation in vitro by antiplatelet antibodies in chronic immune thrombocytopenic purpura. Br J Haematol. 1986;63(2):293–300.
17. Dameshek W, Miller EB. The megakaryocytes in idiopathic thrombocytopenic purpura, a form of hypersplenism. Blood. 1946;1:27–51.
18. Diggs LW, Hewlitt JS. A study of the bone marrow from thirty-six patients with idiopathic hemorrhagic (thrombopenic) purpura. Blood. 1948;3:1090–104.
19. Houwerzijl EJ, Blom NR, van der Want JJ, Esselink MT, Koornstra JJ, Smit JW, Louwes H, Vellenga E, de Wolf JT. Ultrastructural study shows morphologic features of apoptosis and para-apoptosis in megakaryocytes from patients with idiopathic thrombocytopenic purpura. Blood. 2004;103:500–6.
20. Pisciotta AV, Stefanini M, Dameshek W. Studies on platelets. X. Morphologic characteristics of megakaryocytes by phase contrast microscopy in normals and in patients with idiopathic thrombocytopenic purpura. Blood. 1953;8:703–23.

21. Rolovic Z, Baldini M, Dameshek W. Megakaryocytopoiesis in experimentally induced immune thrombocytopenia. Blood. 1970;35:173–88.
22. McMillan R, Wang L, Tomer A, Nichol J, Pistillo J. Suppression of in vitro megakaryocyte production by antiplatelet autoantibodies from adult patients with chronic ITP. Blood. 2004;103:1364–9.
23. Nicol JL. Endogenous TPO (eTPO) levels in health and disease: possible clues for therapeutic intervention. Stem Cells. 1998;16(2):165–75.
24. Zhou B, Zhao H, Yang RC, Han ZC. Multi-dysfunctional pathophysiology in ITP. Crit Rev Oncol Hematol. 2005;54:107–16.
25. Filion MC, Proulx C, Bradley AJ, Devine DV, Sékaly RP, Décary F, Chartrand P. Presence in peripheral blood of healthy individuals of autoreactive T cells to a membrane antigen present on bone marrow derived cells. Blood. 1996;88:2144–50.
26. Semple JW, Milev Y, Cosgrave D, Mody M, Hornstein A, Blanchette V, Freedman J. Difference in serum cytokine levels in acute and chronic autoimmune thrombocytopenic purpura: relationship to platelet phenotype and antiplatelet T-cell reactivity. Blood. 1996;87(10):4245–54.
27. Garcia-Suarez J, Prieto A, Reyes E, Manzano L, Arribalzaga K, Alvarez-Mon M. Abnormal gamma IFN and aTNF secretion in purified CD2+ cells from autoimmune thrombocytopenic purpura (ATP) patients: their implication in the clinical course of the disease. Am J Hematol. 1995;49:271–6.
28. Abboud MR, Laver J, Xu F, Weksler B, Bussel J. Serum levels of GMCSF are elevated in patients with thrombocytopenia. Br J Haematol. 1996;92:486–8.
29. Lazarus AH, Ellis J, Semple JW, Mody M, Crow AR, Freedman J. Comparison of platelet immunity in patients with SLE and ITP. Transfus Sci. 2000;22:19–27.
30. Yoshimura C, Nomura S, Nagahama M, Ozaki Y, Kagawa H, Fukuhara S. Plasma-soluble Fas (APO-1, CD95) and soluble Fas ligand in immune thrombocytopenic purpura. Eur J Haematol. 2000;64:219–24.
31. Mouzaki A, Theodoropoulou M, Gianakopoulos I, Vlaha V, Kyrtsonis MC, Maniatis A. Expression patterns of Th1 and Th2 cytokine genes in childhood idiopathic thrombocytopenic purpura (ITP) at presentation and their modulation by intravenous immunoglobulin G (IVIg) treatment: their role in prognosis. Blood. 2002;100:1774–9.
32. Semple JW. T cell and cytokine abnormalities in patients with autoimmune thrombocytopenic purpura. Transfus Apher Sci. 2003;28:237–42.
33. Crossley AR, Dickinson AM, Proctor SJ, Calvert JE. Effects of interferon alpha therapy on immune parameters in immune thrombocytopenic purpura. Autoimmunity. 1996;24:81–100.
34. Webber NP, Mascarenhas JO, Crow MK, Bussel J, Schattner EJ. Functional properties of lymphocytes in idiopathic thrombocytopenic purpura. Hum Immunol. 2001;62:1346–55.
35. Talaat RM, Mohamed SF, Bassyouni IH, Raouf AA. Th1/Th2/Th17/Treg cytokine imbalance in systemic lupus erythematosus (SLE) patients: correlation with disease severity. Cytokine. 2015;72(2):146–53.
36. Culic S, Labar B, Marusic A, Salamunic I. Correlations among age, cytokines, lymphocyte subtypes, and platelet counts in autoimmune thrombocytopenic purpura. Pediatr Blood Cancer. 2006;47:671–4.
37. Afzali B, Lombardi G, Lechler RI, Lord GM. The role of T helper 17 (Th17) and regulatory T cells (Treg) in human organ transplantation and autoimmune disease. Clin Exp Immunol. 2007;1:32–46.
38. McKenzie CG, Guo L, Freedman J, Semple JW. Cellular immune dysfunction in immune thrombocytopenia. Br J Haematol. 2013;163:10–23.
39. Semple JW, Provan D. The immunopathogenesis of immune thrombocytopenia: T cells still take center-stage. Curr Opin Hematol. 2012;12(5):357–62.
40. Yoh K, Morito N, Ojima M, Shibuya K, Yamashita Y, Morishima Y, Ishii Y, Kusakabe M, Nishikii H, Fujita A, Matsunaga E, Okamura M, Hamada M, Suto A, Nakajima H, Shibuya A, Yamagata K, Takahashi S. Overexpression of RORγt under control of the CD2 promoter induces polyclonal plasmacytosis and autoantibody production in transgenic mice. Eur J Immunol. 2012;42(8):1999–2009.

41. Saitoh T, Tsukamoto N, Koiso H, Mitshui T, Yokohama A, Handa H, Karasawa M, Ogawara H, Nojima Y, Murakami H. Interleukin-17F gene polymorphism in patients with chronic immune thrombocytopenia. Eur J Haematol. 2011;87:253–8.
42. Cao J, Chen C, Zeng L, Li L, Li X, Li Z, Xu K. Elevated plasma IL-22 levels correlated with Th1 and Th22 cells in patients with immune thrombocytopenia. Clin Immunol. 2011;141:121–3.
43. Cao J, Chen C, Li L, Ling-yu Z, Zhen-yu L, Zhi-ling Y, Wei C, Hai C, Sang W, Kai-lin X. Effects of high-dose dexamethasone on regulating interleukin-22 production and correcting Th1 and Th22 polarization in immune thrombocytopenia. J Clin Immunol. 2012;32:523–9.
44. Zhang J, Ma D, Zhu X, Qu X, Ji C, Hou M. Elevated profile of Th17, Th1 and Tc1 cells in patients with immune thrombocytopenic purpura. Haematologica. 2009;94:1326–8. https://doi.org/10.3324/haematol.2009.007823
45. Olsson B, Andersson PO, Jernås M, Jacobsson S, Carlsson B, Carlsson LM, Wadenvik H. T-cell-mediated cytotoxicity toward platelets in chronic idiopathic thrombocytopenic purpura. Nat Med. 2003;9(9):1123–4.
46. Sakaguchi S, Miyara M, Costantino CM, Hafler DA. FOXP3+ regulatory T cells in the human immune system. Nat Rev Immunol. 2010;10(7):490–500.
47. David R. Regulatory T cells: fine-tuning TReg cells. Nat Rev Immunol. 2009;9:226–7.
48. Yazdanbakhsh K. Imbalance immune homeostasis in immune thrombocytopenia. Semin Hematol. 2016;53(Suppl 1):S16–9.
49. Kuwana M, Ikeda Y. The role of autoreactive T cells in the pathogenesis of idiopathic thrombocytopenic purpura. Int J Hematol. 2005;81(2):106–12.
50. André S, Tough DF, Lacroix-Desmazes S, Kaveri SV, Bayry J. Surveillance of antigen-presenting cells by CD4+ CD25+ regulatory T cells in autoimmunity: immunopathogenesis and therapeutic implications. Am J Pathol. 2009;174(5):1575–87.
51. Semple JW, Provan D, Garvey MB, Freedman J. Recent progress in understanding the pathogenesis of immune thrombocytopenia. Curr Opin Hematol. 2010;17(6):590–5.
52. Nishimoto T, Satoh T, Takeuchi T, Ikeda Y, Kuwana M. Critical role of CD4(+)CD25(+) regulatory T cells in preventing murine autoantibodymediated thrombocytopenia. Exp Hematol. 2012;40(4):279–89.
53. Emmerich F, Bal G, Barakat A, Milz J, Mühle C, Martinez-Gamboa L, Dörner T, Salama A. High-level serum B cell activating factor and promoter polymorphisms in patients with idiopathic thrombocytopenic purpura. Br J Haematol. 2007;136(2):309–14.
54. Yang Q, Xu S, Li X, Wang B, Wang X, Ma D, Yang L, Peng J, Hou M. Pathway of Toll-like receptor 7/B cell activating factor/B cell activating factor receptor plays a role in immune thrombocytopenia in vivo. PLoS One. 2011;6(7):e22708.
55. Abdel-Hamid SM, Al-Lithy HN. B cell activating factor gene polymorphisms in patients with risk of idiopathic thrombocytopenic purpura. Am J Med Sci. 2011;342(1):9–14.
56. Olsson B, Ridell B, Jernås M, Wadenvik H. Increased number of B cells in the red pulp of the spleen in ITP. Ann Hematol. 2012;91(2):271–7.
57. Daridon C, Loddenkemper C, Spieckermann S, Kühl AA, Salama A, Burmester GR, Lipsky PE, Dörner T. Splenic proliferative lymphoid nodules distinct from germinal centers are sites of autoantigen stimulation in immune thrombocytopenia. Blood. 2012;120(25):5021–31.
58. Aslam R, Segel GB, Burack R, Spence SA, Speck ER, Guo L, Semple JW. Splenic lymphocyte subtypes in immune thrombocytopenia: increased presence of a subtype of B-regulatory cells. Br J Haematol. 2016;173(1):159–60.
59. Guo Y, Zhang X, Qin M, Wang X. Changes in peripheral CD19+ Foxp3+ and CD19+ TGFb+ regulatory B cell populations in rheumatoid arthritis patients with interstitial lung disease. J Thorac Dis. 2015;7:471–7.
60. Draghiciu O, Lubbers J, Nijman HW, Daemen T. Myeloid derived suppressor cells—an overview of combat strategies to increase immunotherapy efficacy. Oncoimmunology. 2015;4(1):e954829.
61. Kartylewski M, Moreira D. Myeloid cells as target for oligonucleotide therapeutics: turning obstacles into opportunities. Cancer Immunol Immunother. 2017;66(8):979–88. epub ahead of print.

62. Hou Y, Feng Q, Xu M, Li GS, Liu XN, Sheng Z, Zhou H, Ma J, Wei Y, Sun YX, Yu YY, Qiu JH, Shao LL, Liu XG, Hou M, Peng J. High-dose dexamethasone corrects impaired myeloid-derived suppressor cell function via Ets1 in immune thrombocytopenia. Blood. 2016;127(12):1587–97.
63. Aslam R, Burack WR, Segel GB, McVey M, Spence SA, Semple JW. Intravenous immunoglobulin treatment of spleen cells from patients with immune thrombocytopenia significantly increases the percentage of myeloid-derived suppressor cells. Br J Haematol. 2017. https://doi.org/10.1111/bjh.14542.
64. Jernås M, Hou Y, Strömberg Célind F, Shao L, Nookaew I, Wang Q, Ju X, Mellgren K, Wadenvik H, Hou M, Olsson B. Differences in gene expression and cytokine levels between newly diagnosed and chronic pediatric ITP. Blood. 2013;122(10):1789–92.
65. Zhang B, Lo C, Shen L, Sood R, Jones C, Cusmano-Ozog K, Park-Snyder S, Wong W, Jeng M, Cowan T, Engelman EG, Zehner JL. The role of vanin-1 and oxidative stress-related pathways in distinguishing acute and chronic pediatric ITP. Blood. 2011;117(17):4569–79.
66. Bergmann AK, Grace RF, Neufeld EJ. Genetic studies in pediatric ITP: outlook, feasibility and requirements. Ann Hematol. 2010;89(Suppl 1):S95–103.
67. Wang D, Hu SL, Cheng XL, Yang JY. FCGR2A rs1801274 polymorphism is associated with risk of childhood-onset idiopathic (immune) thrombocytopenic purpura: evidence from a meta-analysis. Thromb Res. 2014;134(6):1323–7.
68. Nomura S, Matsuzaki T, Ozaki Y, Yamaoka M, Yoshimura C, Katsura K, Xie GL, Kagawa H, Ishida T, Fukuhara S. Clinical significance of HLA-DRB1*0410 in Japanese patients with idiopathic thrombocytopenic purpura. Blood. 1998;91:3616–22.
69. Takahashi T, Yujiri T, Shinohara K, Inoue Y, Sato Y, Fujii Y, Okubo M, Zaitsu Y, Ariyoshi K, Nakamura Y, Nawata R, Oka Y, Shirai M, Tanizawa Y. Molecular mimicry by Helicobacter pylori CagA protein may be involved in the pathogenesis of H. pylori associated chronic idiopathic thrombocytopenic purpura. Br J Haematol. 2004;124:91–6.
70. Stasi R, Sarpatwari A, Segal JB, Osborn J, Evangelista ML, Cooper N, Provan D, Newland A, Amadori S, Bussel JB. Effects of eradication of Helicobacter pylori infection in patients with immune thrombocytopenic purpura: a systematic review. Blood. 2009;113:1231–40.
71. Wright JG. Severe thrombocytopenia secondary to asymptomatic cytomegalovirus infection in an immunocompetent host. J Clin Pathol. 1992;45:1037–8.
72. Psaila B, Bussel JB. Refractory immune thrombocytopenic purpura: current strategies for investigation and management. Br J Haematol. 2008;143:16–26.
73. Verdonck LF, van Heugten H, de Gast GC. Delay in platelet recovery after bone marrow transplantation: impact of cytomegalovirus infection. Blood. 1985;66:921–5.
74. Yeager AM, Zinkham WH. Varicella-associated thrombocytopenia: clues to the etiology of childhood idiopathic thrombocytopenic purpura. Johns Hopkins Med J. 1980;146:270–4.
75. Mayer JL, Beardsley DS. Varicella-associated thrombocytopenia: autoantibodies against platelet surface glycoprotein V. Pediatr Res. 1996;40:615–9.
76. Zhang W, Nardi MA, Borkowsky W, Karpatkin S. Role of molecular mimicry of hepatitis C virus (HCV) protein with platelet GPIIIa in hepatitis-C related immunologic thrombocytopenia. Blood. 2009;113:4086–409.
77. Pileri P, Uematsu Y, Campagnoli S, Galli G, Falugi F, Petracca R, Weiner AJ, Houghton M, Rosa D, Grandi G, Abrignani S. Binding of hepatitis C virus to CD81. Science. 1998;282:938–41.
78. Charles ED, Green RM, Marukian S, Talal AH, Lake-Bakaar GV, Jacobson IM, Rice CM, Dustin LB. Clonal expansion of immunoglobulin M+CD27+B cells in HCV-associated mixed cryoglobulinemia. Blood. 2008;111:1344–56.
79. Servais J, Nkoghe D, Schmit JC, Arendt V, Robert I, Staub T, Moutschen M, Schneider F, Hemmer R. HIV associated hematologic disorders are correlated with plasma viral load and improve under highly active antiretroviral therapy. J Acquir Immune Defic Syndr. 2001;28:221–5.
80. Carbonara S, Fiorentino G, Serio G, Maggi P, Ingravallo G, Monno L, Bruno F, Coppola S, Pastore G, Angarano G. Response of severe HIV-associated thrombocytopenia to highly active antiretroviral therapy including protease inhibitors. J Infect. 2001;42:251–6.

81. Kunzi MS, Groopman JE. Identification of a novel human immunodeficiency virus strain cytopathic to megakaryocytic cells. Blood. 1993;81:3336–42.
82. Nardi M, Karpatkin S. Antiidiotype antibody against platelet anti-gpIIIa contributes to the regulation of thrombocytopenia in HIV-1-ITP patients. J Exp Med. 2000;191:2093–100.
83. Zucker-Franklin D, Termin CS, Cooper MC. Structural changes in the megakaryocytes of patients infected with the human immune deficiency virus (HIV-1). Am J Pathol. 1989;134:1295–303.
84. Visco C, Ruggeri M, Laura Evangelista M, Stasi R, Zanotti R, Giaretta I, Ambrosetti A, Madeo D, Pizzolo G, Rodeghiero F. Impact of immune thrombocytopenia on the clinical course of chronic lymphocytic leukemia. Blood. 2008;111:1110–6.
85. Hamblin TJ. Autoimmune complications of chronic lymphocytic leukemia. Semin Oncol. 2006;33:230–9.
86. Akbar AN, Salmon M, Ivory K, Taki S, Piling D, Janossy G. Human CD4+CD45R0+ and CD4+CD45RA+ T cells synergize in response to alloantigens. Eur J Immunol. 1991;21(10):2517–22.
87. Lai DW, Loughran TP Jr, Maciejewski JP, Sasu S, Song SX, Epling-Burnett PK, Paquette RL. Acquired amegakaryocytic thrombocytopenia and pure red cell aplasia associated with an occult large granular lymphocyte leukemia. Leuk Res. 2008;32:823–7.
88. Fogarty PF, Stetler-Stevenson M, Pereira A, Dunbar CE. Large granular lymphocytic proliferation-associated cyclic thrombocytopenia. Am J Hematol. 2005;79:334–6.
89. Nakamura M, Tanaka Y, Satoh T, Kawai M, Hirakata M, Kaburaki J, Kawakami Y, Ikeda Y, Kuwana M. Autoantibody to CD40 ligand in systemic lupus erythematosus: association with thrombocytopenia but not thromboembolism. Rheumatology (Oxford). 2006;45:150–6.
90. Kuwana M, Okazaki Y, Kajihara M, Kaburaki J, Miyazaki H, Kawakami Y, Ikeda Y. Autoantibody to cMpl (thrombopoietin receptor) in systemic lupus erythematosus. Arthritis Rheum. 2002;46:2148–59.
91. Nossent JC, Swaak AJG. Prevalence and significance of haematological abnormalities in patients with systemic lupus erythematosus. Q J Med. 1991;80:605–12.
92. Treachy DT, Manno CS, Axsom KM, Andrews T, Choi JK, Greenbaum BH, McMann JM, Sullivan KE, Travis SF, Grupp SA. Unmasking Evans syndrome T-cell phenotype and apoptotic response reveal autoimmune lymphoproliferative syndrome (ALPS). Blood. 2005;105(6):2443–8.
93. Norton A, Roberts I. Management of Evans syndrome. Br J Haematol. 2005;132:125–37.

Chapter 3
Presentation and Evaluation of Immune Thrombocytopenia

Vicky R. Breakey

Introduction

Thrombocytopenia is a common clinical issue in both pediatric and adult medicine. An assessment of the platelet count is routinely sought when there are clinical signs of excessive bruising or bleeding. In addition, thrombocytopenia may be diagnosed incidentally from a complete blood count (CBC) in an asymptomatic patient. While immune thrombocytopenia (ITP) is one of the most common etiologies for a low platelet count, the lack of a specific and sensitive confirmatory diagnostic test makes it a diagnosis of exclusion. This chapter will review the common clinical presentations of ITP and focus on the approach to diagnosis.

Clinical Presentation

The clinical presentation of ITP varies based on the age of the patient and the severity of the thrombocytopenia. In children, ITP usually has an acute onset and often follows a viral illness that occurred in the weeks prior to presentation, resulting in seasonal peaks for diagnosis in the spring and fall [1]. In adulthood, ITP generally has a more insidious onset. The peak pediatric age is 2–6 years, but ITP can occur at any age. In the first year of life, ITP is atypical and is more likely to become chronic. Similarly, ITP in adolescents often behaves more like adult-onset ITP. In children, males and females are equally affected, unlike adults where the incidence of ITP is two- to threefold higher in females.

V. R. Breakey, MD, MEd, FRCPC (Peds) (✉)
Department of Pediatrics, McMaster University, Hamilton, ON, Canada
e-mail: breakev@mcmaster.ca

© Springer International Publishing AG, part of Springer Nature 2018
J. M. Despotovic (ed.), *Immune Hematology*,
https://doi.org/10.1007/978-3-319-73269-5_3

In the setting of newly diagnosed ITP, the patient often presents with petechiae and ecchymoses. Bleeding is a less common presenting symptom of ITP, possibly a result of large, functional young platelets that circulate prior to antibody attack and removal from the circulation [2]. Many studies show that the severity of bleeding does not correlate consistently with the platelet count [3–5]. A recent systemic review of bleeding in ITP showed that intracranial hemorrhage (ICH) is a very rare event in both children (0.4%) and adults (0.6%) [6]. Non-ICH severe bleeding occurred in approximately 10% of adults and 20% of children in the acute presentation with ITP [6]. Significant bleeding is rare and generally occurs only when platelets are $<30 \times 10^9/\mu L$.

History

On the first presentation, a detailed history can assist in determining the etiology of the clinical symptoms (Table 3.1). The bleeding history should document the type, pattern, and timing of bruising and/or bleeding. Common sites of bleeding secondary to abnormal primary hemostasis include predominantly skin and mucocutaneous bleeding (epistaxis, oral, GI bleeding, and menorrhagia). Thrombocytopenia is generally not associated with spontaneous muscle or joint bleeding, so the presence of these findings should instigate additional work-up to assess coagulation factors. The onset and timing of bleeding and its relation to triggers such as surgeries and dental extractions can help to determine the severity as well as the chronicity of the condition.

A review of the family history is also important for patients with thrombocytopenia. Although there is no known genetic cause of ITP, several clusters of ITP in families have been documented suggesting there may be a genetic link [7, 8]. In some cases, multiple family members may be affected with ITP and/or other auto-

Table 3.1 Bleeding history to differentiate causes of thrombocytopenia

Key point	Newly diagnosed ITP	Inherited/genetic thrombocytopenia
Onset of bleeding/bruising	Recent	Early in life
Viral prodrome	Often, especially in children	No
Constitutional symptoms	No	No
History of bleeding with triggers (surgery, dental extractions, minor cuts/trauma)	Usually spontaneous onset of bleeding with no significant past bleeding	Yes, often significant
Evidence of congenital anomalies	No	Sometimes (see Table 3.2)
Consanguinity in parents	No	Sometimes (increased in recessive conditions)
Personal history of low platelet counts	No	Yes
Family members with low platelets	Rarely	Often

Table 3.2 Conditions associated with secondary ITP

Autoimmune disorders	Evans syndrome Autoimmune lymphoproliferative syndrome (ALPS) Systemic lupus erythematosus (SLE)
Immunodeficiencies	Combined variable immunodeficiency (CVID)
Infections	*Helicobacter pylori* HIV Hepatitis C Cytomegalovirus Varicella zoster
Drug effects	Strong evidence for quinine, quinidine, trimethoprim/sulfamethoxazole, vancomycin, penicillin, rifampin, carbamazepine, ceftriaxone, ibuprofen, mirtazapine, oxaliplatin, suramin, glycoprotein IIb/IIIa inhibitors (abciximab, tirofiban, eptifibatide), heparin
Others	Vaccine side effect (MMR) Post-bone marrow or solid organ transplantation Antiphospholipid syndrome (APS)

immune disorders suggesting an underlying immunodeficiency or autoimmune predisposition. More commonly, however, a family history positive for ITP suggests an underlying familial thrombocytopenia that is not immune in nature. Inherited thrombocytopenias should be considered and ruled out in families with multiple people that have low platelets [9] (see Chap. 1).

A detailed review of systems may suggest an underlying condition that may have predisposed to ITP. Common comorbid conditions include primary immunodeficiencies, rheumatologic conditions, and other autoimmune conditions (see Table 3.2). The presence of constitutional symptoms is not in keeping with ITP and may suggest a malignancy. A review of current medications is essential as drug-induced thrombocytopenia may be misdiagnosed as primary ITP. A list of drugs that have been shown to cause immune thrombocytopenia can be found in Table 3.2 and have been reviewed in detail recently [10]. Similarly, a complete vaccination review, including timing of the most recent vaccinations, is important as there is evidence to suggest that ITP may occur subsequent to either natural infection with measles or rubella or after the inoculation for measles, mumps, and rubella (MMR) [11].

Physical Examination

The physical examination serves to document the degree of petechiae and ecchymoses, as well as other types of bleeding, and to ensure that the patient is otherwise well without other abnormalities. In typical ITP, there are no other abnormal physical findings. It is important to confirm the absence of clinically significant lymphadenopathy and hepatosplenomegaly. Familial thrombocytopenias may be associated with specific physical findings related to the causative genetic mutation (Table 3.3).

Table 3.3 Physical findings associated with inherited thrombocytopenias

Condition	Inheritance pattern	Gene implicated	Unique clinical/lab findings (in addition to bleeding symptoms)
Small platelets			
Wiskott-Aldrich syndrome	X-linked	*WAS*	Infections secondary to combined immunodeficiency, autoimmune conditions, eczema, cancer predisposition
X-linked thrombocytopenia	X-linked	*WAS*	None
Normal size platelets			
Congenital amegakaryocytic thrombocytopenia (CAMT)	Autosomal recessive	*MPL*	Pancytopenia/bone marrow failure in childhood
Amegakaryocytic thrombocytopenia with radioulnar synostosis	Autosomal dominant	*HOXA11*	Proximal radioulnar synostosis ± other skeletal anomalies, some with sensorineural deafness
Thrombocytopenia absent radii (TAR)	Autosomal recessive	Unknown	Shortened/absent radii bilaterally
Familial platelet disorder/AML		*AML1*	Early onset myelodysplasia, acute myelogenous leukemia
Large platelets			
MYH9-related disorders	Autosomal dominant	*MYH9*	Sensorineural hearing loss, glomerulonephritis, cataracts
Gray platelet syndrome	Autosomal dominant and recessive types	Unknown	Alpha-granules absent, making platelets appear grey in blood smear, some develop myelofibrosis
X-linked thrombocytopenia with dyserythropoiesis	X-linked	*GATA-1*	Variable anemia ± evidence of hemolysis, hypercellular marrow with erythro- and myelodysplasia
Bernard-Soulier syndrome	Autosomal recessive	*GP1BA, GPIBB, GP9*	Bleeding due to platelet dysfunction
Velocardiofacial syndrome (DiGeorge)	Autosomal dominant	22q deletion	Dysmorphism, developmental and growth delay, cardiac anomalies, cleft lip/palate, hypoparathyroidism, immunodeficiencies
Paris-Trousseau/Jacobsen syndrome	Autosomal dominant	*11q23 (FLI1)*	Congenital impairment, dysmorphic features, cardiac anomalies, growth issues

Bleeding Assessment

Together, the history and physical examination findings can be incorporated into a bleeding score. As the platelet number is often not well correlated with bleeding severity in ITP, the use of a standardized bleeding score can be helpful to quantify bleeding symptoms at the time of diagnosis and to monitor over time. A recent systematic review identified ten ITP-specific bleeding assessment tools in the literature, two of which have been validated [6]. In clinical practice, some of these tools are felt to be onerous to administer, and their utility is reserved to assess response to therapies in research studies.

Initial Diagnostic Investigations

The complete blood count (CBC) confirms and quantifies thrombocytopenia. Patients with ITP have an isolated thrombocytopenia with preservation of normal white and red blood cell counts. It is important to ensure that the low platelet count is genuine; automated counters may underestimate platelet number when platelet size is abnormal. The mean platelet volume (MPV) is an indicator of platelet size and may be inaccurate with devices that count giant platelets as red cells or in counters with settings that exclude platelets at both extremes of size from the MPV calculation. Platelet size is variable to large in ITP, and MPV may help to differentiate ITP from inherited thrombocytopenias. The size of the platelets can be confirmed on a blood smear, which can rule out platelet clumping and pseudothrombocytopenia (Fig. 3.1). Other than fewer than expected platelets of normal-to-large size, no additional findings are typical on the blood smear in patients with ITP, but other abnormalities may give clues to inherited thrombocytopenias, such as the Dohle-like inclusions seen in the neutrophils of patients with macrothrombocytes due to

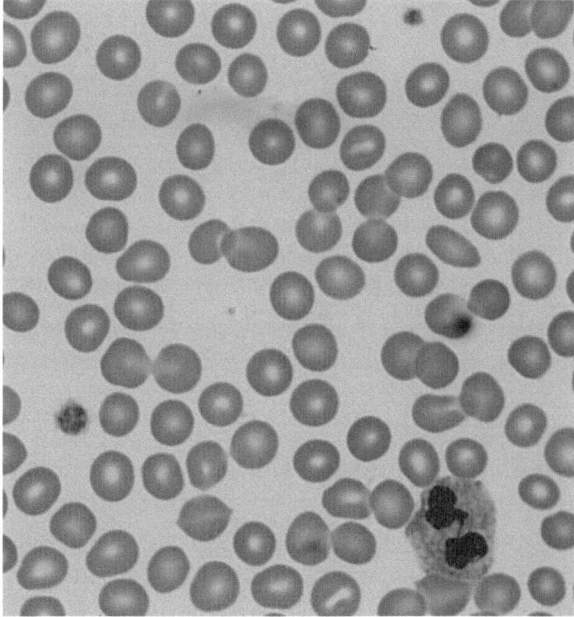

Fig. 3.1 Blood smear in ITP (Image provided by Dr. Jenny Despotovic)

MYH9-related thrombocytopenia. Newer automated machines may report the immature platelet fraction (IPF), which is high in ITP due to high platelet turnover and low in thrombocytopenias due to decreased production. Early studies have suggested that IPF may be useful in deciphering etiology of thrombocytopenia and may be predictive of the development of chronic ITP [12].

In addition to the platelet parameters, other elements of the CBC should be considered. In patients with ITP, the white cell count and differential should be within normal range. Anemia warrants additional consideration, as iron deficiency is prevalent and may be comorbid. In the setting of typical hypochromic, microcytic anemia, iron indices may be sought to confirm iron deficiency anemia. A high MCV and moderate thrombocytopenia should raise the suspicion of possible underlying bone marrow dysfunction, including bone marrow aplasia/dysplasia or inherited bone marrow failure syndromes such as Fanconi anemia. Macrocytic anemia in the setting of thrombocytopenia without a clear etiology warrants bone marrow investigation.

Diagnostic Approach

Taken together, the patient's history, physical examination, and initial investigations are instrumental in considering the differential diagnosis of thrombocytopenia and help in determining if additional testing is necessary. Typical ITP is a diagnosis of exclusion. In addition to the inherited thrombocytopenias mentioned already, other inherited and acquired causes of thrombocytopenia should be considered (see Chap. 1).

Additional Testing for Suspected ITP

The role of additional testing in asymptomatic patients with presumed ITP remains controversial. An International Working Group (IWG) panel of ITP experts published their international consensus on the diagnosis and treatment of ITP in 2010 [13]. Shortly following, the American Society of Hematology (ASH) published an evidence-based practice guideline that summarized the relevant literature using the GRADE system [14]. While these reports are generally in agreement, there are small differences, and their rationales are reviewed here briefly.

The Role of Bone Marrow Testing

The ASH ITP guideline recommends that routine bone marrow examination is not indicated for the diagnosis of typical ITP in children or adolescents, even in those who do not respond to intravenous immunoglobulin (IVIG) therapy. Furthermore, they suggest that bone marrow examination is not needed prior to initiating steroid therapy or prior to splenectomy for typical ITP in children. Similarly, the ASH guidelines suggest that no bone marrow testing is needed in adults with typical ITP, regardless of the age of the patient [14] (Table 3.4).

Conversely, the IWG panel report suggests a bone marrow examination is recommended in children who show no improvement after 3–6 months with no prior response to therapy. For adult patients >60 years of age, a bone marrow evaluation is recommended at presentation of suspected ITP, based on a higher chance of subclinical marrow dysplasia or malignancy.

Table 3.4 Comparison of recommendations from the ASH ITP guidelines (2011) and the International Consensus Panel (2010) for the investigation of suspected ITP

Investigation	International Consensus Panel (2010)	American Society of Hematology ITP Guideline (2011)
Bone marrow examination for children	• Only when atypical features (not just isolated thrombocytopenia in CBC, systemic features, splenomegaly) • Consider in patients who respond minimally or not at all to first-line therapies • Recommend testing if no improvement in >3–6 months	• Not for patients with typical ITP • Not necessary in cases who fail to respond to IVIG therapy • Suggest not needed prior to steroids or splenectomy
Bone marrow examination for adults	• >60 years and/or systemic symptoms/signs • Prior to splenectomy	• Not at any age for typical ITP
H. pylori testing adults	• Screen with the urea breath test or stool antigen test	• Screen patients who would be treated for a positive *H. pylori* result
H. *pylori* testing—children	• May be of benefit in children with persistent or chronic ITP	• No evidence to test children
HIV and hepatitis C testing	• Recommend testing adults for both at diagnosis • Test children with persistent/chronic ITP in regions where there is a high prevalence	• Recommend testing adults for both at diagnosis
Platelet antibody testing	• Describe the glycoprotein-specific antibody testing as "potentially useful" but do not recommend routine analysis as platelet-associated IgG is elevated in both immune and nonimmune thrombocytopenia	• Insufficient evidence for platelet antibody testing
Screening for autoimmune conditions	• Recommend ANA testing in children with persistent/chronic ITP	• No good evidence to screen all patients with ANA
Screening for immunodeficiency	• Suggest baseline Igs studies in all adult patients with acute ITP and for surveillance in children with persistent or chronic ITP	• Utility of screening all patients with baseline Igs is unclear

Platelet Antibody Testing

Many assays have been developed to measure the antiplatelet antibodies that cause platelet destruction in ITP. Unfortunately, these assays lack sensitivity and/or specificity. The IWG panel describes glycoprotein-specific antibody testing as "potentially useful" but does not recommend routine analysis as platelet-associated IgG is elevated in both immune and nonimmune thrombocytopenia. The ASH ITP guidelines suggest there is insufficient evidence to support the routine use of antiplatelet antibodies as a diagnostic test for ITP in children and adults [14].

Screening Tests for Associated Conditions

Infectious Triggers for ITP: Hepatitis C, HIV, and *H. pylori*

There are no recommended screening tests for infections in children with acute ITP. In adults, both ASH and the IWG expert panel recommend screening adults with new-onset ITP for both hepatitis C and HIV. Treatment of these viral infections is recommended if they are confirmed, as it may lead to resolution of the ITP. The IWG suggests screening children in whom ITP persists >3–6 months in regions there is a high prevalence of these infections.

   H. pylori has been implicated in adult ITP, and screening with the urea breath test or stool antigen test has been recommended by the IWG panel. The ASH group also supports screening in adult ITP patients who would be treated for a positive *H. pylori* result. They note that eradication is most successful in patients with less severe ITP and in countries where *H. pylori* is more prevalent. In children, ASH does not recommend *H. pylori* testing for acute or chronic ITP due to a lack of compelling evidence. The IWG group suggests that testing may be of benefit in children with persistent or chronic ITP.

Autoimmune Conditions

Autoimmune hemolytic anemia may occur with ITP, and together they are labeled as Evans syndrome [15]. One study found 22% of all ITP patients tested had a positive direct antiglobulin test (DAT), but the clinical significance of this is unclear [16]. The IWG recommends screening DAT in all patients with ITP. At minimum, a DAT is recommended in patients with anemia, reticulocytosis, and/or evidence of hemolysis. A DAT is also needed prior to therapy with anti-D (see Chap. 4 for more details).

   The ASH ITP guidelines do not support screening with antinuclear antibodies (ANA) in children or adults with typical ITP, while the IWG panel suggests that a positive ANA may be a predictor of chronic ITP developing in children [17].

Similarly, the IWG panel suggests screening for antithyroid antibodies/thyroid function as well as antiphospholipid antibodies to be of potential utility in ITP, while the ASH group points out the lack of evidence for the routine use of these tests in the absence of clinical symptoms in both children and adults with ITP.

Immunodeficiencies

Due to an association between combined variable immunodeficiency (CVID) and ITP, it is common practice to check quantitative immunoglobulins in patients with ITP. While the IWG panel supports baseline studies in all patients with acute ITP and for surveillance in children with persistent/chronic ITP, the ASH guideline is less clear, suggesting that the utility of screening all patients is unclear. It is important to consider an assessment of baseline immunologic function prior to embarking on immunosuppressive therapies for ITP.

Summary

The diagnosis of ITP requires a thorough history, careful physical examination, and minimal investigations to rule out other causes of thrombocytopenia. The approach to diagnostic work-up should follow the evidence whenever possible to minimize unnecessary tests and discomfort to the patient. However, it is reasonable to consider baseline screening to detect underlying causes and/or additional antibodies as recommended by expert consensus guidelines.

References

1. Kuhne T, Imbach P, Bolton-Maggs PH, Berchtold W, Blanchette V, Buchanan GR, et al. Newly diagnosed idiopathic thrombocytopenic purpura in childhood: an observational study. Lancet. 2001;358(9299):2122–5.
2. Kenet G, Lubetsky A, Shenkman B, Tamarin I, Dardik R, Rechavi G, et al. Cone and platelet analyser (CPA): a new test for the prediction of bleeding among thrombocytopenic patients. Br J Haematol. 1998;101(2):255–9.
3. Page LK, Psaila B, Provan D, Hamilton JM, Jenkins JM, Elish AS, et al. The immune thrombocytopenic purpura (ITP) bleeding score: assessment of bleeding in patients with ITP. Br J Haematol. 2007;138(2):245–8.
4. Khellaf M, Michel M, Schaeffer A, Bierling P, Godeau B. Assessment of a therapeutic strategy for adults with severe autoimmune thrombocytopenic purpura based on a bleeding score rather than platelet count. Haematol-Hematol J. 2005;90(6):829–32.
5. Pansy J, Minkov M, Dengg R, Quehenberger F, Lackner H, Nebl A, et al. Evaluating bleeding severity in children with newly diagnosed immune thrombocytopenia: a pilot study. Klin Padiatr. 2010;222(6):374–7.

6. Neunert C, Noroozi N, Norman G, Buchanan GR, Goy J, Nazi I, et al. Severe bleeding events in adults and children with primary immune thrombocytopenia: a systematic review. J Thromb Haemost. 2015;13(3):457–64.

7. Patel AP. Idiopathic autoimmune thrombocytopenia and neutropenia in siblings. Eur J Haematol. 2002;69(2):120–1.

8. Rischewski JR, Imbach P, Paulussen M, Kühne T. Idiopathic thrombocytopenic purpura (ITP): is there a genetic predisposition? Pediatr Blood Cancer. 2006;47(S5):678–80.

9. Drachman JG. Inherited thrombocytopenia: when a low platelet count does not mean ITP. Blood. 2004;103(2):390–8.

10. Arnold DM, Kukaswadia S, Nazi I, Esmail A, Dewar L, Smith JW, et al. A systematic evaluation of laboratory testing for drug-induced immune thrombocytopenia. J Thromb Haemost. 2013;11(1):169–76.

11. Mantadakis E, Farmaki E, Buchanan GR. Thrombocytopenic purpura after measles-mumps-rubella vaccination: a systematic review of the literature and guidance for management. J Pediatr. 2010;156(4):623–8.

12. Serrando M, Marull A, Ruiz M, Perez Del Campo D, Puig-Pey I, Munoz JM, et al. Clinical significance of IPF% measurement in diagnosing thrombocytopenic disorders: distinguishing primary immune thrombocytopenia from other disorders. Int J Lab Hematol. 2016;38(3):e65–8.

13. Provan D, Stasi R, Newland AC, Blanchette VS, Bolton-Maggs P, Bussel JB, et al. International consensus report on the investigation and management of primary immune thrombocytopenia. Blood. 2010;115(2):168–86.

14. Neunert C, Lim W, Crowther M, Cohen A, Solberg L Jr, Crowther MA, et al. The American Society of Hematology 2011 evidence-based practice guideline for immune thrombocytopenia. Blood. 2011;117(16):4190–207.

15. Evans RS, Takahashi K, Duane RT, Payne R, Liu C. Primary thrombocytopenic purpura and acquired hemolytic anemia; evidence for a common etiology. AMA Arch Intern Med. 1951;87(1):48–65.

16. Aledort LM, Hayward CP, Chen MG, Nichol JL, Bussel J, Group ITPS. Prospective screening of 205 patients with ITP, including diagnosis, serological markers, and the relationship between platelet counts, endogenous thrombopoietin, and circulating antithrombopoietin antibodies. Am J Hematol. 2004;76(3):205–13.

17. Altintas A, Ozel A, Okur N, Okur N, Cil T, Pasa S, et al. Prevalence and clinical significance of elevated antinuclear antibody test in children and adult patients with idiopathic thrombocytopenic purpura. J Thromb Thrombolysis. 2007;24(2):163–8.

Chapter 4
The Treatment of Immune Thrombocytopenia

Kandace L. Gollomp and Michele P. Lambert

Introduction

The treatment of patients with immune thrombocytopenia (ITP) has evolved rapidly over the past 20 years. Many of these advances have been based on an improved understanding of the disease, the development of a more nuanced disease classification system, and a recognition that patients, especially children, without significant bleeding can often be safely observed irrespective of platelet count. Newer therapeutics that target platelet production or specific parts of the immune response have changed the landscape of treatment and allowed for increased use of steroid-sparing treatment strategies. As our understanding of disease pathophysiology continues to improve and as more data emerges about the efficacy and safety of novel therapeutics, new questions arise about how to best tailor treatment strategies to individual patients. In 2010–2011, the American Society of Hematology (ASH) [1] and a report from an International Working Group (IWG) [2] sought to address these questions with new guidelines for the diagnosis and management of ITP. In the years since the publication of these seminal papers, the use of thrombopoietin receptor agonists (TPO-RAs) has emerged for the management of chronic disease, and other targeted therapies have been developed. Still, uncertainty remains with respect to which patients require treatment, clarifying the role of splenectomy, and managing children and adults with refractory disease. This chapter addresses these areas of uncertainty by reviewing current ITP therapy, summarizing recent treatment guidelines, examining emerging therapeutic strategies, and highlighting areas of controversy.

K. L. Gollomp, MD (✉) · M. P. Lambert, MD
Division of Hematology, The Children's Hospital of Philadelphia, Philadelphia, PA, USA
e-mail: gollompk@email.chop.edu

© Springer International Publishing AG, part of Springer Nature 2018   45
J. M. Despotovic (ed.), *Immune Hematology*,
https://doi.org/10.1007/978-3-319-73269-5_4

General Treatment Considerations

Before deciding on an appropriate course of treatment, practitioners caring for patients with ITP need to consider numerous factors including bleeding symptoms, risk of future bleeding, the likelihood of spontaneous remission, patient age, medical comorbidities, level of activity, underlying immune function, access to medical care, and concerns related to quality of life. Current guidelines prioritize treating bleeding symptoms over achieving specific platelet thresholds. Recent studies suggest that observation alone is appropriate for the majority of pediatric patients at the time of presentation [3] and may be appropriate for select groups of adult patients with newly diagnosed ITP [4, 5]. When treatment is indicated, first-line therapy for ITP currently includes corticosteroids, intravenous immunoglobulin (IVIG), and intravenous anti-D immunoglobulin (IV anti-D). The list of standard second-line therapies addressed in guidelines include splenectomy, rituximab, and (for adults) TPO-RAs. Data is emerging for the use of a variety of oral immunosuppressants and TPO-RAs in pediatric ITP [1, 2], and new forthcoming updated guidelines are likely to provide additional guidance on the role of these agents in children.

Who Should Be Treated?

The primary goal of treatment for adults and children with ITP is to achieve adequate hemostasis rather than reaching a specific platelet threshold. With this management strategy, it is critical to understand the underlying determinants of severe bleeding, such as intracranial hemorrhage (ICH) or visceral bleeding, in order to recognize patients who require pharmacologic therapy even at higher platelet counts.

Adults: Previous studies have suggested that low platelet counts, increased patient age, newly diagnosed disease, comorbidities (severe hypertension, renal insufficiency, gastritis or peptic ulcer disease), the use of concurrent medications (anticoagulants, antiplatelet agents), and male sex are associated with increased rates of bleeding [6, 7]. Current guidelines recommend treating newly diagnosed adult patients with platelet counts below 30×10^9/L irrespective of individual characteristics or associated bleeding symptoms [1]. Work is being done to develop more nuanced risk stratification to accurately determine which patients will benefit from treatment. For example, preliminary studies suggest that platelet function measurements can be used to predict the risk of future bleeding [8]. Much research is also being done to define risk factors that contribute to intracranial hemorrhage (ICH) because it can have such devastating clinical consequences. This work is difficult as ICH in the setting of ITP is fortunately rare. In 2015, Neunert and colleagues conducted a systematic review, including 118 studies and 908 patients, and found that ICH occurs in 1.4% of adult ITP patients [9]. In 2016, Altomare et al.

used a large medical claims database to identify 6651 patients with primary ITP and found that ICH was reported in 1% of the cohort [10]. To more accurately identify risk factors for ICH, Melboucy-Belkhir and colleagues studied a cohort of 27 cases of adult patients with ITP and ICH. They found that 37% presented with ICH within 3 months of diagnosis and 74% of these patients had received treatment prior to the event [11]. Compared to control ITP patients, those who developed ICH were more likely to have had prior bleeding symptoms, such as hematuria and visceral hemorrhage, and a history of head trauma [11, 12]. Older adults with ITP have also been found to have a significantly higher risk of bleeding. A meta-analysis of 17 clinical case series including 1817 patients showed that the rates of fatal hemorrhage ranged from 0% to 4% per year for patients younger than 40 years, to 13% per year for those 60 years and older [13]. These patients may also be at a greater risk of injury from falls and are more likely to have medical comorbidities that require treatment with antithrombotic agents. In light of these considerations, experts recommend adopting an individualized multidisciplinary treatment approach for older adults with platelet counts between 30 and $50 \times 10^9/L$ [7].

Pediatrics: The rates of bleeding in children with ITP are extremely low, and published treatment guidelines recommend that children with ITP and no bleeding or mild skin bleeding, such as bruising or petechiae, be managed with observation alone irrespective of platelet counts [1]. This recommendation is based on the fact that 70–80% of children achieve spontaneous remission within 6 months of diagnosis [5], and observed rates of significant hemorrhage, such as gastrointestinal bleeding, severe epistaxis, and ICH, are exceedingly low. In a prospective study that followed 505 newly diagnosed children with no bleeding symptoms and platelet counts less than $20 \times 10^9/L$ for 28 days, severe hemorrhage was seen in 0.6% ($n = 3$) of children, all due to mucosal bleeding with no cases of ICH. No relationship was found between the initial mode of treatment and the risk of future bleeding [14]. A 2015 study summarizing data pooled from administrative databases, clinical studies, and ITP registries showed that the frequency of ICH was 0.5% in children. Interestingly, in children with platelet counts below $30 \times 10^9/L$, the severity of thrombocytopenia correlated poorly with the risk of bleeding, indicating that thrombocytopenia is necessary but not sufficient to cause severe hemorrhage [15]. Other risk factors for ICH in children were found to be mucosal bleeding, gross hematuria, acute disease, and head trauma [15]. Due to the low prevalence of severe bleeding events, prior studies have not clarified whether upfront treatment reduces the risk of subsequent hemorrhage in pediatric patients. A randomized trial powered to address this question would require 900 patients per treatment arm and is unlikely to be performed [5]. As the benefits of therapeutic intervention remain unclear, side effect profiles are significant, and the risk of significant bleeding is extremely low in minimally symptomatic children, most experts agree that observation alone is appropriate for these patients who do not have additional risk factors. There is no clear age at which the ASH guidelines recommend treating adolescents like adults [1]. However, it is worth noting that the risk of life-threatening bleeding remains close to the pediatric rate in adults younger than 40 [7].

First-Line Management

The goal of first-line therapy for ITP is the rapid cessation of bleeding and/or bleeding risk. These therapies are not designed to provide durable platelet response. Current first-line options for ITP include corticosteroids, IV immunoglobulin (IVIG), and intravenous anti-D immunoglobulin (IV anti-D). Guidelines recommend treating newly diagnosed adults with platelet counts $<30 \times 10^9/L$ and pediatric or adult patients with moderate to severe bleeding symptoms including oral/mucosal bleeding, epistaxis, menorrhagia, visceral hemorrhage, or ICH.

Corticosteroids

Corticosteroids have been used routinely in the treatment of ITP since the 1960s [16]. In fact, platelet rise following steroid exposure has been used to help confirm the diagnosis of ITP. Corticosteroids generally lead to elevation in platelet count (although onset of action may be slower than IVIG and anti-D, generally ~48–72 h to onset of action) and reduction in bleeding symptoms in roughly two thirds of patients with ITP, but these effects are usually transient, and platelet counts fall with discontinuation of treatment [17]. Steroids are thought to improve immune thrombocytopenia through multiple mechanisms. However, steroid use leads to many common adverse effects including weight gain, hypertension, hyperglycemia, mood changes, growth retardation, cataracts, osteoporosis, and immunosuppression. Even short-term therapy with steroids can have significant side effects including an impact on mood, sleep, and hypertension. Therefore, it is advisable to try to limit steroid exposure in all age groups.

Mechanism of Action

It has been proposed that steroids contribute to prolonged platelet survival by suppressing antibody production, leading to decreased peripheral platelet destruction [18]. They also suppress B- and T-cell reactivity, alter cytokine levels, lead to reduced antibody production, inhibit phagocytosis, and enhance microvascular endothelial stability [19]. However, in the late 1980s, Gernsheimer et al. performed studies that suggested steroid treatment may also influence ITP by increasing platelet production [20]. Their group measured survival time and localization of radiolabeled autologous platelets before and after initiation of prednisone in 12 patients with ITP. In 11 individuals (92%) who had increased platelet counts, they found no changes in the length of platelet survival but did observe a marked increase in platelet production [19]. A 2008 study performed by Houwerzijl et al. found that rates of platelet production may predict responsiveness to steroid treatment in ITP. They examined a group of 75 patients with platelets less than $20 \times 10^9/L$ and performed kinetic studies that demonstrated decreased, normal, and increased platelet production in 33%, 48%, and 19% of individuals, respectively. Sixty-four percent of patients with decreased platelet production responded to prednisone, whereas only 34% of patients with normal to increased rates of platelet production responded to treatment [21]. While these findings could suggest that steroids directly affect thrombopoiesis, other studies demonstrate that they may suppress the production of autoantibodies that bind to megakaryocyte surface glycoproteins and lead to impaired maturation and reduced platelet release [22, 23].

More recent work has shown that steroids may ameliorate ITP by inducing immune tolerance. In 2007, Ling and colleagues examined a group of 24 patients with chronic ITP and found they had decreased regulatory T cells (Tregs) compared to healthy controls. In 2013, Li et al. observed that treatment of chronic ITP with high-dose dexamethasone (HDD) led to normalization of the Th1/Th2 ratio along with a decrease in Th17 levels and restoration of normal numbers of Tregs [24]. Treatment with HDD has also been found to cause a rise in numbers of tolerogenic myeloid dendritic cells [25]. More recently, treatment with HDD has been found to increase the numbers of circulating myeloid-derived suppressor cells (MDSCs) that regulate adaptive immunity by inhibiting T-cell proliferation [26].

Interestingly, following the initiation of corticosteroids, bleeding symptoms often abate before the platelet count rises. Evidence suggests this may occur because antiplatelet antibodies impair microvascular stability by directly activating endothelial cells [27]. Additionally, platelets play an important role in maintaining vascular hemostasis by releasing proangiogenic cytokines and growth factors, and thrombocytopenia can lead to thinning of the endothelium and capillary fragility [28]. Kitchens and colleagues investigated this hypothesis in a study of five patients with ITP, and they found that treatment with a 5-day course of prednisone led to a restoration of normal capillary wall thickness prior to platelet count recovery [29].

Steroid Treatment Recommendations

For many years, prednisone 1 mg/kg/day for 2–4 weeks followed by a taper has been the standard first-line treatment for ITP [5, 30]. This recommendation is based on the results of a randomized controlled trial (RCT), conducted in 2002 by Godeau and colleagues, that examined the use of prednisolone vs. placebo following high-dose methylprednisone or IVIG that showed higher platelet counts in the arm treated with a longer steroid course [31]. Since the publication of the ASH guidelines in 2011, there has been much interest in optimizing steroid therapy. Some experts recommend treating with prednisone 1 mg/kg/day for 4 days followed by a 6 week taper to minimize steroid-related adverse effects [4]. Others report that high-dose short courses of steroids may lead to more durable platelet responses. For example, a group at Royal Manchester Children's Hospital recently found that a 4-day pulse of higher-dose prednisone (4 mg/kg/day) was associated with a 6-week platelet response compared to a 4-week response observed following conventional prednisone treatment [32]. Other groups are investigating whether dexamethasone may be superior to prednisone in the treatment of ITP. Dexamethasone has an anti-inflammatory effect that is 6 times more potent than prednisone and a longer bio-logic half-life of 36–72 h compared to 12–36 h [33]. Laboratory studies have shown that HDD can more effectively modulate T-cell function, correct aberrant T-cell subsets, and alter cytokine secretion [34]. In 2002, a randomized clinical trial com-pared six 3-week cycles of pulsed HDD (0.6 mg/kg/day for 4 days) with standard prednisone therapy in 26 patients with newly diagnosed ITP. The complete response rate (platelet count $\geq 150 \times 10^9/L$) was higher in the HDD arm with 77% of patients achieving a "long-term" remission (median follow-up was 46 months) [30].

To determine if HDD is more likely to lead to a sustained response, a trial was performed with 192 adults with newly diagnosed ITP randomized to receive 1–2 cycles of HDD or standard therapy with 4 weeks of prednisone. While those who received 2 cycles of HDD had a more rapid rise in platelet counts, the 6-month sustained response rates were equivalent in both groups at 40% in the HDD arm and 41.2% in the prednisone arm [35] Mithoowani and colleagues added to these data with a systematic review and meta-analysis including nine randomized trials com-paring different corticosteroid regimens. Five studies (n = 533) compared one to three cycles of HDD to standard prednisone dosing. Fourteen days after the initia-tion of treatment, the platelet count was higher in adults treated with HDD regi-mens, but 6-month durable response rates were found to be similar in all groups. Based on these results, the authors concluded that HDD might be better for treat-ment in adults with acute bleeding who require a rapid rise in platelets counts [33]. This is still controversial, however, because given the increased potency of HDD, the side effect profile can also be significantly higher.

Intravenous Immunoglobulin

IVIG is a serum-precipitated immunoglobulin product prepared from plasma pooled from several thousand healthy donors containing predominantly polyclonal IgG antibodies directed against several million antigens. It was initially developed in the 1950s to treat infections in patients with underlying immunodeficiency and subse-quently found to be effective in the treatment of various autoimmune diseases [36]. It was first found to be useful in the treatment of ITP in 1980 when it was adminis-tered to a child with refractory ITP and Wiskott-Aldrich syndrome who had devel-oped hypogammaglobulinemia and recurrent infections due to prolonged treatment with immunosuppressive agents. Within 24 h of the first infusion (0.4 mg/kg), a significant rise in his platelet count was observed [37]. Numerous studies subse-quently confirmed that this finding was reproducible in children and adults with ITP and normal immunoglobulin levels [38, 39]. Responses are seen in up to 80% of patients, and half of those who respond achieve normal platelet counts. The platelet rise is rapid, occurring within 24 h in some patients with the peak typically seen within 2–4 days of treatment [2]. Studies suggest that IVIG leads to a more rapid platelet rise compared to IV methylprednisone [40]. These characteristics make IVIG the first choice of many clinicians when patients present with acute bleeding symptoms.

Each IVIG product has unique characteristics that may affect efficacy and treatment tolerability. In order to ensure the safety of the final product, donors are carefully selected, and measures are taken to inactivate viruses and minimize the risk of bacterial contamination. There is no recent evidence of IVIG transmission of HIV, HCV, HBV, or HTLV-1 [2]. Adverse effects occur in 24–36% of patients exposed to high-dose IVIG. Most are benign infusion reactions, consisting of fever, chills, myalgias, mild headache, flushing, nausea, changes in blood pressure, and tachycardia [41]. These events most commonly occur within 30 min of the start of treatment and can be curtailed by slowing the infusion rate. Pretreatment with analgesics, antihistamines, and IV glucocorticoids may also help to prevent infusion reactions [41]. True anaphylactoid reactions are very uncommon and usually occur in patients with IgA deficiency who react to small quantities of IgA present in some IVIG preparations. These patients can safely be treated with IgA-depleted IVIG [2, 42]. Severe toxicities such as hemolytic anemia, renal failure, and thrombosis are also rare, although the US FDA label carries two boxed warnings, for renal failure and thrombosis, for many IVIG products. Headaches are commonly reported 6–12 h after the administration of IVIG, and aseptic meningitis has been reported in 1% of patients [43]. When a severe headache occurs, it often leads to re-presentation to medical care, at which time it can be difficult to clinically distinguish aseptic meningitis from ICH, and neuroimaging may be required.

Mechanism of Action

Despite extensive research, the mechanism of action of IVIG is not yet completely understood. The rise in platelet count is thought to be due in part to the inhibition of peripheral immune-mediated platelet destruction [44]. In the early 1980s, Fehr et al. showed that IVIG treatment in non-splenectomized patients delayed the clearance of radiolabeled antibody-sensitized red blood cells. Based on this finding, they proposed that saturation of Fc receptors on splenic macrophages and monocytes in the mononuclear phagocyte system (MPS) (formerly called the reticuloendothelial system) leads to competitive downregulation of the phagocytosis of opsonized platelets [38]. Subsequent studies in murine models of ITP have demonstrated that Fc receptor blockade reverses thrombocytopenia [45–47], and in human trials, a murine monoclonal anti-FcγRIII antibody was found to transiently increase platelet counts in patients with refractory HIV-related ITP [48]. Preliminary studies showed that a humanized anti-FcγRIII antibody (GMA161) increased platelet counts in patients who failed IVIG therapy and is now under investigation in humans (clinicaltrials. gov; NCT00244257).

Other studies have raised questions about the contribution of Fc receptor blockade to the therapeutic effect of IVIG. For example, treatment with F(ab')$_2$ fragments, which have no Fc receptor-binding activity, was shown to improve thrombocytopenia in some patients with acute and chronic ITP [49, 50]. Studies performed by Samuelsson et al. revealed that IVIG is ineffective in the treatment of ITP mice lacking the sole inhibitory Fc receptor, FcγRIIB [46], that decreases B lymphocyte autoantibody production [51] and reduces antigen-presenting cell function [52]. Subsequent experiments showed that FcγRIIB-deficient mice with persistent thrombocytopenia following treatment with IVIG have delayed clearance of antibody-sensitized RBCs, indicating that MPS blockade continues to occur in these animals [53]. These findings have led to the theory that activation and upregulation of FcγRIIB on macrophages, monocytes, and lymphocytes are central to the therapeutic effect of IVIG.

IVIG has also been shown to modulate many other aspects of the immune response. For example, it interacts with various T-cell antigens including the T-cell receptor and can influence maturation of T-cell subtypes leading to higher proportion of suppressive Tregs and a decreased percentage of pro-inflammatory Th17 cells [54, 55]. Several studies have also found that IVIG leads to rapid changes in cytokine levels including tumor necrosis factor (TNF)-α, IL-6, IL-8, and IL-10 and regulation of B-cell inflammatory cytokines such as IFN-γ [56]. Other groups have hypothesized that IVIG leads to increased antibody clearance by saturating the neonatal Fc receptor (FcRn). The FcRn prolongs IgG half-life by transporting endocytosed antibodies out of the cell to protect them from intracellular degradation. They posit that IVIG outcompetes pathogenic antibodies for FcRn binding, leaving them more vulnerable to rapid clearance [57]. It has also been proposed that IVIG contains a subset of antibodies, termed anti-idiotypic antibodies, that bind to the antigen-combining region of autoantibodies, thereby neutralizing them [53]. Finally, there are reports that IVIG can attenuate complement activation by preventing the generation of the C5-9a membrane attack complex, binding C3a and C5a, and inhibit complement-dependent platelet clearance [58, 59].

IVIG Treatment Recommendations

Current guidelines suggest administering IVIG as a one-time infusion of 1 g/kg because it is more likely to lead to a significant platelet increase within 24 h compared to the historical treatment regimen of 0.4 g/kg/day for 5 days [1, 2]. The duration of response is typically 2–4 weeks but it can persist for several months. Of note, it is still effective in individuals who have undergone splenectomy. IVIG is often the preferred first-line therapy in children with bleeding symptoms because it leads to a more rapid platelet response than steroids [60]. It is also recommended as the first-line therapy in any patient for whom steroids are contraindicated. When given in combination with a short course of prednisone, IVIG has been found to lead to a more rapid and more durable platelet response in adults with newly diagnosed ITP with platelet counts less than $20 \times 10^9/L$ [61]. Nevertheless, corticosteroids are preferred as the first-line therapy in adults with new onset disease in the current guidelines because IVIG treatment is expensive, requires a prolonged infusion, and is associated with a high frequency of adverse effects. There is also concern about the use of IVIG in elderly patients for whom the risk of arterial and venous thrombosis is particularly high [7]. IVIG is thought to be safe and effective in pregnancy because it does not cross the placenta and there are no reports of adverse effects in neonates. Of note, it has no effect on fetal or neonatal platelet counts and has not been found to reduce the likelihood of neonatal ITP [62, 63].

Anti-D Immunoglobulin

Patients with ITP who are RhD antigen positive (Rh+) can be treated with Rh(D) immunoglobulin, also called polyclonal anti-D. Anti-D is derived from the plasma of RhD antigen-negative (Rh−) individuals who develop high anti-D titers following immunization with the D antigen. It was developed in the 1960s to prevent Rh isoimmunization in Rh-negative mothers [41] and found to be an effective treatment for ITP in the early 1980s by Salama and colleagues while they were investigating the mechanism underlying the effect of IVIG. To prove that MPS Fc receptor saturation decreases platelet destruction, they infused Rh + ITP patients with IV anti-D and observed a significant platelet increase in the majority of subjects [39, 64, 65]. These findings generated interest in the use of anti-D as a therapy for ITP and led to several clinical studies, the largest of which was performed in 1997 by Scaradavou et al. that included 261 patients treated with 50 μg/kg of anti-D [66]. The treatment response rate was 70% with a median duration of 21 days. Those who were Rh negative and splenectomized had minimal to no response.

Based on these results, anti-D was established as a first-line treatment for patients with ITP and received licensure in 1995. It is generally well tolerated at intravenous doses of 75 μg/kg and leads to a response in approximately 70–80% in Rh-positive patients. The effect typically lasts for 1–5 weeks and occasionally results in long-term remission [67].

At doses of 50 μg/kg, anti-D takes slightly longer than corticosteroids and IVIG to achieve its full effect, but doses of 75 μg/kg have been found to work as quickly as IVIG in pediatric patients [68]. Furthermore, anti-D is usually less expensive than IVIG with an estimated 35% cost saving per episode of treatment [69]. Donor exposure is substantially lower than IVIG (~500 donors per dose compared to ~20,000 in IVIG). Infusion reactions with headache, chills, fever, dizziness, and emesis are seen in 3% of patients [68], a significantly lower rate than that seen in patients treated with IVIG. These reactions can be prevented with premedication regimens including antihistamines, acetaminophen, and corticosteroids (prednisolone 50 mg). There is also a risk of anaphylaxis, usually seen in individuals with IgA deficiency [70].

Extravascular hemolysis is expected following anti-D administration in Rh + patients, and the average drop in hemoglobin of 0.5–2 g/dL is well tolerated in most cases [68]. However, in 2000, Gaines et al. published a report of 15 patients who developed life-threatening hemolysis following anti-D exposure [71]. Six patients required red cell transfusions, eight experienced exacerbation of renal insufficiency, two required dialysis, and two died from pulmonary edema and respiratory distress. Post-marketing surveillance from 1999 to 2004 revealed six cases of anti-D-related disseminated intravascular coagulation (DIC) with a median drop in hemoglobin of 7 g/dL. One pediatric patient in this group survived, but five adults died, and four deaths were associated with renal failure [72]. This information led the Food and Drug Administration (FDA) to issue a black box warning in 2010 [73] stating that anti-D can cause life-threatening hemolysis, clinically compromising anemia, organ failure, and acute respiratory distress syndrome [73]. Following the release of this warning, the use of anti-D declined [73, 74].

In 2012, an expert panel was convened to thoroughly investigate the adverse effects related to the use of anti-D. It concluded that patients at greatest risk of severe side effects where those over 65, those with active infections such as EBV and hepatitis C, those with cancer, and those with autoimmune disease. The panel stressed that the rate of severe hemolytic reactions was extremely low, occurring at a stable rate of 0.02–0.04% in exposed patients [75, 73]. It consequently endorsed the continued use of anti-D as a first-line treatment option for adults and children with ITP but recommended pretreatment with steroids, antihistamines, and acetaminophen. As severe hemolytic reactions occurred within 4 h of administration in 94% of cases, the panel also recommended observation for signs or symptoms of hemolysis for 8 h following drug administration [75]. Anti-D should also be avoided in patients with blood loss, evidence of preexisting hemolysis, cytokine storm/sepsis, or renal impairment. Nevertheless, many studies suggest it can be administered safely and effectively in carefully chosen pediatric and adult patients [76, 77].

Mechanism of Action

Initially, anti-D was thought to act through competitive inhibition of the MPS. This theory is supported by the fact that anti-D is minimally effective in Rh-negative individuals and patients who have undergone splenectomy. A more recent study, performed by Barsam et al. found no increase in immature platelet fraction (IPF) following treatment with anti-D, indicating that it works by decreasing platelet destruction rather than increased platelet production [44]. Using a murine model of ITP, Song et al. found that treatment with anti-RBC antibodies led to improvement in thrombocytopenia in both WT and FcγIIb knockout mice. They also noted that anti-D led to downregulation of the activating Fc receptor, FcγRIIIA, on splenic macrophages [78]. Cooper et al. performed a study comparing changes in cytokine levels in patients following IVIG and anti-D and found that IL-6, TNF-α, MCP-1, IL-10, and transforming growth factor (TGF)-β levels were significantly higher following anti-D than IVIG. These changes were found to be significantly influenced by FcγRIIa genotype, suggesting that anti-D exerts its effect through Fc receptor engagement [79]. These results suggest that anti-D and IVIG act through different mechanisms, with IVIG upregulating the inhibitory FcγRIIb receptor and anti-D inhibiting the activating Fc receptors, FcγRIIA and FcγRIIIA. Adding further support to this hypothesis, Bussel et al. have found that there is no relationship between clinical response to IVIG and response to anti-D. In fact, patients who are refractory to one treatment may be responsive to the other [80].

Anti-D Treatment Recommendations

Current guidelines support the first-line use of anti-D in patients who are Rh positive and have not undergone a splenectomy who require treatment for their ITP. Anti-D has many advantages when compared to IVIG including its moderate cost, its lower rate of infusion reactions [77], its comparable efficacy, and its possible increased duration of action [66]. A baseline complete blood count, reticulocyte count, and direct antiglobulin test (DAT) must be obtained prior to treatment to ensure that no patients with blood loss or hemolysis receive anti-D [75]. Patients over 65 and those with evidence of an acute infection should be treated with extreme caution, and anti-D should not be given to patients with renal disease. Following the infusion, clinicians should monitor all patients for evidence of hemolysis and obtain posttreatment complete blood counts and urinalyses [75]. The authors of the ASH guidelines concluded that there was insufficient evidence to recommend a specific dose of anti-D, and IV infusions of 50–75 µg/kg are acceptable. Although not a standard therapy, intramuscular and subcutaneous routes of administration have also been found to be effective and are associated with decreased severity of hemolysis [81]. Other benefits of these modes of treatment include decreased cost, ease of administration, and increased availability in developing countries [82, 83]. Subcutaneous anti-D can also be tolerated over many years without loss of efficacy, making it useful as maintenance therapy for patients with chronic disease [84].

Second-Line Therapy

Current guidelines for the management of ITP discuss only three strategies for second-line therapy for ITP—splenectomy, rituximab, and TPO-RAs. Significant progress in the study of TPO-RAs has been made since the publication of these guidelines leading to an increasing preference for medical therapy and decreased prevalence of splenectomy [85].

Splenectomy

In 1916, Paul Kaznelson, then a medical student, suggested that ITP resulted from increased platelet destruction in the spleen. He convinced his tutor to perform a splenectomy on a 36-year-old woman with chronic ITP, and she had a prompt rise in her platelet count from 2 to over 500 with a resolution of her purpura, menorrhagia, and epistaxis [16]. However, the two next patients that underwent splenectomy only had a temporary improvement in their platelet count, and the debate regarding the underlying cause of ITP remained unresolved. Nevertheless, by the 1920s, splenectomy had become the mainstay of therapy for severe refractory ITP [16]. After the introduction of steroids in the 1950s, splenectomy continued to be considered the gold standard for treatment because it led to a sustained response in the majority of patients. A study published in 2016 reported that approximately 25% of adults continue to undergo splenectomy as their initial second-line therapy. Five to ten years after surgery, 60% of the patients in this group continue to have a sustained platelet response and require no additional therapy [86, 87].

Although most patients will tolerate a splenectomy with minimal complications, there are risks associated with the surgery. Perioperative mortality is less than 1% in the hands of an experienced surgeon, and the risk of portal vein thrombosis is also low at 0.1–4 events per 100 patient years [7, 88]. However, the spleen is a secondary lymphoid organ that plays an important role in the immune response, and splenectomy leads to an increased risk of bacterial infections, with a particular increased susceptibility to encapsulated organisms [89]. There is a 5–30-fold increased risk of infection in the first 90 days following surgery and a 1–3-fold lifelong increased risk of invasive infection or sepsis [90]. Overall, risk of mortality from overwhelming postsplenectomy infection has been found to be 0.73 per 1000 patient years [91]. The spleen also plays an important role as a filter for senescent platelets and red blood cells which may explain the finding that splenectomy is associated with a 30-fold increased risk of venous thromboembolism (VTE). There are also reports of increased rates of myocardial infarction, stroke, and pulmonary hypertension [92].

To better understand the risks related to splenectomy, Thai and colleagues published an observational study comparing 83 patients with ITP who were at least 10 years status post splenectomy to 83 age and gender-matched non-splenectomized ITP controls [85]. On average, splenectomy was performed 16 months following the diagnosis of ITP. There were slightly more infections in the patients who had undergone splenectomy, and those infections were more likely to necessitate hospitalization, although they were not associated with increased mortality. However, the most significant difference between the groups was the risk of VTE, observed in 16% of the splenectomy patients ($n = 13$) compared to 2% of the control patients ($n = 2$). The risk of thrombosis was not found to be related to the platelet number, the severity of disease, or the patients bleeding score. The mechanism underlying the increased rate of thrombosis remains unclear, but laboratory work suggests it may involve increased endothelial activation, increased platelet reactivity, and decreased clearance of platelet microparticles [92, 93]. Despite these factors, 1 year following the surgery, patients who underwent splenectomy have a comparable to reduced risk of mortality compared to non-splenectomized patients [5]. These data support the conclusion that splenectomy is relatively safe, but not without immediate risks or potential long-term complications.

Mechanism of Action

The spleen is thought to be the major site of platelet phagocytosis and autoantibody production, and removal of the organ has been shown to lead to a reduction in platelet destruction [19]. Studies done in the 1970s showed that following splenectomy, patients had an increased platelet life span associated with decrease in rates of platelet production [94]. In the 1990s, Lamy and colleagues infused 111 ITP patients with autologous indium-labeled platelets and confirmed that platelet life span was reduced in most of these individuals. They also observed that the majority of their patients had platelet sequestration in the spleen rather than the liver and found that patients with splenic sequestration were significantly more likely to have normalization of their platelet counts following splenectomy compared to those with hepatic sequestration [95]. Fujisawa and colleagues examined six ITP patients who underwent splenectomy and found that those who responded to the surgery had decreased platelet autoantibody levels while those with refractory disease had persistent platelet antibody production [96]. These findings suggest that prolonged platelet survival following splenectomy is likely the combined result of diminished autoantibody production and decreased platelet clearance.

Splenectomy Treatment Recommendations

Current guidelines recommend that splenectomy be deferred for at least 6 months following ITP diagnosis in adults [1]. In children, splenectomy is only recommended in patients with bleeding symptoms, and attempts should be made to defer surgery for at least 12 months following diagnosis because of the high rate of delayed spontaneous remission [1]. However, it may be performed earlier in children with severe disease that is refractory to other therapies and detrimental to quality of life [1]. Of note, splenectomy is associated with a higher risk of sepsis in pediatric patients, particularly those younger than 5 [97]. In all age groups, laparoscopic splenectomy is preferred over open splenectomy because it requires a smaller incision, is associated with less pain, and has a more rapid recovery time. Preoperatively, therapies such as corticosteroids, IVIG, and anti-D can be used to transiently increase platelet counts, while platelet transfusions are typically reserved for patients with perioperative bleeding.

Approximately 80% of patients with ITP will have a significant rise in platelet counts following surgery, with over 60% having a durable response [92]. As there are risks associated with the surgery, there is great interest in identifying the patients most likely to respond. Patient age, duration of illness, response to IVIG, response to steroids, primary site of platelet sequestration, and preoperative platelet count have all been proposed as predictive factors [98]. A systematic literature review performed by Kojouri et al. showed that younger age was most reliably associated with a good response but did not find consistent results regarding the other variables [87].

In order to prevent infection with encapsulated organisms, all patients undergoing splenectomy should receive vaccinations to *Pneumococcus*, *Haemophilus influenzae* type b, and *Meningococcus*, ideally, at least 2 weeks prior to surgery. Patient's younger than 5 should be started on penicillin prophylaxis following the surgery. There is not yet sufficient evidence to determine if prophylaxis is indicated in older patients [99], although many practitioners recommend penicillin prophylaxis for at least some period of time after surgery.

Rituximab

Rituximab is a genetically engineered chimeric murine/human monoclonal antibody directed against the CD20 antigen, present on premature and mature B lymphocytes. Following administration, it leads to the rapid depletion of circulating premature and mature B cells with a return to normal levels within 6–12 months [100]. It is used in the treatment of various hematologic malignancies and autoimmune conditions and first found to be effective in the treatment of chronic ITP in adults in the early 2000s [101, 102]. Rituximab is generally well tolerated. Infusion reactions are common (~10%) following the first treatment, including fever, headache, nausea, and pruritis [103]. Fortunately, reactions are rare following subsequent treatments and can be prevented in most patients by slowing the infusion rate and pretreating with corticosteroids, antihistamines, and acetaminophen. Rituximab also impairs the response to *Streptococcus pneumoniae* and *Haemophilus influenzae* type b vaccinations for at least 6 months [104]. This is of particular concern in unvaccinated patients who may require future treatment with splenectomy. The risk of infection following treatment with rituximab is quite low but is more significant in patients receiving additional immunosuppressive agents and those with underlying immune dysfunction. In these patients, there is also concern for the risk of the reactivation of latent viruses such as hepatitis B. Prolonged hypogammaglobulinemia develops in 1–2% of patients and further increases the risk of infection [105]. Other toxicities include serum sickness which occurs infrequently in adults but is seen in 5–10% of children [106] and rare complications such as prolonged neutropenia and progressive multifocal leukoencephalopathy, which is usually seen in patients with underlying immune dysregulation or rheumatologic disease [107].

Many hematologists favor rituximab as a second-line agent because it is generally well tolerated, there is a high initial overall response rate of approximately 60%, and it is thought to offer the possibility of cure in certain patients [108]. In 2015, Ghanima and colleagues published the first randomized placebo-controlled study to assess the efficacy of rituximab as a second-line treatment for adult ITP. The goal was to determine if rituximab monotherapy can lead to durable responses that may decrease the need for splenectomy. The study included 112 steroid-refractory patients, and while 81% of patients responded to rituximab, the duration of response was typically less than 12 months, with platelet counts greater than $20–30 \times 10^9/L$ in 30–50% of patients at 1 year, in 20–40% of patients at 2 years, and in only 20% of patients at 5 years. Compared to placebo, there was no significant benefit observed at 1.5 years. However, within the first 15 months, the rituximab group were more likely to maintain platelet counts above $30 \times 10^9/L$, and these remissions were longer lasting compared to placebo (36 weeks vs. 7 weeks). Overall, the study identified a 10% difference in the long-term response rates between the two groups [109]. Although rituximab did not significantly reduce the rate of long-term treatment failure, these results demonstrate that it is a good treatment option for patients who respond poorly to or are unable to tolerate corticosteroids.

Mechanism of Action

The precise mechanism by which rituximab leads to clinical improvement in ITP remains unclear. Initially, researchers proposed that the depletion of CD20-expressing memory cells and autoreactive B-cell clones would lead to a reduction in levels of antiplatelet antibodies. However, rituximab largely spares humoral immunity because CD20 is not present on plasma cells, which are a main source of antibody production [103]. Therefore, while peripheral B-cell depletion occurs rapidly and consistently, mature plasma cells are unaffected. IgG and IgM depletion eventually occurs in a small subset of patients 5–11 months after therapy, presumably when the preexisting plasma cells expire and the patient is unable to generate new ones [110]. To better characterize the ability of rituximab to decrease antiplatelet autoantibodies, Arnold and colleagues examined a cohort of ITP patients randomized to receive rituximab vs. placebo and measured autoantibody levels before and after treatment. Forty-five percent of their patients had detectable autoantibodies directed against platelet surface glycoproteins GPIIbIIIa and GPIb-IX. However the presence of an autoantibody was not predictive of treatment response. Although rituximab led to a significant decrease in anti-GPIIbIIIa antibodies, with a nadir 6 months following treatment, it did not impact levels of anti-GPIb-IX antibodies. Furthermore, the disappearance of platelet autoantibodies was not associated with a rise in platelet counts. These findings indicate that antibody depletion is not the only mechanism by which rituximab induces improvement in ITP [108].

There has been considerable interest in the role of T lymphocytes in the pathogenesis of ITP, and it has been suggested that rituximab may act by indirectly regulating T-cell behavior [111]. Stasi and colleagues observed that patients who respond to rituximab have normalization of T-cell subsets with an increase in the Th1/Th2 ratio [112]. They also found that rituximab responders have increased numbers and improved function of regulatory T cells [113]. Based on these finding, they posit that B cells play a role in sustaining autoreactive T cells, which is why B-cell depletion leads to normalization of T-cell populations.

Rituximab Treatment Recommendations

As patients with underlying immune dysfunction are at a higher risk of hypogammaglobulinemia and infectious complications following rituximab administration, many experts recommend sending lymphocyte subsets and immunoglobulin levels before starting treatment [4]. Treatment is also contraindicated in patients with active hepatitis B infection [114]. Most studies have examined the effect of 4 weekly infusions at doses of 375 mg/m^2, but similar response rates have been reported in patients treated with 1 g/m^2 × 2 doses 2 weeks apart [115]. Two clinical trials have examined rituximab in combination with HDD in newly diagnosed patients with ITP. Remission rates were higher in patients treated with combination therapy vs. rituximab monotherapy at 6 months (58–63% vs. 36–37% [116, 117]) and 1 year (53 vs. 33%) [117]. However improved remission rates occurred at the cost of increased grade 3 and 4 toxicity [116, 117]. In an attempt to reduce adverse effects and improve long-term remission rates, investigators have combined HDD with lower-dose rituximab (100 mg/m^2 × 4 doses) and additional immunosuppressive medications. One study treated 20 adults with chronic ITP with a regimen of HDD, oral cyclosporine, and IV low-dose rituximab. The cohort tolerated the treatment well, and there was a 75% rate of 12-month treatment-free survival, with 30% of patients demonstrating a complete response (platelet count >100 × 10^9/L) for at least 6 months [118]. Many patients who initially respond to rituximab can respond to subsequent doses. However, the safety and efficacy of repeated dosing of rituximab has not been systematically evaluated.

Thrombopoietin Receptor Agonists (TPO-RAs)

The most recent clinical development that has changed second-line ITP therapy is the emergence of TPO-RAs. Several medications in this class have been studied and eltrombopag and romiplostim are FDA approved for the treatment of adults with chronic ITP. Eltrombopag is also approved for use in children >1 year. A recent meta-analysis of eltrombopag use in ITP, including 6 randomized controlled trials, demonstrated that eltrombopag significantly improved platelet counts (RR 3.42; 95% CI, 2.51–4.65) and decreased incidence of bleeding (RR 0.74; 95% CI, 0.66–0.83) [119]. In the reported clinical trials of eltrombopag and romiplostim, over 80% of patients had at least one platelet count >50 × 10^9/L, even among highly refractory and multiply treated patients [120]. In clinical practice, the response rate is slightly lower (74–94%), reflecting perhaps the increased heterogeneity of a nonclinical trial population [121–123]. The literature also suggests that patients who are unresponsive to one TPO-RA may successfully switch to the other [124].

Mechanism of Action

Thrombopoietin (TPO) is a cytokine produced at a constant rate by the liver and kidneys, which functions as the primary regulator of megakaryocyte development and platelet production. After it is released from hepatocytes and enters the circulation, TPO binds to the c-Mpl receptor (CD110), constitutively expressed on hematopoietic progenitor cells, and stimulates Janus kinase (Jak)-2, signal transducer and activators of transcription (STAT)-5, the mitogen-activated protein kinase pathway (MAPK), and anti-apoptotic pathways that lead to the production of mature mega-karyocytes and platelets [125]. Although the concept of a hematopoietic growth factor that regulated platelet production was first proposed in 1958 [126], thrombo-poietin was not discovered until 1994, when it was identified nearly simultaneously by five separate groups [127–131]. This breakthrough led to the synthesis of full-length recombinant human TPO along with a truncated form of the protein still capable of binding to the c-Mpl receptor. Both molecules were clinically evaluated in the late 1990s and found to lead to a dose-dependent increase in circulating plate-let counts accompanied by a rise in megakaryocytes. Unfortunately, some healthy individuals developed neutralizing antibodies directed against these drugs that cross-reacted with endogenous TPO, paradoxically leading to increased thrombocy-topenia [132]. To avoid this complication, researchers subsequently developed TPO receptor agonists that did not share epitopes with endogenous human TPO, and this work led to the generation of the second-generation TPO receptor agonists.

Romiplostim is composed of two short peptides coupled to an Fc receptor domain that yields four c-Mpl-binding sites. Its half-life is prolonged by endothelial neona-tal Fc receptor (FcRn) recycling, and it is administered weekly by subcutaneous injection [126]. A dose-dependent platelet rise is observed 5 days following treat-ment that peaks on days 12–14 and returns to baseline levels by day 28 [133]. It is cleared by the MPS, and renal or hepatic dysfunction has not been shown to affect its half-life or function [126]. Romiplostim has no sequence homology to endoge-nous human TPO, and although there are reports of neutralizing antibody forma-tion, they have never been found to cross-react with endogenous TPO [134].

Eltrombopag is an orally available small organic nonpeptide that selectively binds to the transmembrane domain of the c-Mpl receptor and activates it through a different mechanism than recombinant TPO or romiplostim that also leads to increased platelet production [135]. As it binds to a distinct region of the c-Mpl receptor, it does not compete with endogenous TPO for binding. Studies suggest that it complements the effect of endogenous TPO and therefore remains effective in disease states associated with increased TPO levels and may provide additional ben-efit when used concurrently with romiplostim [126]. Eighty-five percent of patients with ITP respond to eltrombopag, with median platelet counts increasing to $>50 \times 10^9/L$ after 2 weeks of therapy, with persistent elevation in approximately 60% of patients [136]. Of note, eltrombopag has no sequence homology with endog-enous TPO, and due to its small size, it is considered to be non-immunogenic. To date, there are no reports of the development of anti-eltrombopag neutralizing anti-bodies. Enteral absorption of eltrombopag is significantly reduced by polyvalent cations and certain medications, and it should ideally be taken on an empty stomach [137].

Avatrombopag is an orally administered nonpeptide TPO-RA developed in 2008 [138]. Like eltrombopag, it binds to the transmembrane domain of the TPO receptor and does not interfere with the activity of endogenous TPO. Unlike eltrombopag, it does not interact significantly with food and does not have to be taken on an empty stomach [139]. In phase 2 trials, it has been found to be well tolerated and effective in the treatment of chronic ITP and of thrombocytopenia due to cirrhosis [140, 141]. Additional studies are underway to evaluate the efficacy and safety of avatrombopag compared to the other TPO-RAs.

TPO-RA Adverse Effects

There has been great progress in the study of TPO-RAs since the publication of the most recent ITP treatment guidelines in 2011. At that time, there was emerging data regarding drug efficacy, but there were limited results regarding adverse effects including thromboembolism, cataract formation, and bone marrow fibrosis. Long-term follow-up data is now available for eltrombopag and romiplostim treatment in adult patients. The EXTEND trial (Eltrombopag eXTENDed dosing) has published data on 299 patients with chronic ITP treated with eltrombopag, 104 of whom have data available for ≥2 years of follow-up [136]. The long-term safety of romiplostim was evaluated by Cines and colleagues in an integrated analysis of 14 trials including 924 patients with a mean study duration of 75–77 weeks [142]. Both romiplostim and eltrombopag have been found to be well tolerated, and the most common adverse events observed with either medication are nasopharyngitis, headache, and fatigue [143]. Recent data from the EXTEND trial reveals that eltrombopag is associated with hepatic enzyme elevation in 15% of patients that resolves with discontinuation of treatment [144].

Epidemiologic evidence suggests that patients with ITP are at increased risk for venous and arterial thromboembolism despite their thrombocytopenia [145]. Based on preclinical data, there is concern that TPO-RA therapy may further increase the thrombotic risk in ITP patients by raising platelet counts and by increasing platelet reactivity [135, 146]. Fortunately, to date, clinical studies have not demonstrated a strong risk of thrombosis associated with TPO-RA use. In a meta-analysis of 924 patients, Cines et al. observed that the rate of thrombosis was equivalent (5.5 per 100 patient years) in patients receiving romiplostim and those receiving placebo or standard of care [142]. In the EXTEND trial, approximately 3% of patients with chronic ITP had a history of thrombosis prior to the initiation of eltrombopag, while 6.3% of patients experienced thromboembolic events after starting the medication. Based on these results, the researchers were not able to determine if the increased risk of thrombosis was attributable to the therapy or the underlying disease state [136, 144]. Of note, patients at the greatest thrombotic risk, those with atherosclerotic disease or a history of venous thromboembolism, have been excluded from many TPO-RA trials. Therefore, it is not possible to determine the true thrombotic risk in this population, and TPO-RAs should be used with caution in patients with these comorbidities.

Based on human and animal data, there is also concern that TPO-RAs may lead to an increase in bone marrow fibrosis. In rodent models, overexpression of endogenous TPO or administration of romiplostim induces dose-dependent marrow fibrosis [147]. In a study of 15 patients with acute myeloid leukemia, 8 out of 9 patients treated with recombinant human TPO developed increased marrow reticulin fibrosis that resolved following drug discontinuation [148]. Romiplostim therapy has been associated with increased reticulin deposition in the marrow at a rate of 1.3 events per 100 patient years with higher rates and grades in patients who exceed the currently recommended maximum dose of 10 µg/kg [142]. Prior retrospective studies that have attempted to examine the risk of marrow fibrosis in ITP patients treated with TPO-RAs have been limited by the low rate of bone marrow examination. To address this concern, in 2017, Brynes et al. published a 2-year longitudinal prospective study of the effect of eltrombopag on the bone marrow of patients with chronic ITP that included 93 patients who received bone marrow biopsies prior to the initiation of eltrombopag, followed by marrow examination after 1 and 2 years of TPO-RA therapy. They observed that most patients had little to no fibrosis at the time of diagnosis. After 2 years of therapy, 89% of patients had no increase in reticulin or collagen formation, and 11% (10 patients) had minimally increased reticulin deposition [149]. In the EXTEND trial, bone marrow reticulin fiber was assessed in 147 bone marrow biopsies obtained from patients treated for a median of 12 months. Eight percent of patients ($n = 11$) were found to have grade 2 reticulin fiber formation without collagen fiber formation. Bone marrow biopsies obtained over ≥ 2 years of follow-up showed 8/11 with no change in grade, 1/11 with an increase from grade 1 to grade 2, and 2/11 with a decrease in grade [136]. A systematic investigation of bone marrow fibrosis has not yet been undertaken in children.

Eltrombopag is hepatically metabolized and leads to the development of liver function test (LFT) abnormalities in 13% of adults. Therefore, routine liver function testing is recommended in all patients, and reduced dosing should be considered in patients with preexisting liver disease [136]. In preclinical toxicology studies, high doses of eltrombopag were found to induce cataract formation in juvenile rodents [143]. In the EXTEND trial, 5% of patients ($n = 15$) treated with eltrombopag for over 6 months reported cataracts, with 4 patients developing new cataracts and 10 patients having progression of preexisting cataracts [136]. However, these results are difficult to interpret because steroid use, a known risk factor for cataract formation, was reported in 13/15 of these patients. Although more data is needed to assess the contribution of eltrombopag to the risk of cataract formation and most experts recommend annual ophthalmology screening in all patients treated with eltrombopag; the most recent data does not support a significant increased risk above baseline. Finally, some biological data suggests that eltrombopag can chelate intracellular iron [150], and a recent retrospective case review demonstrated significant iron deficiency in eltrombopag-treated patients which was not present in a romiplostim-treated cohort (although some patients overlapped) [150].

Eltrombopag and romiplostim can both induce thrombocytosis, sometimes causing platelets to rise above 1000×10^9/L. Although this finding has not been associated with an increased risk of thrombosis [126], the prescribing information recommends holding treatment when platelet counts reach 400×10^9/L. This recommendation should be interpreted cautiously because abrupt medication discontinuation can lead to rebound thrombocytopenia in 8–10% of patients, with platelet counts dropping below baseline for 1–3 weeks before returning to pretreatment levels, exposing patients to a significant bleeding risk [151]. It has been suggested that this drop occurs because the expanded megakaryocyte population induced by TPO-RA therapy more rapidly clears endogenous TPO. Another contributing factor may be the prior discontinuation or dose reduction of concurrent ITP therapy [143]. Although the etiology of rebound thrombocytosis remains unclear, in order to maintain adequate platelet counts most experts recommend decreasing TPO-RA dose by 25–50%, rather than stopping the medication abruptly [126].

Treatment Recommendations

The 2011 ASH guidelines recommend that TPO-RAs only be used in patients at risk of bleeding who relapse after splenectomy or have contraindications to the surgery and have failed at least one other therapy [1]. Since that time, TPO-RA use has become much more common, and these agents are often used to prevent or delay splenectomy. The decision about which TPO-RA to use is typically based on patient-specific factors. Romiplostim injections are not yet approved for home administration, and while some patients prefer not having to take a daily medication, others find it difficult to travel to clinic for weekly treatments. On the other hand, patients treated with eltrombopag need to pay attention to the timing of meals and may require adjustments in the doses of their other medications and supplements. Most practitioners will start romiplostim treatment at doses of 2–3 μg/kg and titrate weekly to a maximum dose of 10 μg/kg to achieve the desired platelet count. Eltrombopag is taken orally once a day at a starting doses of 50 mg/day and titrated to effect. In the East Asian population, a common polymorphism results in higher plasma levels due to decreased clearance and a lower starting dose of 25 mg/day is recommended in this population [3]. For children less than 6 years old, the recommended starting dose is 25 mg/day. Eltrombopag should be taken 1 h before or 2 h after a meal. A 4-h interval is required between eltrombopag and calcium-rich foods and mineral supplements because interaction with polyvalent cations, such as iron and calcium, leads to decreased absorption. It also decreases the metabolism of certain drugs, including statins, and doses of concomitant medications may need to be reduced [137].

Use of TPO-RAs in Pediatric ITP

Prior to the publication of both the IWG and ASH guidelines, none of the TPO-RAs had been approved for use in children, and there was very little published literature regarding their safety or efficacy in pediatric patients. Since then, two randomized, double-blind phase III trials (PETIT and PETIT2) have been published studying eltrombopag in pediatric patients with ITP >6 months duration [152, 153]. The medication was well tolerated, and approximately 50% of enrolled patients achieved a sustained response and were able to discontinue their baseline ITP medications. These results form the basis for the FDA approval of eltrombopag for use in children [153]. Additionally, three smaller randomized placebo-controlled trials evaluating romiplostim in children have been published, the largest of which reported a durable platelet response in 52% of patients with a single treatment-related adverse event including headache and thrombocytosis [154–156]. The ITP Consortium of North America (ICON) recently reported on the real-world use of TPO-RAs in pediatric patients with ITP [157]. In this study, 79 children received 87 treatments (28 eltrombopag, 43 romiplostim, 8 both). Sixty percent had chronic ITP, 18% were newly diagnosed, and 22% had persistent disease. Most physicians started treatment because of bleeding symptoms, and all patients had received previous therapies, including steroids, IVIG, splenectomy, and rituximab. Within 3 months, 89% achieved platelet counts above 50×10^9/L. Average response time was 6.4 weeks with romiplostim and 7 weeks with eltrombopag. Both romiplostim and eltrombopag were well tolerated with minimal adverse effects. However, only 40% of patients had a consistent response with stable dosing, while the remainder of patients responded intermittently and required dose titration. Thirteen percent had an initial response that waned over the course of the study. Notably, there were two thrombotic events and one patient developed neutralizing antibodies to romiplostim [157]. Based on the results of published pediatric trials, it is evident that fluctuating platelet counts are to be expected in patients treated with TPO-RAs, and this effect may be more pronounced in children than adults.

Use of TPO-RAs in Newly Diagnosed ITP

Two small studies have examined TPO-RA use in newly diagnosed patients with ITP. The first was a 12-month study of romiplostim in 75 patients with ITP for <6 months. Dosing was tapered if the platelet count was $\geq 50 \times 10^9$/L by the end of the observation period [158]. Thirty-two percent of patients met the primary endpoint which was defined as a platelet count $\geq 50 \times 10^9$/L for 24 consecutive weeks following discontinuation of therapy [158]. A second study, enrolling 12 adults, looked at the combination of HDD × 4 days, followed by eltrombopag 50 mg/day for days 5–32. Nine out of twelve patients (75%) had a platelet count $\geq 30 \times 10^9$/L at 6 months and 8/12 (67%) maintained their counts for 12 months [159]. These preliminary data are interesting, but additional studies with more patients are needed to evaluate the long-term outcomes and better characterize toxicities with up-front TPO-RA treatment.

Management of Life-Threatening Bleeding

In the setting of trauma, emergent surgery, or severe unprovoked hemorrhage, it is typically necessary to use a combination of treatments to control bleeding by inducing a rapid and sustained increase in platelet counts. Most experts recommend starting with IVIG with high-dose steroids because this regimen has a quick onset of action, observed within hours to days [1]. However, in order to achieve more immediate hemostasis, frequent platelet transfusions may be administered to overwhelm antibody-mediated destruction, although there is no consensus regarding the optimal dose. In 2008, Salama et al. treated ten refractory ITP patients with hemorrhage with massive platelet transfusions (1 Unit/30 min) leading to cessation of bleeding in all patients without any observed adverse effects including thrombosis [160]. In order to further suppress antibody-mediated platelet destruction, one group recommended concomitant infusion of continuous IVIG (1 g/kg) over 24 h. In a retrospective review of 40 adults with life-threatening hemorrhage treated with continuous IVIG and platelet transfusions every 4–8 h, all had resolution of their bleeding [161].

Alternative agents that may be considered as adjunctive therapies in patients with ITP and uncontrolled bleeding include recombinant factor VIIa, antifibrinolytics such as aminocaproic acid and tranexamic acid, and vincristine. The use of recombinant factor VIIa for the control of bleeding or preparation for surgery has been reported in 18 ITP patients. Hemorrhage was controlled in all patients, but three died despite cessation of bleeding [162]. Due to limited data and concerns for potential thrombosis, recombinant factor VIIa should be used with caution in ITP. Alternatively, antifibrinolytics are associated with a low risk of adverse effects, and there are reports that they may be helpful in the treatment of mucosal bleeding in ITP [163], but their efficacy in ITP has not been studied in any randomized controlled trials [1]. Vincristine has been shown to be effective in refractory ITP [164], and it has been recommended as an adjunctive therapy in the management of emergent bleeding [2, 165], but it does not lead to a rise in platelet counts for 5–7 days [164] and should only be used in conjunction with more rapidly acting therapies. There is emerging interest in the early initiation of TPO mimetics in patients with life-threatening bleeding [166], but there is scant data on their utility in this setting, and treatment for several days is required before platelet counts begin to rise.

Finally, emergent splenectomy may be considered in patients with truly life-threatening hemorrhage. The surgery may be done in concert with IVIG and corticosteroids and is usually performed with platelet transfusions [1]. According to the 2011 ASH treatment guidelines, emergent splenectomy should be considered heroic as unplanned major abdominal surgery is risky in all patients, but especially so in those with thrombocytopenia [1]. Furthermore, because there is no time to administer appropriate vaccinations against encapsulated organisms, these patients may be at an increased risk of bacterial infection.

Other Agents

Several additional therapies have been used in the management of patients with refractory ITP requiring ongoing treatment with inadequate responses to standard first- and second-line therapies. Each of these agents have been studied in small numbers of patients and limited efficacy data is available. However, many have been used for other indications providing sufficient safety information. Generally, these agents have limited efficacy for most patients with ITP but may be reasonable options for secondary ITP or refractory primary ITP patients with inadequate response to other therapies.

Antimetabolites

Mycophenolate mofetil (MMF): Is a prodrug of mycophenolic acid, an inhibitor of purine biosynthesis. This drug causes cell cycle arrest and reduced proliferation in B and T lymphocytes because they cannot recycle purine nucleotides. MMF also impacts T-cell function by depleting guanosine triphosphate (GTP), which plays an important role in T-cell activation [167]. MMF was first introduced in the use of renal transplant patients in the 1990s and has been shown to have a favorable safety profile [168]. It is now licensed for prophylaxis of acute rejection in solid organ transplant but is also widely used as an immunomodulatory agent in the treatment of autoimmune disease. Although there are no RCTs of MMF in ITP [4], retrospective studies show a 50% response rate in adults with refractory ITP, although it appears to have minimal effect in viral-associated disease [169]. Experts recommend adult starting doses of 500 mg twice a day, titrating up to 1000–1500 g twice a day as tolerated. Patients may require treatment for 6–8 weeks before they achieve a sustained response [4], and there is variability in duration of response after discontinuation [167]. Side effects include headaches, gastrointestinal toxicity, LFT abnormalities, and increased risk of infection [4]. MMF is also a known teratogen, leading to abnormalities in 21–27% of pregnancies, and cannot be administered during pregnancy (www.toxbase.org).

Azathioprine (AZA): Is one of the first drugs shown to be effective in the treatment of chronic ITP [170]. It is a prodrug whose active metabolite, 6-mercaptopurine (6-MP), is a purine analog that blocks purine synthesis and DNA repair, leading to inhibition of cellular proliferation in rapidly dividing cells such as lymphocytes [171]. Small studies have showed that AZA leads to an improvement in platelet counts in refractory ITP and the combination with corticosteroids may be synergistic [172, 173]. The largest study of AZA in ITP included 53 adults with refractory disease and showed a complete response rate of 45% and an overall response rate of 64%. Patients who had undergone splenectomy were just as likely to respond to AZA. After drug discontinuation, 42% remained in remission for a variable follow-up of time of 7–43 months [174]. Based on the results of this study, most providers recommend treating patients with 150 mg per day. As the platelet rise may be delayed, AZA should be continued for 4 months before a patient is considered unresponsive. AZA toxicities include myelosuppression, hepatotoxicity, and pancreatitis [3]. Although there has been no direct comparison between MMF and AZA, many providers believes that AZA is not as well tolerated. However, AZA may be preferred in women of childbearing age because it is not teratogenic [4].

Cyclophosphamide: Is an alkylating agent that induces apoptosis by creating DNA cross-linking. Although this mechanism is cell cycle independent, rapidly proliferating cells are the most sensitive. Lymphocytes are particularly vulnerable to cyclophosphamide because they have low levels of aldehyde dehydrogenase, which is required for drug detoxification [175]. Although cyclophosphamide is commonly used to treat malignancies, it has also been used extensively in the treatment of autoimmune disease. It can be given orally (1–2 mg/kg once per day) or intravenously (500–100 mg/m^2 once every 3–4 weeks × 2–3 courses). Two studies have evaluated its use in the treatment of ITP, and it has been found to be effective in splenectomy refractory patients, leading to a complete response in 50% of patients and a partial response in 20% of patients [176, 177]. However, cyclophosphamide can be difficult to tolerate, and toxicities include hemorrhagic cystitis, myelosuppression, infertility, and secondary malignancy [3]. Patients taking cyclophosphamide should have their blood counts monitored every week and be instructed to drink at least 2 L of fluid a day to prevent hemorrhagic cystitis [3].

Cyclosporine A: Is a calcineurin inhibitor that suppresses T-cell function by selectively inhibiting antigen-induced CD4+ activation and interleukin 2-induced CD4+ differentiation. These effects indirectly reduce B lymphocyte growth and differentiation [178]. Several studies have shown that it is helpful in the treatment of refractory ITP [179]. The largest study included 20 adult patients and reported a response rate of 50–60%, with efficacy observed in individuals who had undergone splenectomy and occasional durable remissions following drug discontinuation [178]. A recent retrospective review of cyclosporine treatment in 30 children with chronic ITP revealed a 57% response rate with a sustained response in 23% of patients [180]. Adverse effects include hypertension, nephrotoxicity, and immunosuppression that can be difficult for many patients to tolerate [178].

Rapamycin (also known as Sirolimus): Is a mammalian target of rapamycin (mTor) inhibitor which blocks the activation of B and T lymphocytes by inhibiting cytokine receptor-dependent signal transduction [181]. Some research also suggests that it selectively expands functional Tregs [182]. It is most commonly used to prevent rejection of solid organ transplants but has also been found to be effective in the treatment of autoimmune lymphoproliferative syndrome (ALPS) and refractory immune cytopenias [183]. A retrospective study of its use in 12 patients with ITP showed that 78% achieved a complete response [183]. A separate observational study of 43 patients treated with a combination rapamycin and low-dose prednisone revealed an overall response rate of 58% associated with a significant rise in Tregs [184]. Rapamycin is generally well tolerated, and the main side effects include hypercholesterolemia, hypertension, decreased glucose tolerance, and immunosuppression.

Vinca Alkaloids: Vincristine and vinblastine are believed to disrupt phagocytosis of opsonized platelets by binding to tubulin and inhibiting microtubule polymerization [185]. Vincristine was first used in 1969 for treatment of refractory disease. Based on evidence generated in the 1970s–1980s, it came to be recommended as a second-line therapy [3]. Most studies report a rapid rise in platelet counts in 50–90% of adult patients [164], which occurs within 5–7 days of treatment but declines rapidly after completion of therapy [3, 186]. Vinca alkaloids continue to be effective in patients who have undergone splenectomy [185]. Vincristine and vinblastine are administered as 4 weekly infusions at doses of 1.5 mg/m^2 and 6 mg/m^2, respectively.

Vinblastine can cause myelosuppression, and both agents can induce constipation and peripheral neuropathy. Vinca alkaloids may be considered in patients who do not respond to conventional therapy but require a rapid rise in platelet counts, especially in the setting of emergencies [2].

Danazol: Is an attenuated androgen with mild virilizing effects found to be effective in ITP in 1983 [187]. Its mechanism of action remains unclear, but there are reports that it acts by influencing Fc receptor levels on phagocytic cells [188], reducing the proliferation of lymphocytes [189], decreasing pro-inflammatory cytokine levels, and promoting Treg differentiation [190]. Response rates vary widely between studies from 10% to 70%, although this may reflect heterogeneity in dosing with some trials using low-dose danazol (50 mg daily) and others using standard dosage (400–800 mg divided twice a day) [3, 187]. As responses are sometimes delayed, many practitioners recommend treating for at least 6 months. Furthermore, danazol appears to be more effective at inducing a sustainable response if patients can tolerate prolonged treatment for at least a year [191]. Some practitioners believe that patients who are responsive to steroids are more likely to respond to danazol and recommend avoiding therapy in steroid-refractory patients [3]. Alternatively, splenectomized patients [192] and older adults are thought to have a high rate of response [7]. Danazol is generally well tolerated, although it is rarely used at full doses in younger women due to its virilizing effects. There are also rare reports of hepatomas and hepatic peliosis, and patients should be monitored for signs of liver toxicity [174]. Other toxicities include an increased risk of venous thrombosis and accelerated growth of prostate cancer [7].

Dapsone: Is an antibiotic with anti-inflammatory and immunomodulatory effects that was first used in the treatment of ITP in the 1990s [193]. Its mechanism of action remains unclear, although it has been proposed that drug-induced hemolysis limits the phagocytosis of opsonized platelets [193]. This hypothesis is indirectly supported by the fact that there is a greater degree of hemolysis in patients who respond to treatment and a lower response rate in those who have undergone splenectomy [194]. There are no RCTs evaluating the efficacy of dapsone, and treatment recommendations are based on prospective and retrospective cohort studies [194, 195]. In the literature, the overall response rates range from 40% to 75%, and the typical time to response is 6–8 weeks [196]. Dapsone is an attractive treatment option because it is inexpensive, orally administered (100 mg daily), and generally well tolerated [197]. Toxicities include methemoglobinemia, cutaneous hypersensitivity, agranulocytosis, anemia, gastrointestinal complications, and hemolysis. Most individuals experience a 1–2 g/dL drop in hemoglobin, but the drop can be severe in patients with G6PD deficiency. Males should therefore be screened for G6PD deficiency before treatment initiation [3].

Novel Therapies

Several novel agents are on the horizon for the management of ITP in patients who fail conventional first- and second-line treatment [198]. These therapies include antibodies targeting the interaction between CD40 and CD154 that block communication between antigen-presenting cells and T cells [199, 200], treatments targeting Fc receptor binding [201], Syk kinase inhibitors that modify downstream signaling following Fc receptor activation [202], medications that decrease pathologic IgG half-life by blocking the neonatal Fc receptor [198], and novel agents that increase platelet production, including new TPO-RAs such as avatrombopag and the cytoprotective agent amifostine [203]. Hopefully, therapies designed based on our evolving understanding of this complex and heterogeneous disease will lead to a reduction in treatment-related morbidities and an overall improvement in patient health outcomes.

References

1. Neunert C, Lim W, Crowther M, Cohen A, Solberg L Jr, Crowther MA, et al. The American Society of Hematology 2011 evidence-based practice guideline for immune thrombocytopenia. Blood. 2011;117(16):4190–207.
2. Provan D, Stasi R, Newland AC, Blanchette VS, Bolton-Maggs P, Bussel JB, et al. International consensus report on the investigation and management of primary immune thrombocytopenia. Blood. 2010;115(2):168–86.
3. Cuker A, Neunert CE. How I treat refractory immune thrombocytopenia. Blood. 2016;128(12):1547–54.
4. Cooper N. State of the art—how I manage immune thrombocytopenia. Br J Haematol. 2017;177(1):39–54.
5. Cuker A, Cines DB, Neunert CE. Controversies in the treatment of immune thrombocytopenia. Curr Opin Hematol. 2016;23(5):479–85.
6. Rodeghiero F, Stasi R, Gernsheimer T, Michel M, Provan D, Arnold DM, et al. Standardization of terminology, definitions and outcome criteria in immune thrombocytopenic purpura of adults and children: report from an international working group. Blood. 2009;113(11):2386–93.
7. Mahevas M, Michel M, Godeau B. How we manage immune thrombocytopenia in the elderly. Br J Haematol. 2016;173(6):844–56.
8. Middelburg RA, Carbaat-Ham JC, Hesam H, Ragusi MA, Zwaginga JJ. Platelet function in adult ITP patients can be either increased or decreased, compared to healthy controls, and is associated with bleeding risk. Hematology. 2016;21(9):549–51.
9. Neunert C, Arnold DM. Severe bleeding events in adults and children with primary immune thrombocytopenia: a systematic review: reply. J Thromb Haemost. 2015;13(8):1522–3.
10. Altomare I, Cetin K, Wetten S, Wasser JS. Rate of bleeding-related episodes in adult patients with primary immune thrombocytopenia: a retrospective cohort study using a large administrative medical claims database in the US. Clin Epidemiol. 2016;8:231–9.
11. Melboucy-Belkhir S, Khellaf M, Augier A, Boubaya M, Levy V, Le Guenno G, et al. Risk factors associated with intracranial hemorrhage in adults with immune thrombocytopenia: a study of 27 cases. Am J Hematol. 2016;91(12):E499–501.
12. Cortelazzo S, Finazzi G, Buelli M, Molteni A, Viero P, Barbui T. High risk of severe bleeding in aged patients with chronic idiopathic thrombocytopenic purpura. Blood. 1991;77(1):31–3.
13. Cohen YC, Djulbegovic B, Shamai-Lubovitz O, Mozes B. The bleeding risk and natural history of idiopathic thrombocytopenic purpura in patients with persistent low platelet counts. Arch Intern Med. 2000;160(11):1630–8.
14. Neunert CE, Buchanan GR, Imbach P, Bolton-Maggs PH, Bennett CM, Neufeld EJ, et al. Severe hemorrhage in children with newly diagnosed immune thrombocytopenic purpura. Blood. 2008;112(10):4003–8.

15. Neunert CE. Individualized treatment for immune thrombocytopenia: predicting bleeding risk. Semin Hematol. 2013;50(Suppl 1):S55–7.
16. Stasi R, Newland AC. ITP: a historical perspective. Br J Haematol. 2011;153(4):437–50.
17. Provan D, Newland A. Fifty years of idiopathic thrombocytopenic purpura (ITP): management of refractory itp in adults. Br J Haematol. 2002;118(4):933–44.
18. Zen M, Canova M, Campana C, Bettio S, Nalotto L, Rampudda M, et al. The kaleidoscope of glucocorticoid effects on immune system. Autoimmun Rev. 2011;10(6):305–10.
19. Gernsheimer T, Stratton J, Ballem PJ, Slichter SJ. Mechanisms of response to treatment in autoimmune thrombocytopenic purpura. N Engl J Med. 1989;320(15):974–80.
20. Thachil J. Alternate considerations for current concepts in ITP. Hematology. 2014;19(3):163–8.
21. Houwerzijl EJ, Louwes H, Sluiter WJ, Smit JW, Vellenga E, de Wolf JT. Platelet production rate predicts the response to prednisone therapy in patients with idiopathic thrombocytopenic purpura. Ann Hematol. 2008;87(12):975–83.
22. Nugent D, McMillan R, Nichol JL, Slichter SJ. Pathogenesis of chronic immune thrombocytopenia: increased platelet destruction and/or decreased platelet production. Br J Haematol. 2009;146(6):585–96.
23. McMillan R, Wang L, Tomer A, Nichol J, Pistillo J. Suppression of in vitro megakaryocyte production by antiplatelet autoantibodies from adult patients with chronic ITP. Blood. 2004;103(4):1364–9.
24. Li J, Wang Z, Hu S, Zhao X, Cao L. Correction of abnormal T cell subsets by high-dose dexamethasone in patients with chronic idiopathic thrombocytopenic purpura. Immunol Lett. 2013;154(1-2):42–8.
25. Ling Y, Cao X, Yu Z, Ruan C. Circulating dendritic cells subsets and CD4+Foxp3+ regulatory T cells in adult patients with chronic ITP before and after treatment with high-dose dexamethasone. Eur J Haematol. 2007;79(4):310–6.
26. Hou Y, Feng Q, Xu M, Li GS, Liu XN, Sheng Z, et al. High-dose dexamethasone corrects impaired myeloid-derived suppressor cell function via Ets1 in immune thrombocytopenia. Blood. 2016;127(12):1587–97.
27. Goerge T, Ho-Tin-Noe B, Carbo C, Benarafa C, Remold-O'Donnell E, Zhao BQ, et al. Inflammation induces hemorrhage in thrombocytopenia. Blood. 2008;111(10):4958–64.
28. Nachman RL, Rafii S. Platelets, petechiae, and preservation of the vascular wall. N Engl J Med. 2008;359(12):1261–70.
29. Kitchens CS, Pendergast JF. Human thrombocytopenia is associated with structural abnormalities of the endothelium that are ameliorated by glucocorticosteroid administration. Blood. 1986;67(1):203–6.
30. Matschke J, Muller-Beissenhirtz H, Novotny J, Vester I, Hertenstein B, Eisele L, et al. A randomized trial of daily prednisone versus pulsed dexamethasone in treatment-naive adult patients with immune thrombocytopenia: EIS 2002 study. Acta Haematol. 2016;136(2):101–7.
31. Godeau B, Chevret S, Varet B, Lefrere F, Zini JM, Bassompierre F, et al. Intravenous immunoglobulin or high-dose methylprednisolone, with or without oral prednisone, for adults with untreated severe autoimmune thrombocytopenic purpura: a randomised, multicentre trial. Lancet. 2002;359(9300):23–9.
32. Grainger J, Bolton-Maggs P, Elizabeth P. Response to first line treatment in childhood ITP. 2016 ASH abstract 1372
33. Mithoowani S, Gregory-Miller K, Goy J, Miller MC, Wang G, Noroozi N, et al. High-dose dexamethasone compared with prednisone for previously untreated primary immune thrombocytopenia: a systematic review and meta-analysis. Lancet Haematol. 2016;3(10):e489-e96.
34. Liu Z, Wang M, Zhou S, Ma J, Shi Y, Peng J, et al. Pulsed high-dose dexamethasone modulates Th1-/Th2-chemokine imbalance in immune thrombocytopenia. J Transl Med. 2016;14(1):301.
35. Wei Y, Ji XB, Wang YW, Wang JX, Yang EQ, Wang ZC, et al. High-dose dexamethasone vs prednisone for treatment of adult immune thrombocytopenia: a prospective multicenter randomized trial. Blood. 2016;127(3):296–302. quiz 70

36. Bonilla FA. Intravenous immunoglobulin: adverse reactions and management. J Allergy Clin Immunol. 2008;122(6):1238–9.
37. Imbach P. Treatment of immune thrombocytopenia with intravenous immunoglobulin and insights for other diseases. A historical review. Swiss Med Wkly. 2012;142:w13593.
38. Fehr J, Hofmann V, Kappeler U. Transient reversal of thrombocytopenia in idiopathic thrombocytopenic purpura by high-dose intravenous gamma globulin. N Engl J Med. 1982;306(21):1254–8.
39. Salama A, Mueller-Eckhardt C, Kiefel V. Effect of intravenous immunoglobulin in immune thrombocytopenia. Lancet. 1983;2(8343):193–5.
40. Ancona KG, Parker RI, Atlas MP, Prakash D. Randomized trial of high-dose methylprednisolone versus intravenous immunoglobulin for the treatment of acute idiopathic thrombocytopenic purpura in children. J Pediatr Hematol Oncol. 2002;24(7):540–4.
41. Katz U, Achiron A, Sherer Y, Shoenfeld Y. Safety of intravenous immunoglobulin (IVIG) therapy. Autoimmun Rev. 2007;6(4):257–9.
42. Orbach H, Katz U, Sherer Y, Shoenfeld Y. Intravenous immunoglobulin: adverse effects and safe administration. Clin Rev Allergy Immunol. 2005;29(3):173–84.
43. Cherin P, Marie I, Michallet M, Pelus E, Dantal J, Crave JC, et al. Management of adverse events in the treatment of patients with immunoglobulin therapy: a review of evidence. Autoimmun Rev. 2016;15(1):71–81.
44. Barsam SJ, Psaila B, Forestier M, Page LK, Sloane PA, Geyer JT, et al. Platelet production and platelet destruction: assessing mechanisms of treatment effect in immune thrombocytopenia. Blood. 2011;117(21):5723–32.
45. Song S, Crow AR, Freedman J, Lazarus AH. Monoclonal IgG can ameliorate immune thrombocytopenia in a murine model of ITP: an alternative to IVIG. Blood. 2003;101(9):3708–13.
46. Samuelsson A, Towers TL, Ravetch JV. Anti-inflammatory activity of IVIG mediated through the inhibitory Fc receptor. Science. 2001;291(5503):484–6.
47. Yu X, Menard M, Prechl J, Bhakta V, Sheffield WP, Lazarus AH. Monovalent Fc receptor blockade by an anti-Fcgamma receptor/albumin fusion protein ameliorates murine ITP with abrogated toxicity. Blood. 2016;127(1):132–8.
48. Soubrane C, Tourani JM, Andrieu JM, Visonneau S, Beldjord K, Israel-Biet D, et al. Biologic response to anti-CD16 monoclonal antibody therapy in a human immunodeficiency virus-related immune thrombocytopenic purpura patient. Blood. 1993;81(1):15–9.
49. Tovo PA, Miniero R, Fiandino G, Saracco P, Messina M. Fc-depleted vs intact intravenous immunoglobulin in chronic ITP. J Pediatr. 1984;105(4):676–7.
50. Debre M, Bonnet MC, Fridman WH, Carosella E, Philippe N, Reinert P, et al. Infusion of Fc gamma fragments for treatment of children with acute immune thrombocytopenic purpura. Lancet. 1993;342(8877):945–9.
51. Nikolova KA, Tchorbanov AI, Djoumerska-Alexieva IK, Nikolova M, Vassilev TL. Intravenous immunoglobulin up-regulates the expression of the inhibitory FcgammaIIB receptor on B cells. Immunol Cell Biol. 2009;87(7):529–33.
52. Kondo N, Ozawa T, Mushiake K, Motoyoshi F, Kameyama T, Kasahara K, et al. Suppression of immunoglobulin production of lymphocytes by intravenous immunoglobulin. J Clin Immunol. 1991;11(3):152–8.
53. Crow AR, Song S, Siragam V, Lazarus AH. Mechanisms of action of intravenous immunoglobulin in the treatment of immune thrombocytopenia. Pediatr Blood Cancer. 2006;47(5 Suppl):710–3.
54. Gilardin L, Bayry J, Kaveri SV. Intravenous immunoglobulin as clinical immune-modulating therapy. CMAJ. 2015;187(4):257–64.
55. Kessel A, Ammuri H, Peri R, Pavlotzky ER, Blank M, Shoenfeld Y, et al. Intravenous immunoglobulin therapy affects T regulatory cells by increasing their suppressive function. J Immunol. 2007;179(8):5571–5.
56. Pang SJ, Lazarus AH. Mechanisms of platelet recovery in ITP associated with therapy. Ann Hematol. 2010;89(Suppl 1):31–5.

57. Hansen RJ, Balthasar JP. Intravenous immunoglobulin mediates an increase in anti-platelet antibody clearance via the FcRn receptor. Thromb Haemost. 2002;88(6):898–9.
58. Lutz HU, Stammler P, Bianchi V, Trueb RM, Hunziker T, Burger R, et al. Intravenously applied IgG stimulates complement attenuation in a complement-dependent autoimmune disease at the amplifying C3 convertase level. Blood. 2004;103(2):465–72.
59. Basta M, Van Goor F, Luccioli S, Billings EM, Vortmeyer AO, Baranyi L, et al. F(ab)′2-mediated neutralization of C3a and C5a anaphylatoxins: a novel effector function of immuno-globulins. Nat Med. 2003;9(4):431–8.
60. Beck CE, Nathan PC, Parkin PC, Blanchette VS, Macarthur C. Corticosteroids versus intra-venous immune globulin for the treatment of acute immune thrombocytopenic purpura in children: a systematic review and meta-analysis of randomized controlled trials. J Pediatr. 2005;147(4):521–7.
61. Godeau B. High-dose dexamethasone or oral prednisone for immune thrombocytopenia? Lancet Haematol. 2016;3(10):e453-e4.
62. Sun D, Shehata N, Ye XY, Gregorovich S, De France B, Arnold DM, et al. Corticosteroids compared with intravenous immunoglobulin for the treatment of immune thrombocytopenia in pregnancy. Blood. 2016;128(10):1329–35.
63. Cooper N. Intravenous immunoglobulin and anti-RhD therapy in the management of immune thrombocytopenia. Hematol Oncol Clin North Am. 2009;23(6):1317–27.
64. Salama A, Kiefel V, Amberg R, Mueller-Eckhardt C. Treatment of autoimmune thrombocyto-penic purpura with rhesus antibodies (anti-Rh0(D)). Blut. 1984;49(1):29–35.
65. Becker T, Kuenzlen E, Salama A, Mertens R, Kiefel V, Weiss H, et al. Treatment of child-hood idiopathic thrombocytopenic purpura with Rhesus antibodies (anti-D). Eur J Pediatr. 1986;145(3):166–9.
66. Scaradavou A, Woo B, Woloski BM, Cunningham-Rundles S, Ettinger LJ, Aledort LM, et al. Intravenous anti-D treatment of immune thrombocytopenic purpura: experience in 272 patients. Blood. 1997;89(8):2689–700.
67. Cooper N, Woloski BM, Fodero EM, Novoa M, Leber M, Beer JH, et al. Does treatment with intermittent infusions of intravenous anti-D allow a proportion of adults with recently diag-nosed immune thrombocytopenic purpura to avoid splenectomy? Blood. 2002;99(6):1922–7.
68. Tarantino MD, Young G, Bertolone SJ, Kalinyak KA, Shafer FE, Kulkarni R, et al. Single dose of anti-D immune globulin at 75 microg/kg is as effective as intravenous immune globulin at rapidly raising the platelet count in newly diagnosed immune thrombocytopenic purpura in children. J Pediatr. 2006;148(4):489–94.
69. Simpson KN, Coughlin CM, Eron J, Bussel JB. Idiopathic thrombocytopenia purpura: Treatment patterns and an analysis of cost associated with intravenous immunoglobulin and anti-D therapy. Semin Hematol. 1998;35(1 Suppl 1):58–64.
70. Berger M. Adverse effects of IgG therapy. J Allergy Clin Immunol Pract. 2013;1(6):558–66.
71. Gaines AR. Acute onset hemoglobinemia and/or hemoglobinuria and sequelae following Rh(o)(D) immune globulin intravenous administration in immune thrombocytopenic purpura patients. Blood. 2000;95(8):2523–9.
72. Gaines AR. Disseminated intravascular coagulation associated with acute hemoglobinemia or hemoglobinuria following Rh(0)(D) immune globulin intravenous administration for immune thrombocytopenic purpura. Blood. 2005;106(5):1532–7.
73. Thompson JC, Klima J, Despotovic JM, O'Brien SH. Anti-D immunoglobulin therapy for pediatric ITP: before and after the FDA's black box warning. Pediatr Blood Cancer. 2013;60(11):E149–51.
74. Long M, Kalish LA, Neufeld EJ, Grace RF. Trends in anti-D immune globulin for child-hood immune thrombocytopenia: usage, response rates, and adverse effects. Am J Hematol. 2012;87(3):315–7.
75. Despotovic JM, Neunert CEI. anti-D immunoglobulin still a frontline treatment option for immune thrombocytopenia? Hematology Am Soc Hematol Educ Program. 2013;2013:283–5.

76. Yacobovich J, Abu-Ahmed S, Steinberg-Shemer O, Goldberg T, Cohen M, Tamary H. Anti-D treatment for pediatric immune thrombocytopenia: Is the bad reputation justified? Semin Hematol. 2016;53(Suppl 1):S64–6.
77. Eghbali A, Azadmanesh P, Bagheri B, Taherahmadi H, Sadeghi Sedeh B. Comparison between IV immune globulin (IVIG) and anti-D globulin for treatment of immune thrombocytopenia: a randomized open-label study. Fundam Clin Pharmacol. 2016;30(4):385–9.
78. Song S, Crow AR, Siragam V, Freedman J, Lazarus AH. Monoclonal antibodies that mimic the action of anti-D in the amelioration of murine ITP act by a mechanism distinct from that of IVIg. Blood. 2005;105(4):1546–8.
79. Cooper N, Heddle NM, Haas M, Reid ME, Lesser ML, Fleit HB, et al. Intravenous (IV) anti-D and IV immunoglobulin achieve acute platelet increases by different mechanisms: modulation of cytokine and platelet responses to IV anti-D by FcgammaRIIa and FcgammaRIIIa polymorphisms. Br J Haematol. 2004;124(4):511–8.
80. Bussel JB, Kaufmann CP, Ware RE, Woloski BM. Do the acute platelet responses of patients with immune thrombocytopenic purpura (ITP) to IV anti-D and to IV gammaglobulin predict response to subsequent splenectomy? Am J Hematol. 2001;67(1):27–33.
81. Meyer O, Kiesewetter H, Hermsen M, Salama A. Efficacy and safety of anti-D given by subcutaneous injection to patients with autoimmune thrombocytopenia. Eur J Haematol. 2004;73(1):71–2.
82. Gringeri A, Cattaneo M, Santagostino E, Mannucci PM. Intramuscular anti-D immunoglobulins for home treatment of chronic immune thrombocytopenic purpura. Br J Haematol. 1992;80(3):337–40.
83. Sirachainan N, Anurathapan U, Chuansumrit A, Songdej D, Wongwerawattanakoon P, Hutspardol S, et al. Intramuscular anti-D in chronic immune thrombocytopenia children with severe thrombocytopenia. Pediatr Int. 2013;55(6):e146–8.
84. Trebo MM, Frey E, Gadner H, Minkov M. Subcutaneous anti-D globulin application is a safe treatment option of immune thrombocytopenia in children. Ann Hematol. 2010;89(4):415–8.
85. Thai LH, Mahevas M, Roudot-Thoraval F, Limal N, Languille L, Dumas G, et al. Long-term complications of splenectomy in adult immune thrombocytopenia. Medicine (Baltimore). 2016;95(48):e5098.
86. Palandri F, Polverelli N, Sollazzo D, Romano M, Catani L, Cavo M, et al. Have splenectomy rate and main outcomes of ITP changed after the introduction of new treatments? A monocentric study in the outpatient setting during 35 years. Am J Hematol. 2016;91(4):E267–72.
87. Kojouri K, Vesely SK, Terrell DR, George JN. Splenectomy for adult patients with idiopathic thrombocytopenic purpura: a systematic review to assess long-term platelet count responses, prediction of response, and surgical complications. Blood. 2004;104(9):2623–34.
88. Park YH, Yi HG, Kim CS, Hong J, Park J, Lee JH, et al. Clinical outcome and predictive factors in the response to splenectomy in elderly patients with primary immune thrombocytopenia: a multicenter retrospective study. Acta Haematol. 2016;135(3):162–71.
89. O'Neal HR Jr, Niven AS, Karam GH. Critical illness in patients with asplenia. Chest. 2016;150(6):1394–402.
90. Rodeghiero F, Ruggeri M. Short- and long-term risks of splenectomy for benign haematological disorders: should we revisit the indications? Br J Haematol. 2012;158(1):16–29.
91. Ahmed R, Devasia AJ, Viswabandya A, Lakshmi KM, Abraham A, Karl S, et al. Long-term outcome following splenectomy for chronic and persistent immune thrombocytopenia (ITP) in adults and children : splenectomy in ITP. Ann Hematol. 2016;95(9):1429–34.
92. Crary SE, Buchanan GR. Vascular complications after splenectomy for hematologic disorders. Blood. 2009;114(14):2861–8.
93. Frey MK, Alias S, Winter MP, Redwan B, Stubiger G, Panzenboeck A, et al. Splenectomy is modifying the vascular remodeling of thrombosis. J Am Heart Assoc. 2014;3(1):e000772.
94. Branehog I. Platelet kinetics in idiopathic thrombocytopenic purpura (ITP) before and at different times after splenectomy. Br J Haematol. 1975;29(3):413–26.

95. Lamy T, Moisan A, Dauriac C, Ghandour C, Morice P, Le Prise PY. Splenectomy in idiopathic thrombocytopenic purpura: its correlation with the sequestration of autologous indium-111-labeled platelets. J Nucl Med. 1993;34(2):182–6.

96. Fujisawa K, Tani P, Piro L, McMillan R. The effect of therapy on platelet-associated autoantibody in chronic immune thrombocytopenic purpura. Blood. 1993;81(11):2872–7.

97. Stasi R, Provan D. Management of immune thrombocytopenic purpura in adults. Mayo Clin Proc. 2004;79(4):504–22.

98. Katkhouda N, Grant SW, Mavor E, Friedlander MH, Lord RV, Achanta K, et al. Predictors of response after laparoscopic splenectomy for immune thrombocytopenic purpura. Surg Endosc. 2001;15(5):484–8.

99. Kaplinsky C, Spirer Z. Post-splenectomy antibiotic prophylaxis--unfinished story: to treat or not to treat? Pediatr Blood Cancer. 2006;47(5 Suppl):740–1.

100. Cooper N, Stasi R, Cunningham-Rundles S, Feuerstein MA, Leonard JP, Amadori S, et al. The efficacy and safety of B-cell depletion with anti-CD20 monoclonal antibody in adults with chronic immune thrombocytopenic purpura. Br J Haematol. 2004;125(2):232–9.

101. Saleh MN, Gutheil J, Moore M, Bunch PW, Butler J, Kunkel L, et al. A pilot study of the anti-CD20 monoclonal antibody rituximab in patients with refractory immune thrombocytopenia. Semin Oncol. 2000;27(6 Suppl 12):99–103.

102. Stasi R, Pagano A, Stipa E, Amadori S. Rituximab chimeric anti-CD20 monoclonal antibody treatment for adults with chronic idiopathic thrombocytopenic purpura. Blood. 2001;98(4):952–7.

103. Garvey B. Rituximab in the treatment of autoimmune haematological disorders. Br J Haematol. 2008;141(2):149–69.

104. Nazi I, Kelton JG, Larche M, Snider DP, Heddle NM, Crowther MA, et al. The effect of rituximab on vaccine responses in patients with immune thrombocytopenia. Blood. 2013;122(11):1946–53.

105. Levy R, Mahevas M, Galicier L, Boutboul D, Moroch J, Loustau V, et al. Profound symptomatic hypogammaglobulinemia: a rare late complication after rituximab treatment for immune thrombocytopenia. Report of 3 cases and systematic review of the literature. Autoimmun Rev. 2014;13(10):1055–63.

106. Cooper N, Bussel JB. The long-term impact of rituximab for childhood immune thrombocytopenia. Curr Rheumatol Rep. 2010;12(2):94–100.

107. Sokol J, Lisa L, Zelenakova J, Balharek T, Plamenova I, Stasko J, et al. Rituximab-associated progressive multifocal leukoencephalopathy. Vnitr Lek. 2017;63(1):60–4.

108. Arnold DM, Vrbensky JR, Karim N, Smith JW, Liu Y, Ivetic N, et al. The effect of rituximab on anti-platelet autoantibody levels in patients with immune thrombocytopenia. Br J Haematol. 2017;178(2):302–7.

109. Ghanima W, Khelif A, Waage A, Michel M, Tjonnfjord GE, Romdhan NB, et al. Rituximab as second-line treatment for adult immune thrombocytopenia (the RITP trial): a multicentre, randomised, double-blind, placebo-controlled trial. Lancet. 2015;385(9978):1653–61.

110. Audia S, Mahevas M, Samson M, Godeau B, Bonnotte B. Pathogenesis of immune thrombocytopenia. Autoimmun Rev. 2017;16(6):620–32.

111. Zufferey A, Kapur R, Semple JW. Pathogenesis and therapeutic mechanisms in immune thrombocytopenia (ITP). J Clin Med. 2017;6(2):pii: E16.

112. Stasi R, Del Poeta G, Stipa E, Evangelista ML, Trawinska MM, Cooper N, et al. Response to B-cell depleting therapy with rituximab reverts the abnormalities of T-cell subsets in patients with idiopathic thrombocytopenic purpura. Blood. 2007;110(8):2924–30.

113. Stasi R, Cooper N, Del Poeta G, Stipa E, Laura Evangelista M, Abruzzese E, et al. Analysis of regulatory T-cell changes in patients with idiopathic thrombocytopenic purpura receiving B cell-depleting therapy with rituximab. Blood. 2008;112(4):1147–50.

114. Schmajuk G, Tonner C, Trupin L, Li J, Sarkar U, Ludwig D, et al. Using health-system-wide data to understand hepatitis B virus prophylaxis and reactivation outcomes in patients receiving rituximab. Medicine (Baltimore). 2017;96(13):e6528.

115. Provan D, Butler T, Evangelista ML, Amadori S, Newland AC, Stasi R. Activity and safety profile of low-dose rituximab for the treatment of autoimmune cytopenias in adults. Haematologica. 2007;92(12):1695–8.
116. Zaja F, Baccarani M, Mazza P, Bocchia M, Gugliotta L, Zaccaria A, et al. Dexamethasone plus rituximab yields higher sustained response rates than dexamethasone monotherapy in adults with primary immune thrombocytopenia. Blood. 2010;115(14):2755–62.
117. Gudbrandsdottir S, Birgens HS, Frederiksen H, Jensen BA, Jensen MK, Kjeldsen L, et al. Rituximab and dexamethasone vs dexamethasone monotherapy in newly diagnosed patients with primary immune thrombocytopenia. Blood. 2013;121(11):1976–81.
118. Choi PY, Roncolato F, Badoux X, Ramanathan S, Ho SJ, Chong BH. A novel triple therapy for ITP using high-dose dexamethasone, low-dose rituximab, and cyclosporine (TT4). Blood. 2015;126(4):500–3.
119. Elgebaly AS, Ashal GE, Elfil M, Menshawy A. Tolerability and efficacy of eltrombopag in chronic immune thrombocytopenia: meta-analysis of randomized controlled trials. Clin Appl Thromb Hemost. 2016;23(8):928–37.
120. Provan D, Newland AC. Current management of primary immune thrombocytopenia. Adv Ther. 2015;32(10):875–87.
121. Mazza P, Minoia C, Melpignano A, Polimeno G, Cascavilla N, Di Renzo N, et al. The use of thrombopoietin-receptor agonists (TPO-RAs) in immune thrombocytopenia (ITP): a "real life" retrospective multicenter experience of the Rete Ematologica Pugliese (REP). Ann Hematol. 2016;95(2):239–44.
122. Gonzalez-Lopez TJ, Alvarez-Roman MT, Pascual C, Sanchez-Gonzalez B, Fernandez-Fuentes F, Jarque I, et al. Eltrombopag safety and efficacy for primary chronic immune thrombocytopenia in clinical practice. Eur J Haematol. 2016;97(3):297–302.
123. Khellaf M, Michel M, Quittet P, Viallard JF, Alexis M, Roudot-Thoraval F, et al. Romiplostim safety and efficacy for immune thrombocytopenia in clinical practice: 2-year results of 72 adults in a romiplostim compassionate-use program. Blood. 2011;118(16):4338–45.
124. Gonzalez-Porras JR, Mingot-Castellano ME, Andrade MM, Alonso R, Caparros I, Arratibel MC, et al. Use of eltrombopag after romiplostim in primary immune thrombocytopenia. Br J Haematol. 2015;169(1):111–6.
125. Kuter DJ, Begley CG. Recombinant human thrombopoietin: basic biology and evaluation of clinical studies. Blood. 2002;100(10):3457–69.
126. Kuter DJ. The biology of thrombopoietin and thrombopoietin receptor agonists. Int J Hematol. 2013;98(1):10–23.
127. Lok S, Kaushansky K, Holly RD, Kuijper JL, Lofton-Day CE, Oort PJ, et al. Cloning and expression of murine thrombopoietin cDNA and stimulation of platelet production in vivo. Nature. 1994;369(6481):565–8.
128. Bartley TD, Bogenberger J, Hunt P, Li YS, Lu HS, Martin F, et al. Identification and cloning of a megakaryocyte growth and development factor that is a ligand for the cytokine receptor Mpl. Cell. 1994;77(7):1117–24.
129. de Sauvage FJ, Hass PE, Spencer SD, Malloy BE, Gurney AL, Spencer SA, et al. Stimulation of megakaryocytopoiesis and thrombopoiesis by the c-Mpl ligand. Nature. 1994;369(6481):533–8.
130. Kato T, Ogami K, Shimada Y, Iwamatsu A, Sohma Y, Akahori H, et al. Purification and characterization of thrombopoietin. J Biochem. 1995;118(1):229–36.
131. Kuter DJ, Beeler DL, Rosenberg RD. The purification of megapoietin: a physiological regulator of megakaryocyte growth and platelet production. Proc Natl Acad Sci U S A. 1994;91(23):11104–8.
132. Buchbinder D, Nugent D, Hsieh L. Spotlight on romiplostim in the treatment of children with chronic immune thrombocytopenia: design, development, and potential place in therapy. Drug Des Devel Ther. 2017;11:1055–63.
133. Wang B, Nichol JL, Sullivan JT. Pharmacodynamics and pharmacokinetics of AMG 531, a novel thrombopoietin receptor ligand. Clin Pharmacol Ther. 2004;76(6):628–38.

134. Carpenedo M, Cantoni S, Coccini V, Pogliani EM, Cairoli R. Response loss and development of neutralizing antibodies during long-term treatment with romiplostim in patients with immune thrombocytopenia: a case series. Eur J Haematol. 2016;97(1):101–3.
135. Erhardt JA, Erickson-Miller CL, Aivado M, Abboud M, Pillarisetti K, Toomey JR. Comparative analyses of the small molecule thrombopoietin receptor agonist eltrombopag and thrombopoietin on in vitro platelet function. Exp Hematol. 2009;37(9):1030–7.
136. Saleh MN, Bussel JB, Cheng G, Meyer O, Bailey CK, Arning M, et al. Safety and efficacy of eltrombopag for treatment of chronic immune thrombocytopenia: results of the long-term, open-label EXTEND study. Blood. 2013;121(3):537–45.
137. Novartis. Promacta(eltrombopag) dosing & administration 2016 [cited 2017]. https://www. hcp.novartis.com/products/promacta/chronic-immune-idiopathic-thrombocytopenia/?site=4 3700019327523549&source=01030&irmasrc=prmwb25351.
138. Fukushima-Shintani M, Suzuki K, Iwatsuki Y, Abe M, Sugasawa K, Hirayama F, et al. AKR-501 (YM477) in combination with thrombopoietin enhances human megakaryocytopoiesis. Exp Hematol. 2008;36(10):1337–42.
139. Nomoto M, Pastino G, Rege B, Aluri J, Ferry J, Han D. Pharmacokinetics, pharmacodynamics, pharmacogenomics, safety, and tolerability of avatrombopag in healthy Japanese and White subjects. Clin Pharmacol Drug Dev. 2018;7(2):188–95.
140. Bussel JB, Kuter DJ, Aledort LM, Kessler CM, Cuker A, Pendergrass KB, et al. A randomized trial of avatrombopag, an investigational thrombopoietin-receptor agonist, in persistent and chronic immune thrombocytopenia. Blood. 2014;123(25):3887–94.
141. Terrault NA, Hassanein T, Howell CD, Joshi S, Lake J, Sher L, et al. Phase II study of avatrombopag in thrombocytopenic patients with cirrhosis undergoing an elective procedure. J Hepatol. 2014;61(6):1253–9.
142. Cines DB, Gernsheimer T, Wasser J, Godeau B, Provan D, Lyons R, et al. Integrated analysis of long-term safety in patients with chronic immune thrombocytopaenia (ITP) treated with the thrombopoietin (TPO) receptor agonist romiplostim. Int J Hematol. 2015;102(3): 259–70.
143. Cuker A. Toxicities of the thrombopoietic growth factors. Semin Hematol. 2010;47(3): 289–98.
144. Saleh M, Bussel JB, Wong R, Meddeb B, Salama A, Quebe-Fehling E, et al. Hepatobiliary and thromboembolic events during long-term E.X.T.E.N.Ded treatment with eltrombopag in adult patients with chronic immune thrombocytopenia. Blood. 2016;128(12):Abstract 1368.
145. Rodeghiero F. Is ITP a thrombophilic disorder? Am J Hematol. 2016;91(1):39–45.
146. Harker LA, Marzec UM, Hunt P, Kelly AB, Tomer A, Cheung E, et al. Dose-response effects of pegylated human megakaryocyte growth and development factor on platelet production and function in nonhuman primates. Blood. 1996;88(2):511–21.
147. Kuter DJ, Mufti GJ, Bain BJ, Hasserjian RP, Davis W, Rutstein M. Evaluation of bone marrow reticulin formation in chronic immune thrombocytopenia patients treated with romiplostim. Blood. 2009;114(18):3748–56.
148. Douglas VK, Tallman MS, Cripe LD, Peterson LC. Thrombopoietin administered during induction chemotherapy to patients with acute myeloid leukemia induces transient morphologic changes that may resemble chronic myeloproliferative disorders. Am J Clin Pathol. 2002;117(6):844–50.
149. Brynes RK, Wong RS, Thein MM, Bakshi KK, Burgess P, Theodore D, et al. A 2-year, longitudinal, prospective study of the effects of eltrombopag on bone marrow in patients with chronic immune thrombocytopenia. Acta Haematol. 2017;137(2):66–72.
150. Lambert MP, Witmer CM, Kwiatkowski JL. Therapy induced iron deficiency in children treated with eltrombopag for immune thrombocytopenia. Am J Hematol. 2017;92(6):E88–91.
151. Kuter DJ, Bussel JB, Lyons RM, Pullarkat V, Gernsheimer TB, Senecal FM, et al. Efficacy of romiplostim in patients with chronic immune thrombocytopenic purpura: a double-blind randomised controlled trial. Lancet. 2008;371(9610):395–403.

152. Bussel JB, de Miguel PG, Despotovic JM, Grainger JD, Sevilla J, Blanchette VS, et al. Eltrombopag for the treatment of children with persistent and chronic immune thrombocytopenia (PETIT): a randomised, multicentre, placebo-controlled study. Lancet Haematol. 2015;2(8):e315–25.

153. Grainger JD, Locatelli F, Chotsampancharoen T, Donyush E, Pongtanakul B, Komvilaisak P, et al. Eltrombopag for children with chronic immune thrombocytopenia (PETIT2): a randomised, multicentre, placebo-controlled trial. Lancet. 2015;386(10004):1649–58.

154. Tarantino MD, Bussel JB, Blanchette VS, Despotovic J, Bennett C, Raj A, et al. Romiplostim in children with immune thrombocytopenia: a phase 3, randomised, double-blind, placebo-controlled study. Lancet. 2016;388(10039):45–54.

155. Bussel JB, Buchanan GR, Nugent DJ, Gnarra DJ, Bomgaars LR, Blanchette VS, et al. A randomized, double-blind study of romiplostim to determine its safety and efficacy in children with immune thrombocytopenia. Blood. 2011;118(1):28–36.

156. Elalfy MS, Abdelmaksoud AA, Eltonbary KY. Romiplostim in children with chronic refractory ITP: randomized placebo controlled study. Ann Hematol. 2011;90(11):1341–4.

157. Neunert C, Despotovic J, Haley K, Lambert MP, Nottage K, Shimano K, et al. Thrombopoietin receptor agonist use in children: data from the pediatric ITP consortium of North America ICON2 study. Pediatr Blood Cancer. 2016;63(8):1407–13.

158. Newland A, Godeau B, Priego V, Viallard JF, Lopez Fernandez MF, Orejudos A, et al. Remission and platelet responses with romiplostim in primary immune thrombocytopenia: final results from a phase 2 study. Br J Haematol. 2016;172(2):262–73.

159. Gomez-Almaguer D, Herrera-Rojas MA, Jaime-Perez JC, Gomez-De Leon A, Cantu-Rodriguez OG, Gutierrez-Aguirre CH, et al. Eltrombopag and high-dose dexamethasone as frontline treatment of newly diagnosed immune thrombocytopenia in adults. Blood. 2014;123(25):3906–8.

160. Salama A, Kiesewetter H, Kalus U, Movassaghi K, Meyer O. Massive platelet transfusion is a rapidly effective emergency treatment in patients with refractory autoimmune thrombocytopenia. Thromb Haemost. 2008;100(5):762–5.

161. Spahr JE, Rodgers GM. Treatment of immune-mediated thrombocytopenia purpura with concurrent intravenous immunoglobulin and platelet transfusion: a retrospective review of 40 patients. Am J Hematol. 2008;83(2):122–5.

162. Salama A, Rieke M, Kiesewetter H, von Depka M. Experiences with recombinant FVIIa in the emergency treatment of patients with autoimmune thrombocytopenia: a review of the literature. Ann Hematol. 2009;88(1):11–5.

163. Mayer B, Salama A. Successful treatment of bleeding with tranexamic acid in a series of 12 patients with immune thrombocytopenia. Vox Sang. 2017;112(8):767–72.

164. Stirnemann J, Kaddouri N, Khellaf M, Morin AS, Prendki V, Michel M, et al. Vincristine efficacy and safety in treating immune thrombocytopenia: a retrospective study of 35 patients. Eur J Haematol. 2016;96(3):269–75.

165. Boruchov DM, Gururangan S, Driscoll MC, Bussel JB. Multiagent induction and maintenance therapy for patients with refractory immune thrombocytopenic purpura (ITP). Blood. 2007;110(10):3526–31.

166. Okazuka K, Masuko M, Matsuo Y, Miyakoshi S, Tanaka T, Kozakai T, et al. Successful treatment of severe newly diagnosed immune thrombocytopenia involving an alveolar hemorrhage with combination therapy consisting of romiplostim, rituximab and vincristine. Intern Med. 2013;52(11):1239–42.

167. Provan D, Moss AJ, Newland AC, Bussel JB. Efficacy of mycophenolate mofetil as single-agent therapy for refractory immune thrombocytopenic purpura. Am J Hematol. 2006;81(1):19–25.

168. Hogan J, Schwenk MH, Radhakrishnan J. Should mycophenolate mofetil replace cyclophosphamide as first-line therapy for severe lupus nephritis? Kidney Int. 2012;82(12):1256–60.

169. Taylor A, Neave L, Solanki S, Westwood JP, Terrinonive I, McGuckin S, et al. Mycophenolate mofetil therapy for severe immune thrombocytopenia. Br J Haematol. 2015;171(4):625–30.

170. Bouroncle BA, Doan CA. Refractory idiopathic thrombocytopenic purpura treated with aza-thioprine. N Engl J Med. 1966;275(12):630–5.
171. Miller AV, Ranatunga SK. Immunotherapies in rheumatologic disorders. Med Clin North Am. 2012;96(3):475–96. ix–x
172. Sussman LN. Azathioprine in refractory idiopathic thrombocytopenic purpura. JAMA. 1967;202(4):259–63.
173. Goebel KM, Goebel FD. Idiopathic thrombocytopenia after treatment with steroids and immunosuppressives. Chemotherapy. 1973;18(2):112–8.
174. Quiquandon I, Fenaux P, Caulier MT, Pagniez D, Huart JJ, Bauters F. Re-evaluation of the role of azathioprine in the treatment of adult chronic idiopathic thrombocytopenic purpura: a report on 53 cases. Br J Haematol. 1990;74(2):223–8.
175. Ahlmann M, Hempel G. The effect of cyclophosphamide on the immune system: implications for clinical cancer therapy. Cancer Chemother Pharmacol. 2016;78(4):661–71.
176. Reiner A, Gernsheimer T, Slichter SJ. Pulse cyclophosphamide therapy for refractory autoimmune thrombocytopenic purpura. Blood. 1995;85(2):351–8.
177. Verlin M, Laros RK Jr, Penner JA. Treatment of refractory thrombocytopenic purpura with cyclophosphamide. Am J Hematol. 1976;1(1):97–104.
178. Kappers-Klunne MC, van't Veer MB. Cyclosporin A for the treatment of patients with chronic idiopathic thrombocytopenic purpura refractory to corticosteroids or splenectomy. Br J Haematol. 2001;114(1):121–5.
179. Zver S, Zupan IP, Cernelc P. Cyclosporin A as an immunosuppressive treatment modality for patients with refractory autoimmune thrombocytopenic purpura after splenectomy failure. Int J Hematol. 2006;83(3):238–42.
180. Liu AP, Cheuk DK, Lee AH, Lee PP, Chiang AK, Ha SY, et al. Cyclosporin A for persistent or chronic immune thrombocytopenia in children. Ann Hematol. 2016;95(11):1881–6.
181. Emoto C, Fukuda T, Venkatasubramanian R, Vinks AA. The impact of CYP3A5*3 polymorphism on sirolimus pharmacokinetics: insights from predictions with a physiologically-based pharmacokinetic model. Br J Clin Pharmacol. 2015;80(6):1438–46.
182. Battaglia M, Stabilini A, Tresoldi E. Expanding human T regulatory cells with the mTOR-inhibitor rapamycin. Methods Mol Biol. 2012;821:279–93.
183. Jasinski S, Weinblatt ME, Glasser CL. Sirolimus as an effective agent in the treatment of immune thrombocytopenia (ITP) and Evans syndrome (ES): a single institution's experience. J Pediatr Hematol Oncol. 2017;39(6):420–4.
184. Li J, Wang Z, Dai L, Cao L, Su J, Zhu M, et al. Effects of rapamycin combined with low dose prednisone in patients with chronic immune thrombocytopenia. Clin Dev Immunol. 2013;2013:548085.
185. Park YH, Yi HG, Lee MH, Kim CS, Lim JH. Clinical efficacy and tolerability of vincristine in splenectomized patients with refractory or relapsed immune thrombocytopenia: a retrospective single-center study. Int J Hematol. 2016;103(2):180–8.
186. Sikorska A, Slomkowski M, Marlanka K, Konopka L, Gorski T. The use of vinca alkaloids in adult patients with refractory chronic idiopathic thrombocytopenia. Clin Lab Haematol. 2004;26(6):407–11.
187. Ahn YS, Horstman LL. Idiopathic thrombocytopenic purpura: pathophysiology and management. Int J Hematol. 2002;76(Suppl 2):123–31.
188. Schreiber AD, Chien P, Tomaski A, Cines DB. Effect of danazol in immune thrombocytopenic purpura. N Engl J Med. 1987;316(9):503–8.
189. Hill JA, Barbieri RL, Anderson DJ. Immunosuppressive effects of danazol in vitro. Fertil Steril. 1987;48(3):414–8.
190. Uchiyama M, Jin X, Zhang Q, Hirai T, Bashuda H, Watanabe T, et al. Danazol induces prolonged survival of fully allogeneic cardiac grafts and maintains the generation of regulatory CD4(+) cells in mice. Transpl Int. 2012;25(3):357–65.
191. Mylvaganam R, Ahn YS, Garcia RO, Kim CI, Harrington WJ. Very low dose danazol in idiopathic thrombocytopenic purpura and its role as an immune modulator. Am J Med Sci. 1989;298(4):215–20.

192. Maloisel F, Andres E, Zimmer J, Noel E, Zamfir A, Koumarianou A, et al. Danazol therapy in patients with chronic idiopathic thrombocytopenic purpura: long-term results. Am J Med. 2004;116(9):590–4.

193. Durand JM, Lefevre P, Hovette P, Mongin M, Soubeyrand J. Dapsone for idiopathic autoimmune thrombocytopenic purpura in elderly patients. Br J Haematol. 1991;78(3):459–60.

194. Godeau B, Durand JM, Roudot-Thoraval F, Tenneze A, Oksenhendler E, Kaplanski G, et al. Dapsone for chronic autoimmune thrombocytopenic purpura: a report of 66 cases. Br J Haematol. 1997;97(2):336–9.

195. Patel AP, Patil AS. Dapsone for immune thrombocytopenic purpura in children and adults. Platelets. 2015;26(2):164–7.

196. Rodrigo C, Gooneratne L. Dapsone for primary immune thrombocytopenia in adults and children: an evidence-based review. J Thromb Haemost. 2013;11(11):1946–53.

197. Audia S, Godeau B, Bonnotte B. Is there still a place for "old therapies" in the management of immune thrombocytopenia? Rev Med Interne. 2016;37(1):43–9.

198. Shih A, Nazi I, Kelton JG, Arnold DM. Novel treatments for immune thrombocytopenia. Presse Med. 2014;43(4 Pt 2):e87–95.

199. Kuwana M, Nomura S, Fujimura K, Nagasawa T, Muto Y, Kurata Y, et al. Effect of a single injection of humanized anti-CD154 monoclonal antibody on the platelet-specific autoimmune response in patients with immune thrombocytopenic purpura. Blood. 2004;103(4):1229–36.

200. Patel VL, Schwartz J, Bussel JB. The effect of anti-CD40 ligand in immune thrombocytopenic purpura. Br J Haematol. 2008;141(4):545–8.

201. Robak T, Windyga J, Trelinski J, von Depka Prondzinski M, Giagounidis A, Doyen C, et al. Rozrolimupab, a mixture of 25 recombinant human monoclonal RhD antibodies, in the treatment of primary immune thrombocytopenia. Blood. 2012;120(18):3670–6.

202. Podolanczuk A, Lazarus AH, Crow AR, Grossbard E, Bussel JB. Of mice and men: an open-label pilot study for treatment of immune thrombocytopenic purpura by an inhibitor of Syk. Blood. 2009;113(14):3154–60.

203. Fan H, Zhu HL, Li SX, Lu XC, Zhai B, Guo B, et al. Efficacy of amifostine in treating patients with idiopathic thrombocytopenia purpura. Cell Biochem Biophys. 2011;59(1):7–12.

Part II
Autoimmune Hemolytic Anemia (AIHA)

Chapter 5
Background, Presentation and Pathophysiology of Autoimmune Hemolytic Anemia

Shawki Qasim

History of Immune Hemolysis

The earliest described constellation of symptoms suggestive of AIHA dates back to 1769, when Morgagni reported a priest presenting with red urine, fatigue, a pallid color, and an enlarged spleen [1]; however, this could have been consistent with a then more common illness, such as malaria [2]. Another report by Andral in 1843 described a spontaneous anemia, arising without any prior blood loss that he attributed to altered structure of the corpuscles and their "true" destruction [2, 3]. In 1852, Vogel thought that the coloring matter in the urine was the same as that in the blood, suggesting it consisted of a "decomposition of blood discs." He also recorded a connection between fevers, colored urine, decomposition of the blood, and anemia, recognizing an anemia secondary to infection [2].

The association between cold exposure and certain forms of AIHA was first reported in 1854 by Dressler, who described a 10-year-old boy who, after exposure to cold, passed red urine that gradually paled to a natural color; microscopic examination of the urine showed a "dirty brown pigment" and no blood cells [4]. Similar cases were described in the literature in the following years with no major advances in the understanding of AIHA until 1871, when Vanlair and Masius concluded that premature destruction of RBCs leads to jaundice. They described a patient with anemia, splenomegaly, reddish brown urine, and spherical dwarf cells in the peripheral blood they referred to as "microcytes" (likely spherocytes), hence, the name they gave the condition, "microcythemia" [5]. In 1879, Stephen Mackenzie reported a case of paroxysmal cold hemoglobinuria (PCH) with anemia without history of blood loss, dark urine that was negative for red blood cells (RBCs) and demonstra-

S. Qasim, MD
Baylor College of Medicine, Texas Children's Hospital, Houston, TX, USA
e-mail: slqasim@texaschildrens.org

© Springer International Publishing AG, part of Springer Nature 2018   83
J. M. Despotovic (ed.), *Immune Hematology*,
https://doi.org/10.1007/978-3-319-73269-5_5

tion of clinical improvement upon rewarming. He hypothesized that the "proteid" (hemoglobin) was the reason for the dark color of the urine. He hypothesized that the chills and rigors heralding the hemolysis were actually responsible for breaking the RBCs and forcing them through the kidneys [6]. In the late nineteenth century, Hayem and Minkowski contributed to the understanding of the distinction between acquired and congenital forms of hemolysis and differentiated hemolytic from hepatobiliary jaundice [7, 8]. In 1901 Landsteiner discovered the ABO blood group system, leading to an understanding of RBC antigens; then in 1904, along with Donath, they suggested a then novel mechanism for hemolysis, implicating a serum "hemolytic substance" in the development of PCH. This is considered the first study to describe the role of autoantibodies in autoimmune diseases. They later demonstrated that this hemolytic substance (hemolysin) causes RBC agglutination at low temperatures and again upon rewarming in the presence of complement, establishing the basis for the current diagnostic testing for PCH (Donath-Landsteiner Antibody test, see Chap. 6) [9, 10].

Splenectomy then became a standard treatment for AIHA with most other suggested therapeutic measures being less effective.

In 1907, Chauffard introduced the term acute hemolytic icterus to describe patients with AIHA and suggested that hemolysins are endogenous. He demonstrated that affected patients' sera are capable of lysing other RBCs. His group also standardized the osmotic fragility test and described reticulocytosis in congenital hemolytic anemias [11–13].

In 1911 Micheli performed the first splenectomy for acquired hemolytic anemia, while Banti introduced the term hemolytic splenomegaly in 1912, after noticing splenic enlargement and congestion in research animals with hemolysis, which he observed to be milder in splenectomized animals. Banti suggested a role for the splenic endothelium in destroying RBCs, that is shared by their hepatic counterparts (Kupffer cells), but only in severe hemolysis, paving the way for the current understanding of the reticuloendothelial system involvement in extravascular hemolysis [14, 15].

In 1936, Witts recognized that hemoglobinuria is most always the result of intravascular hemolysis and follows hemoglobinemia [16]. Around the same time, Dameshek and Schwartz described patients with splenectomy-responsive acute hemolytic anemia whose sera were able to lyse allogeneic and autologous RBCs with the degree of spherocytosis being proportional to the hemolysin titer [17].

In 1944, Race and Weiner separately suggested that there were two types of Rh antibody, one bound to the RBC surface which drove agglutination (the "complete" antibody; IgM) and one that also adsorbed to the RBC surface but did not cause agglutination (the "incomplete" antibody; IgG) [18, 19]. This conclusion provided the basis for the current distinction between warm and cold AIHA types as described in the following sections.

In 1945, Coombs, Mourant, and Race submitted their landmark paper titled "A New Test for The Detection of Weak and 'Incomplete' Rh Agglutinins," the first described direct antiglobulin test (DAT) using rabbit antihuman sera to detect incomplete antibodies bound to human RBCs [20].

From 1948 to 1950, Evans and Duane proposed that the spleen was the primary production site of the hemolysin, given reduction in RBC sensitization after splenectomy, but suggested there might also be a role for other hemolymphatic organs in the pathogenesis. No evidence was available to suggest a role for complement fixation in hemolysis at that time [21].

Studies in the 1950s supported the theory of autoimmunization as basis for immune hemolysis [22, 23]; therefore, by the 1960s, immunosuppressive therapy became widely used for the treatment of AIHA based on the concept of immune overactivity and failure of immune surveillance. Studies in the 1960s and early 1970s focused on further characterizing the autoantibodies, their subtypes, thermodynamic properties, and their targets [24–26]. In 1972, the mechanisms of complement-mediated hemolysis were described by Schreiber and Frank [27].

By the 1980s, quantitative studies of autoantibodies and complement components were conducted and used to assess the severity of AIHA. In the subsequent years, more studies were performed on the pathogenesis of AIHA, role of antigen-presenting cells, other types of immune cells, major histocompatibility complexes, and opsonization-phagocytosis [28, 29].

Definitions and Classification

AIHA has been classically divided into warm and cold types based on the thermodynamics of antibody-antigen interaction. The term "warm AIHA" has historically been used to describe IgG-mediated hemolysis with optimal antibody-antigen interaction at core body temperature, while "cold AIHA" usually refers to IgM-mediated hemolysis with optimal antibody-antigen interaction at sub-core temperature.

With better understanding of AIHA pathophysiology and the availability of more sensitive assays, the disorder can be divided into four distinct serologic forms [30–36], as detailed in Table 5.1.

The essential laboratory test for diagnosis and differentiation of AIHA is the DAT, formerly known as the Coombs test.

The initial screening DAT is done by the addition of a reagent containing polyspecific antiglobulin antibodies to washed, suspended patient red blood cells (RBCs). This screening antiglobulin reacts to both IgG and C3d (a component of the complement fragment C3b). If agglutination happens after sample centrifugation, this would be consistent with RBC cross-linking, and the test would be considered positive. Furthermore, the positivity of DAT can be graded based on the titer (strength of agglutination) and typically ranges between 0 and 3+; correlation between the strength of DAT positivity and the severity of clinical hemolysis has been demonstrated in a few studies [33, 37].

If the screening test is positive, then more specific antiglobulins are used to differentiate between IgG- and C3d-coated RBCs in a similar manner. Further charac-

Table 5.1 Summary of different serologic forms of AIHA

Type	Incidence	Antibodies-antigens	Optimal reaction temperature	Mechanism of hemolysis	Serology
Warm AIHA	65–70%	Polyclonal IgG targeting Rh polypeptides or less commonly glycophorins	37 °C	**Major:** *Extravascular hemolysis* of IgG-coated RBCs, mostly in the spleen (to a lesser extent in the liver and bone marrow) **Minor:** *Intravascular hemolysis* due to complement activation **Minor:** *Extravascular hemolysis* of C3b-coated RBCs mostly in the liver	IgG-positive +/− C3d-positive DAT IAT positive for pan-agglutinating IgG
Cold AIHA	20–25%	Mono- or oligoclonal IgM pentamers targeting polysaccharide antigens (I, i, Pr, and others)	0–5 °C	**Acutely:** *Intravascular hemolysis* due to complement activation **Chronically:** *Extravascular hemolysis* of C3b-coated RBCs mostly in the liver	C3d-positive DAT High-cold agglutinin titer
Paroxysmal cold hemoglobinuria	1–3% (30–40% in children)	IgG (Donath-Landsteiner antibodies) directed against P-antigen	0–5 °C	**Cold exposure:** IgG attaches to RBC with incomplete fixation of complement **Rewarming:** detachment of antibody and completion of complement activation causing *intravascular hemolysis*	C3b-positive DAT

(continued)

Table 5.1 (continued)

Type	Incidence	Antibodies-antigens	Optimal reaction temperature	Mechanism of hemolysis	Serology
Mixed AIHA	8%	IgG and IgM		A combination of the above mechanisms	Positive direct anti-globulin test for IgG and C3b
DAT-negative warm AIHA	~5%	Low-affinity or titer IgG, IgA, or monomeric IgM	37 °C	*Extravascular hemolysis* of IgG, monoclonal IgM, or IgA-coated RBCs	Negative standard DAT—micro-column DAT is needed to confirm diagnosis

AIHA autoimmune hemolytic anemia, *DAT* direct antiglobulin test, *IAT* indirect antiglobulin test, *RBC* red blood cell

terization of the antibody type can be done by performing an indirect antiglobulin test (IAT or indirect Coombs test) in which the patient's serum or RBC eluate is incubated with a panel of donor RBCs with known surface antigenic characteristics. After incubation, a DAT is performed to identify which particular RBCs in the standardized panel attracted the autoantibody [38].

Warm AIHA

Warm agglutinin immune hemolytic anemia is the most common form of immune hemolysis, accounting for 65–70% of cases [32]. While warm AIHA remains the dominant form in children, its contribution to the etiology of immune hemolytic anemia is lower than that in adults [39]. It is characterized by the production of high concentrations of polyclonal IgG autoantibodies, typically directed against a component of the Rhesus (Rh) protein complex with optimal antibody-antigen interaction at 37 °C (core body temperature).

Pathophysiology

The process of antibody production in warm AIHA is not fully understood, but an interplay of multiple complex mechanisms is suggested, including:

- *Molecular mimicry* due to cross-reactivity of endogenous RBC and exogenous/environmental antigens which could be heteroimmune in nature as in viral infections or alloimmune in nature as in blood product transfusion reactions [32, 40].

- *Dysregulated processing* of autoantigens influenced by acquired factors (infection, malignancy, drugs, etc.), which reduces self-tolerance [32, 33, 41–43].
- *B and T cell dysfunction* including reduced numbers of regulatory T cells [44] and other T cell abnormalities, commonly among patients with immunodeficiency (as in common variable immunodeficiency [CVID], human immunodeficiency virus [HIV], and other infections) or other immune dysregulation, including lymphoproliferative disorders like chronic lymphocytic leukemia (CLL) and autoimmune lymphoproliferative syndrome (ALPS), which are known to be associated with a higher risk of AIHA and DAT positivity [45, 46].

The majority of warm agglutinin immune hemolysis is extravascular with no evidence of complement activation owing to the nature of their most common target, the Rh protein complex. Rh complexes are far apart on the RBC surface and cannot move laterally given their attachment to the cytoskeleton; therefore, the Fc portions of the attached IgG autoantibodies cannot be brought close enough to each other to activate complement, since two IgG molecules are needed to activate C1q and initiate the classical complement pathway cascade [47]. Furthermore, IgG molecules attached to two neighboring RBCs cannot be approximated due to the repelling negative charges on the RBC surface, known as the zeta potential.

However, IgG-sensitized RBCs traveling through the spleen, liver, and bone marrow are recognized by Fc receptors on tissue macrophages with IgG acting as an opsonin and facilitating receptor-mediated phagocytosis. RBCs are typically partially engulfed and digested by lysosomal enzymes, leaving a red cell with decreased surface area to volume ratio, adopting microspherocyte form that is less deformable and easily entrapped, then destroyed in reticuloendothelial organs, especially splenic sinuses. Less commonly, full erythrophagocytosis is seen [48].

Rarely and only with IgG1 and IgG3 subclasses, reactive to glycophorin antigens (epitopes of which are close enough to each other on RBC surface), the classical pathway of complement is activated with formation of C5b-9 membrane attack complex (MAC) resulting in intravascular hemolysis. If complement is activated, C3b-sensitized (opsonized) RBCs are recognized by C3b receptors on tissue macrophages then destroyed through receptor-mediated phagocytosis [49, 50].

The typical serologic picture in warm AIHA shows a DAT that is IgG positive either with or without C3d positivity and an IAT that is usually positive for pan-agglutinating IgG autoantibodies reacting to all panel RBCs.

While the above describes the serology of the majority of warm AIHA patients, about 3–5% of patients with a clinical and laboratory picture consistent with warm AIHA have a negative standard DAT (Coombs-negative warm AIHA). Most of these patients either have a low-titer and/or lower-affinity pan-agglutinating IgG, monoclonal IgM, or rarely IgA autoantibodies that are not detected by standard DAT. A micro-column DAT or flow cytometry can be helpful in confirming the diagnosis if suspicion is high [51].

Confirmation of the diagnosis of AIHA requires the presence of clinical and laboratory evidence of hemolysis along with the positive serology, as 0.1% of blood donors and up to 8% of hospitalized patients may have a positive DAT without clinical or laboratory evidence of hemolysis. Also, it is not uncommon for patients to develop DAT positivity after packed red blood cell (PRBC) transfusions or intravenous immunoglobulin (IVIG) administration with or without significant hemolysis [52].

Etiologically, warm AIHA can be divided into primary (idiopathic) and secondary categories, with the latter being a component or a presenting feature of an underlying disorder to which the immune dysregulation is attributed. These disorders usually fall into the categories of autoimmunity, immunodeficiency, malignancy, infection, and/or drug exposure [32].

Autoimmune diseases, especially systemic lupus erythematosus (SLE), are commonly associated with warm AIHA. Up to 10% of patients with SLE have a clinically significant warm AIHA with moderate-to-severe anemia, reticulocytosis, hyperbilirubinemia, and elevated lactate dehydrogenase (LDH) [53]. The presence of overt hemolytic anemia is typically associated with a subset of SLE patients characterized by a younger age of disease onset and a more severe disease with a higher likelihood of renal involvement, seizures, serositis, and other cytopenias [54].

Conditions with immune dysregulation like HIV infection, ALPS, and CVID are also commonly associated with warm AIHA. Although HIV-related immune hemolysis is usually ascribed to concurrent Epstein-Barr virus (EBV) and/or cytomegalovirus (CMV) infections that are typically associated with cold agglutinins, occasionally warm agglutinins are detected [55]. More commonly, DAT positivity without overt hemolysis is observed in patients with HIV infection; one study reports 18% DAT-positivity rate in patients with HIV [56]. Up to 11% of patients with CVID are reported to have some form of autoimmune cytopenia, in whom 50% present prior to or at CVID diagnosis [57]. Also, nearly 50–70% of patients with ALPS have autoimmune cytopenias, usually a combination of AIHA and immune thrombocytopenia (ITP) that is referred to as Evans syndrome [58] (see Chap. 3).

Among malignancies, CLL is one of the most frequently associated with warm AIHA in adults, with approximately 4–10% of CLL cases being complicated by AIHA. This is usually compounded by the added AIHA risk attributed to CLL chemotherapeutics, especially purine analogs such as fludarabine. About 90% of AIHA occurrences in CLL are due to polyclonal high-affinity IgG autoantibodies produced by nonmalignant B cell clones directed against RBC antigens [45, 59]. Other mechanisms include direct cytokine-mediated inhibition of erythropoiesis by cytotoxic T cells and natural killer (NK) cells in a dysregulated immune microenvironment induced by soluble factors secreted by the malignant CLL clone [60]. Additionally, subclinical DAT positivity is seen in up to 35% of patients with CLL [45].

Medications can cause AIHA with or without underlying immune dysregulation. The number of drugs implicated in causing drug-induced immune hemolytic anemia (DIIHA) has increased over the past few decades to ~125 according to one report [43]. Three groups of drugs predominated: 42% were antimicrobials, 15% were anti-inflammatory, and 11% were antineoplastics. In the 1970s, the most common drug by far to cause DIIHA was alpha-methyldopa, accounting for 67% of all DIIHA cases at some point. High-dose intravenous penicillin accounted for 25% of DIIHA. As these therapies are less commonly used in recent years, the most common causative group of drugs has become the cephalosporins, which account for 70% of the DIIHA encountered since the ~1990s. Among the cephalosporins, cefotetan is the most commonly implicated agent in DIIHA [43, 61]. Mechanisms and examples of DIIHA are outlined below and in Table 5.2.

Table 5.2 Common underlying disorders in secondary warm AIHA

Category	Example		
Autoimmunity	Systemic lupus erythematosus (SLE) Rheumatoid arthritis (RA) Antiphospholipid syndrome (APS) Autoimmune thyroiditis Evans syndrome Inflammatory bowel disease (IBD) Primary biliary cirrhosis (PBC)		
Immunodeficiency	Common variable immunodeficiency (CVID) Autoimmune lymphoproliferative syndrome (ALPS) IgA deficiency Post-transplant		
Malignancy	Chronic lymphocytic leukemia (CLL) Non-Hodgkin lymphoma (NHL) Hodgkin lymphoma		
Infection	Mostly with EBV and HIV		
Drug-induced immune hemolytic anemia (DIIHA)	Mechanisms		Examples
	Antigen alteration (drug-independent autoantibodies)		Alpha-methyldopa Fludarabine Oxaliplatinum
	Haptenization (drug-dependent autoantibodies)	Firmly attached haptens	Penicillin, cefotetan
		Loosely attached haptens	2nd–3rd-generation cephalosporin, piperacillin
	Non-immune protein adsorption (NIPA)		1st generation cephalosporins, b-lactamase inhibitors (clavulanate, sulbactam, tazobactam)

AIHA autoimmune hemolytic anemia, *EBV* Epstein-Barr virus, *HIV* human immunodeficiency virus

There are three general mechanisms proposed to explain different forms of DIIHA:

- *Antigen alteration*: in this case, the culprit drug interacts with a particular target protein on the RBC surface changing its structure, so circulating lymphocytes would consider it foreign and generate antibodies against it. These antibodies in turn would interact with the unaltered, normally expressed copies of the protein on the RBC surface with subsequent RBC destruction. Note that the culprit drug here is neither a part of the antigen epitope nor is it needed for subsequent antibody production (drug-independent autoantibodies), therefore drug discontinuation does not guarantee resolution of AIHA in these patients.

  The classic example from the group of drugs acting via this mechanism is alpha-methyldopa, which is known to induce autoantibody formation in ~ 15% of patients, while 0.5–1% develop clinically significant DIIHA. Alpha-methyldopa is thought to interact and alter one of the components of the Rh protein complex rendering it antigenic [62]. In this case the typical autoantibody response is mediated by IgG; therefore, most of the hemolysis is extravascular. Although IgG1 and IgG3 subclasses are able to activate complement, this is not observed with alpha-methyldopa DIIHA as the target protein complexes are far apart on the RBC surface hindering attached IgG molecules from activating complement [43, 62, 63]. The typical serologic picture here is a DAT that is positive for IgG, negative for C3d, and pan-agglutinating IgG-positive IAT.

- *Haptenization:* A hapten is a small molecule that is not antigenic in itself, but when attached to a particular target protein, it increases the immunogenicity of that protein, such that circulating lymphocytes would consider it foreign. Note that a hapten is an essential component of the antigenic epitope, unlike the alpha-methyldopa example above.

  This mechanism can be further subdivided into two different categories:

  - Firmly (covalently) attached haptens: with the classical example being penicillin, especially when administered in large IV doses. In those who develop DIIHA following penicillin administration, it is thought that the drug firmly attaches to a component in the Rh protein complex rendering the penicillin-Rh combination antigenic. Specific IgG autoantibodies target the haptenized Rh protein complex and tag RBCs for extravascular hemolysis. Again, complement is not activated in this case. Given the inclusion of the culprit drug in the epitope, the autoantibodies only react to the haptenized proteins; therefore drug discontinuation is often successful in resolving the hemolysis within a few days. The typical serologic picture would be an IgG-positive, C3d-negative DAT, while standard IAT is only positive if the panel RBCs are pre-treated with high concentrations of the offending drug [42, 43].
  - Loosely attached haptens: until recently, drugs in this category were thought to provoke an autoantibody response without associating with RBCs, with antibody-antigen complexes formed being deposited on nearby RBCs, causing complement activation and intravascular hemolysis; however, recent

evidence suggests that these drugs loosely associate with RBC surface antigens, forming an epitope which contains both drug and RBC protein—with autoantibodies reacting to both the haptenized protein and the separate drug at times. These reactions are typically IgM mediated, with complement activation and intravascular hemolysis. The typical serologic picture would be a C3d-positive DAT (rarely IgG positive as well) and a negative IAT that only becomes positive if both the drug and a source of complement are added to the reaction [43, 64, 65].

- *Nonimmune protein adsorption (NIPA)*: in this proposed mechanism, the offending drug is thought to induce morphological changes in the RBC surface protein structure in a way which attracts several plasma proteins in a nonimmunologic manner, including IgG, albumin, C3, fibrinogen, and others. Attachment of polyclonal IgG to the surface of RBCs reduces their life-span and can mediate opsonization-phagocytosis, resulting in extravascular hemolysis. Typically, there is no complement activation here, as the antibodies are not immunologically attached but rather adsorbed to the RBC surface. Classic examples of drugs associated with NIPA include first-generation cephalosporins and beta-lactamase inhibitors. Serologically, these patients would have an IgG-positive or IgG-negative, C3d-positive DAT, while IAT is essentially negative [43].

Clinical Features

The clinical manifestations associated with warm AIHA are generally nonspecific and commonly correlate with the severity of anemia. Patients with subclinical DAT positivity are essentially asymptomatic, while most patients with a clear diagnosis of warm AIHA tend to have moderate-to-severe anemia presenting in fatigue, exercise intolerance, palpitations, exertional dyspnea, postural dizziness, and/or headaches. Signs include pallor, jaundice, wide pulse pressure, bounding pulses, tachycardia, hyperdynamic precordium, and/or mild to moderate splenomegaly. Signs of high-output heart failure, like resting tachycardia, bibasilar pulmonary crackles, peripheral edema, and/or jugular venous distension, can be seen in patients with severe anemia, especially those with underlying congenital or acquired heart disease. Additionally, many patients with secondary AIHA would present with symptoms and signs related to the underlying disorder; therefore it is crucial for health-care providers to look for the stigmata of a potential underlying autoimmunity, immunodeficiency, malignancy, and/or infection [32].

Laboratory findings in patients with warm AIHA include:

- *Anemia:* Low hemoglobin with an average of 7–10 g/dL.
- *Macrocytosis:* Increased mean corpuscular volume (MCV) mostly secondary to reticulocytosis.
- *Spherocytosis* and *increased mean corpuscular hemoglobin concentration* (MCHC) due to partial RBC phagocytosis reducing the surface area to volume ratio.

- *Reticulocytosis:* This is observed in 70–80% of patients with warm AIHA, with reticulocyte percentages that are mostly above 5% and a reticulocyte production index >2–3%. Less commonly, 20–30% of patients have inappropriately normal or slightly reduced reticulocyte counts, with explanations including myelosuppression due to drugs or concurrent viral infection or antibodies that are reactive to RBC precursors and reticulocytes causing early destruction in the bone marrow before release [66].
- *Elevated LDH* and *depleted haptoglobin* is observed in the overwhelming majority of patients. A small group of patients (up to 7%) have normal or high haptoglobin levels, especially those in whom AIHA is secondary to an underlying autoimmunity, infection, and/or malignancy, in which baseline haptoglobin levels can be elevated, as an acute phase reactant. On the other hand, absent or low haptoglobin levels are common in full term and premature newborns (up to 3 months of age) [67, 68]. Despite these exceptions, a combination of high LDH and low haptoglobin has a 90% specificity for diagnosing hemolysis [69].
- *Indirect hyperbilirubinemia.*
- *Positive DAT* (IgG-positive, C3d-positive or negative) in the overwhelming majority of patients. As mentioned above, only 3–5% of patients with a clinical picture of warm AIHA are DAT negative, owing to low-titer/low-affinity IgG, IgM monomers, or IgA-mediated hemolysis.
- *Positive IAT for pan-agglutinating IgG autoantibodies* reacting to all panel RBCs with exceptions as detailed above, especially in drug-induced immune hemolytic anemia.
- Laboratory manifestations of intravascular hemolysis including hemoglobinemia, hemoglobinuria, hemosiderinuria, and/or hypocomplementemia are rare in warm AIHA as the overwhelming majority of RBC destruction is extravascular, but rarely complement activation and intravascular hemolysis do happen with warm AIHA, especially when IgG is reactive to RBC surface glycophorins or in cases of drug-induced IgM-mediated warm AIHA.
- *Thrombocytopenia* or *neutropenia* in patients with acute infection or AIHA as part of Evans syndrome.
- *Elevated inflammatory markers* like erythrocyte sedimentation rate (ESR) and C-reactive protein (CRP), especially with underlying autoimmunity, infection, or malignancy.

Cold AIHA (Cold Agglutinin Disease)

Cold agglutinin disease accounts for 20–25% of AIHA cases [41]. It is almost always caused by the production of pathologic amounts of IgM autoantibodies, directed at a variety of polysaccharide RBC surface antigens. Cold agglutinins, like most IgM molecules, exist in a homopentamer state which allows them to attach to multiple RBCs at the same time, evading the repelling negative charges—zeta potential—and maximizing their ability to agglutinate RBCs [70]. Unlike the Fc portions of IgG autoantibodies, IgM Fc fragments are attached to each other by the "J" peptide, and phagocytes do not express receptors for them; therefore, opsonization-phagocytosis does not contribute to hemolysis in acute cold AIHA. On the other hand, IgM pentamers are very potent complement activators, capable of inducing severe and sometimes life-threatening forms of intravascular hemolysis. The severity of hemolysis depends on the autoantibody concentration, the highest temperature at which it reacts with antigen, the degree of inhibition by regulatory complement components on RBC surface, and the specificity of the autoantibody. Most cold agglutinins are optimally reactive at 0–5 °C, but the ones that remain reactive at higher temperatures are more pathogenic since they are more likely to be active at extremity temperature, especially in a cold environment [30, 41].

Pathophysiology

Cold agglutinins loosely attach to RBC surface polysaccharides when their requisite temperature range is reached, but in many instances the duration of time that circulating blood spends in that particular temperature range is very short, so the antibody detaches without complement activation. Sometimes this short-lived attachment results in agglutinating a few RBCs (without hemolysis) at the tips of the digits causing acrocyanosis. In instances where the thermal amplitude of the cold agglutinin is high enough, it is still capable of attaching to RBC surface polysaccharides in sub-core but not necessarily very low temperatures. The duration of that attachment is long enough to allow for complement activation and formation of membrane attack complexes, which create perforations in the RBC membrane and ultimately result in intravascular hemolysis [30, 41, 71].

Given the presence of RBC surface complement inhibitors such as CD55 and CD59, clinically significant intravascular hemolysis is only encountered with large-scale complement activation. Therefore, significant hemolysis is typically seen only during the acute presentation or exacerbation of chronic disease, while most of the hemolysis in the stable chronic form of cold agglutinin disease results from attachment of earlier components of the classical complement pathway, particularly C3b—to a lesser extent C4b—that act as opsonins, mediating RBC phagocytosis by reticuloendothelial macrophages, especially Kupffer cells in the liver (extravascular hemolysis). Notably, complement-mediated opsonization-phagocytosis results in complete RBC engulfment; therefore, unlike warm AIHA, microspherocytosis is not seen [30, 41, 71].

Cold agglutinins are typically divided into four major types based on their in vitro reactivity to different RBC surface polysaccharides [72, 73]:

- *Anti-I autoantibodies:* these react to branched aminyllactose polymers present on almost all adult RBCs and account for the majority of pathogenic cold agglutinins.
- *Anti-i autoantibodies:* these react to linear aminyllactose polymers present on fetal or cord RBCs.

- *Anti-J autoantibodies:* these have equal reactivity to linear and branched aminyl-lactose polymers.
- *Anti-Pr autoantibodies:* these are uncommon, and they react to glycoprotein associated polysaccharides treated with proteases in vitro.

Clinical Features

Cold AIHA commonly develops secondary to an underlying infectious, paraneoplastic, and/or neoplastic process, as shown in Table 5.3, but can also adopt an idiopathic chronic form known as chronic cold agglutinin syndrome.

Infection-related cold AIHA most commonly develops after mycoplasma pneumoniae or EBV infection.

Oligoclonal cold agglutinins form in 50–75% of patients within 1–2 weeks of mycoplasma pneumoniae infection. The incidence is higher in children and gradually declines with age. It is thought that molecular mimicry between mycoplasma surface antigens and RBC surface polysaccharides is the primary mechanism, with most patients developing anti-I type antibodies. Most patients do not develop clinically significant hemolysis given the low autoantibody titers and the presence of strong complement inhibitory mechanisms, but a minority will present with severe hemolysis requiring hospitalization and blood product transfusion [30, 74]. Alternatively, up to 60% of patients with infectious mononucleosis due to EBV develop anti-i antibodies, but only very few develop clinically significant hemolysis,; hence, only 1% of AIHA cases are attributed to EBV infection. Other less common infections associated with cold agglutinin

Table 5.3 Common underlying disorders in secondary cold AIHA

Infection	Oligoclonal	Anti-I	Mycoplasma pneumonia Listeria monocytogenes
		Anti-i	EBV CMV Influenza Varicella Legionella Citrobacter
Neoplastic process	Monoclonal	Anti-I	Chronic lymphocytic leukemia (CLL) Small lymphocytic lymphoma (SLL) Well-differentiated lymphocytic lymphoma Waldenström macroglobulinemia Monoclonal gammopathy of undetermined significance (MGUS) Adenocarcinoma
		Anti-i	Poorly differentiated/aggressive lymphoma

AIHA autoimmune hemolytic anemia, *EBV* Epstein-Barr virus, *CMV* cytomegalovirus formation include CMV, legionella, citrobacter, influenza, and varicella [30, 75, 76].

Infection-related cold AIHA usually presents 1–2 weeks after the onset of primary infection and resolves within 2–4 weeks of primary infection resolution. Antibody titers decline gradually, returning to normal levels within 3–4 months of infection. Unlike the acute, occasionally life-threatening, but ultimately self-limiting nature of infection-related cold AIHA, malignancy-associated cold agglutinin disease adopts a more chronic form with stable pathologic concentrations of monoclonal autoantibodies.

Generally, patients with well-differentiated lymphoid malignancies (as in chronic lymphocytic leukemia and small lymphocytic lymphoma) and those with plasma cell dyscrasias (gammopathies) have a tendency to produce anti-I, while patients with poorly differentiated and aggressive forms of lymphoma tend to produce anti-i cold agglutinins. Although there are some exceptions to this generalization, a patient with persistent anti-i cold agglutinins and no evidence of an underlying infection is very likely to have a poorly differentiated lymphoma [30]. It is thought that malignancy-related cold agglutinin production is due to stimulation of a neoplastic lymphocytic clone, and so their titers tend to correspond with disease activity and can potentially be used as tumor markers or indicators of relapse.

Patients with chronic cold agglutinin syndrome are thought to have a benign monoclonal IgM gammopathy, typically diagnosed in older individuals with persistent anti-I antibodies. These patients may have stable disease for many years, but in up to 10%, the presumed benign lymphoid clone responsible for cold agglutinin production transforms into a malignant gammopathy, presenting with fever, leukocytosis, hypergammaglobulinemia, increased cold agglutinin titer, lymphadenopathy, and/or hepatosplenomegaly [30, 77].

As in warm AIHA, patients with cold agglutinin disease present with some general nonspecific symptoms of anemia like fatigue, exercise intolerance, palpitations, headache, postural dizziness, pallor, and/or jaundice. Unlike warm AIHA though, many patients develop more specific symptoms related to RBC agglutination and intravascular hemolysis, including [30, 77]:

- *Acrocyanosis* which results from non-hemolytic RBC agglutination by IgM pentamers at the tips of the digits, nose, and/or ears when exposed to a cold environment. The purple/gray discoloration and associated pain resolves with rewarming, with minimal reactive hyperemia. Generally, the antibody-antigen interaction is long enough to allow for agglutination, but not complement activation. Other cutaneous manifestations of RBC agglutination include full-blown Raynaud phenomena, livedo reticularis, urticaria, or very early skin necrosis/ulceration.
- *Dark urine* resulting from hemoglobinuria due to intravascular hemolysis followed by glomerular filtration of hemoglobin and eventually formation of hemosiderin.
- *Episodic worsening* of disease manifestations upon cold exposure (including cold water drinking), stress, trauma, surgery, and/or fever. These conditions are

known to induce complement production, fueling the intravascular hemolytic process.

- Clinical manifestations of associated disorders, including lymphadenopathy and hepatosplenomegaly with malignancy, or fever and respiratory symptoms with infection, among others.

Laboratory findings in patients with cold agglutinin disease include [30, 77]:

- Anemia: most patients with chronic cold agglutinin production have a moderate degree of anemia that is essentially ascribed to extravascular hemolysis through C3b opsonization, given the lower titers of circulating cold agglutinins that are not enough to produce frank intravascular hemolysis in the presence of normal levels of surface RBC complement inhibitors. On the other hand, patients with infection-related cold agglutinins and those with exacerbations of chronic disease due to cold exposure or other stressors can have severe forms of anemia ascribed to frank intravascular hemolysis in the presence of overwhelmingly high cold agglutinin titers capable of saturating normal complement inhibitory measures.
- Inaccurate measurement of RBC count and indices due to agglutination, resulting in underestimation of count and overestimation of volume due to clumps of RBCs passing through automated counters. Therefore, blood samples should be warmed, hand delivered to the lab and processed immediately, to avoid agglutination.
- Reticulocytosis is seen in most patients, although just as in warm AIHA, some patients may have antibodies targeting reticulocytes, or viral or drug-induced myelosuppression, resulting in reticulocytopenia.
- RBC clumping and rouleaux formation is typically seen on peripheral blood smear, while unlike warm AIHA, microspherocytosis is not typically encountered.
- Elevated LDH, low haptoglobin, hemoglobinemia, hemoglobinuria, hemosiderinuria, and hyperbilirubinemia are variably seen, especially in acute or exacerbated chronic disease.
- C3d-positive and IgG-negative DAT.
- IAT is usually positive for mono- or oligoclonal IgM reactive to polysaccharide antigens (I, i, Pr, and Others) at temperatures ranging from 0 to 5 °C.
- High titers of cold agglutinins are seen in most patients with cold AIHA, with levels ranging from 1 in 2000 to 50,000.
- Hypocomplementemia (low C3 and C4) is seen in many patients with cold agglutinin disease due to constant consumption in intravascular hemolysis.
- Hypergammaglobulinemia is seen in many patients with monoclonal gammopathy-related cold agglutinin disease.

Paroxysmal Cold Hemoglobinuria

Paroxysmal cold hemoglobinuria (PCH) is a rare form of hemolytic anemia that accounts for 1–3% of AIHA cases. Although PCH accounts for only few cases of AIHA in adults, it is a common cause of childhood AIHA, accounting for as many as 30–40% of cases in some studies [78, 79]. PCH was first described in association with secondary or tertiary syphilis but is now more commonly reported as a post-infectious complication or, more rarely, within the context of autoimmunity or malignancy.

Pathophysiology

PCH is characterized by the production of a cold-reactive polyclonal IgG autoantibody, known as Donath-Landsteiner antibody, typically directed at a very common RBC surface polysaccharide known as the P antigen. The antibody attaches to the RBC surface upon cold exposure, usually in extremities, followed by activation of C1q, then subsequent fixation of C2 and C4, but the process is typically halted until the blood attains core temperature (37 °C) again, when the antibody detaches and the remainder of the classical complement pathway cascade is completed, resulting in MAC formation and intravascular hemolysis [35, 41, 80].

Clinical Features

Most patients with PCH are children who develop symptoms within 1–2 weeks of the onset of a viral infection, most commonly with varicella, but also reported with measles, mumps, EBV, CMV, adenovirus, and influenza A. The illness is typically acute, with moderate-to-severe anemia, jaundice, dark urine (hemoglobinuria), and rarely Raynaud phenomena and/or urticaria. Symptoms usually start within a few minutes of cold exposure and start to improve soon after rewarming. Antibodies are usually persistent for up to 12 weeks, but hemolysis typically subsides within a few weeks to a month [35, 41, 80]. Alternatively, adults with PCH usually have an underlying autoimmune disorder or a lymphoid malignancy (like CLL) and display a more chronic form of the disease.

Laboratory manifestations in PCH include [35]:

- Anemia: this is usually moderate to severe in acute post-infectious PCH seen in children while mild to moderate with intermittent exacerbations in adults with more chronic forms of the disease.
- Reticulocytosis and rarely microspherocytosis.
- Elevated LDH, low haptoglobin, hemoglobinemia, hemoglobinuria, hemosiderinuria, and hyperbilirubinemia.
- Hypocomplementemia.

- C3d-positive and IgG-negative DAT (DAT may be negative depending on processing and temperature excursions).
- Positive Donath-Landsteiner antibody test, in which the patient's serum is incubated with donor RBCs and a source of complement at 4 °C, allowing for antibody attachment and early complement fixation, then warmed back to 37 °C and observed for hemolysis. This test can be challenging to perform, but its sensitivity can be improved if donor RBCs lacking surface complement inhibitors are used instead. These are usually obtained from patients with paroxysmal nocturnal hemoglobinuria (PNH).

Mixed AIHA

A mixed serologic picture with both warm and cold agglutinins is identified in ~8% of patients with AIHA. In many of these patients, the driver of hemolysis is the warm component, as the cold agglutinins are typically of low-thermal amplitude, being only reactive at low temperatures (0–20 °C) and in many instances of low titers. Nevertheless, there are case reports of true mixed AIHA with pathologic titers of both warm and high-thermal amplitude cold agglutinins. Most of these patients have an underlying autoimmune disorder [36, 41, 81].

References

1. Morgagni G, Alexander B. The seats and causes of diseases investigated by anatomy; in five books, containing a great variety of dissections, with remarks. To which are added very accurate and copious indexes of the principal things and names therein contained. London: Printed for A. Millar, and T. Cadell; 1769.
2. Freedman J. Autoimmune hemolysis: a journey through time. Transfus Med Hemother. 2015;42(5):278–85.
3. Andral G. Essai d'hématologie pathologique. Paris: Fortin, Masson et Cie; 1843.
4. Major RH. Classic descriptions of disease. Springfield, IL: C. C. Thomas; 1939.
5. Vanlair C, Masius J. De la microcythémia. Bull Acad R Med Belg. 1871;5:515–612.
6. Mackenzie S. Paroxysmal haemoglobinuria, with remarks on its nature. Lancet. 1879;II:116–7.
7. Minkowski O. Ueber eine hereditäre, unter dem Bilde eines chronischen Icterus mit Urobilinurie, Splenomegalie und Nierensiderosis verlaufende Affection. Verh Krong Inn Med. 1900;1(18):316–21.
8. Hayem G. Sur une variete particuliere d'ictere chronique. Ictere infectieux chronique splenomegalique. Presse Méd. 1898;1(6):121–5.
9. Landsteiner K. Zur Kentniss der antifermentativen, lytischen und agglutinierenden Wirkungen des Blutserums und der Lymphe. Zbl Bakt. 1900;1(27):357–62.
10. Donath JLK. Über paroxysmale Hämoglobinurie. Münch Med Wochenschr. 1904;1(51):1590–5.
11. Chauffard M. Pathogénie de l'ictère congenital de l'adulte. Semaine Med. 1907;1(27):25–9.
12. Chauffard M, Troissier J. Anémie grave avec hémolysinique dans le sérum; ictère hémolysiniqe. Semaine Med. 1908;1(28):345.

13. Chauffard M, Vincent C. Hémoglobinurie hémolysinique avec ictère polycholique aigu. Semaine Med. 1909;1(29):601–4.
14. Micheli F. Unmittelbare Effekte der Splenektomie bei einem Fall von erworbenem hämolytischen splenomegalischen Ikterus Typus Hayem-Widal (spleno-hämolytischer Ikterus). Wien Klin Wochenschr. 1911;1(24):1269–74.
15. Banti G. La esplanomegalia hemolitica. Semaine Med. 1912;1(32):265–8.
16. Witts LJ. The paroxysmal haemoglobinurias. Lancet. 1936;II:115–20.
17. Dameshek W, Schwartz SO. The presence of hemolysins in acute hemolytic anemia. New Engl J Med. 1938;218:75–80.
18. Weiner AS. A new test (blocking test) for Rh sensitization. Proc Soc Exp Biol NY. 1944;56(2):173–6.
19. Race RR. An 'incomplete' antibody in human serum. Nature. 1944;153(3895):771–2.
20. Coombs RR, Mourant AE, Race RR. A new test for the detection of weak and incomplete Rh agglutinins. Br J Exp Pathol. 1945;26:255–66.
21. Evans RS, Duane RT. Acquired hemolytic anemia; the relation of erythrocyte antibody production to activity of the disease; the significance of thrombocytopenia and leukopenia. Blood. 1949;4(11):1196–213.
22. Iafusco F, Buffa V. Autoimmune hemolytic anemia in a newborn infant. Pediatria. 1962;70:1256–64.
23. Pirofsky B. The hemolytic anemias—historical review and classification. The hemolytic anemias—historical review and classification. 1. Baltimore, MA: Williams & Wilkins; 1969. p. 3–21.
24. Schubothe H. Current problems of chronic cold hemagglutinin disease. Annals NY Acad Sci. 1965;124(2):484–90.
25. Dacie JV. Aetiology of the auto-immune haemolytic anaemias. Haematologia. 1971;5(4):351–7.
26. Rosse WF. The autinglobulin test in autoimmune hemolytic anemia. Annu Rev Med. 1975;26:331–6.
27. Schreiber AD, Frank MM. Role of antibody and complement in the immune clearance and destruction of erythrocytes. I. In vivo effects of IgG and IgM complement-fixing sites. J Clin Invest. 1972;51(3):575–82.
28. Engelfriet CP, Borne AE, Beckers D, Van Loghem JJ. Autoimmune haemolytic anaemia: serological and immunochemical characteristics of the autoantibodies; mechanisms of cell destruction. Ser Haematol. 1974;7(3):328–47.
29. von dem Borne AE, Beckers D, Engelfriet CP. Mechanisms of red cell destruction mediated by non-complement binding IgG antibodies: the essential role in vivo of the Fc part of IgG. Br J Haematol. 1977;36(4):485–93.
30. Berentsen S, Randen U, Tjonnfjord GE. Cold agglutinin-mediated autoimmune hemolytic anemia. Hematol Oncol Clin North Am. 2015;29(3):455–71.
31. Engelfriet CP, Overbeeke MA, von dem Borne AE. Autoimmune hemolytic anemia. Semin Hematol. 1992;29(1):3–12.
32. Naik R. Warm autoimmune hemolytic anemia. Hematol Oncol Clin North Am. 2015;29(3):445–53.
33. Quist E, Koepsell S. Autoimmune hemolytic anemia and red blood cell autoantibodies. Arch Pathol Lab Med. 2015 Nov;139(11):1455–8.
34. Segel GB, Lichtman MA. Direct antiglobulin ("Coombs") test-negative autoimmune hemolytic anemia: a review. Blood Cells Mol Dis. 2014;52(4):152–60.
35. Shanbhag S, Spivak J. Paroxysmal cold hemoglobinuria. Hematol Oncol Clin North Am. 2015;29(3):473–8.
36. Shulman IA, Branch DR, Nelson JM, Thompson JC, Saxena S, Petz LD. Autoimmune hemolytic anemia with both cold and warm autoantibodies. Jama. 1985;253(12):1746–8.
37. Kaplan M, Hammerman C, Vreman HJ, Wong RJ, Stevenson DK. Direct antiglobulin titer strength and hyperbilirubinemia. Pediatrics. 2014;134(5):e1340–4.

38. Zantek ND, Koepsell SA, Tharp DR Jr, Cohn CS. The direct antiglobulin test: a critical step in the evaluation of hemolysis. Am J Hcmatol. 2012;87(7):707–9.
39. Habibi B, Homberg JC, Schaison G, Salmon C. Autoimmune hemolytic anemia in children. A review of 80 cases. Am J Med. 1974;56(1):61–9.
40. Barker RN, Hall AM, Standen GR, Jones J, Elson CJ. Identification of T-cell epitopes on the rhesus polypeptides in autoimmune hemolytic anemia. Blood. 1997;90(7):2701–15.
41. Liebman HA, Weitz IC. Autoimmune hemolytic anemia. Med Clin North Am. 2017;101(2):351–9.
42. Petz LD, Fudenberg HH. Coombs-positive hemolytic anemia caused by penicillin administration. N Engl J Med. 1966;274(4):171–8.
43. Garratty G. Drug-induced immune hemolytic anemia. Hematology/the Education Program of the American Society of Hematology American Society of Hematology Education Program. 2009;73–9.
44. Ahmad E, Elgohary T, Ibrahim H. Naturally occurring regulatory T cells and interleukins 10 and 12 in the pathogenesis of idiopathic warm autoimmune hemolytic anemia. J Investig Allergol Clin Immunol. 2011;21(4):297–304.
45. Visco C, Barcellini W, Maura F, Neri A, Cortelezzi A, Rodeghiero F. Autoimmune cytopenias in chronic lymphocytic leukemia. Am J Hematol. 2014;89(11):1055–62.
46. De Angelis V, Biasinutto C, Pradella P, Vaccher E, Spina M, Tirelli U. Clinical significance of positive direct antiglobulin test in patients with HIV infection. Infection. 1994;22(2):92–5.
47. Rosse WF. Fixation of the first component of complement (C'la) by human antibodies. J Clin Invest. 1969;47(11):2430–45.
48. Ravetch JV. Fc receptors. Curr Opin Immunol. 1997;9(1):121–5.
49. Schur PH. IgG subclasses—a review. Ann Allergy. 1987;58(2):89–96.
50. Garratty G, Arndt P, Domen R, Clarke A, Sutphen-Shaw D, Clear J, et al. Severe autoimmune hemolytic anemia associated with IgM warm autoantibodies directed against determinants on or associated with glycophorin A. Vox Sang. 1997;72(2):124–30.
51. Sachs UJ, Roder L, Santoso S, Bein G. Does a negative direct antiglobulin test exclude warm autoimmune haemolytic anaemia? A prospective study of 504 cases. Br J Haematol. 2006;132(5):655–6.
52. Lau P, Haesler WE, Wurzel HA. Positive direct antiglobulin reaction in a patient population. Am J Clin Pathol. 1976;65(3):368–75.
53. Keeling DM, Isenberg DA. Haematological manifestations of systemic lupus erythematosus. Blood Rev. 1993;7(4):199–207.
54. Jeffries M, Hamadeh F, Aberle T, Glenn S, Kamen DL, Kelly JA, et al. Haemolytic anaemia in a multi-ethnic cohort of lupus patients: a clinical and serological perspective. Lupus. 2008;17(8):739–43.
55. Iordache L, Launay O, Bouchaud O, Jeantils V, Goujard C, Boue F, et al. Autoimmune diseases in HIV-infected patients: 52 cases and literature review. Autoimmun Rev. 2014;13(8):850–7.
56. Toy PT, Reid ME, Burns M. Positive direct antiglobulin test associated with hyperglobulinemia in acquired immunodeficiency syndrome (AIDS). Am J Hematol. 1985;19(2):145–50.
57. Wang J, Cunningham-Rundles C. Treatment and outcome of autoimmune hematologic disease in common variable immunodeficiency (CVID). J Autoimmun. 2005;25(1):57–62.
58. Neven B, Magerus-Chatinet A, Florkin B, Gobert D, Lambotte O, De Somer L, et al. A survey of 90 patients with autoimmune lymphoproliferative syndrome related to TNFRSF6 mutation. Blood. 2011;118(18):4798–807.
59. Hamblin TJ, Oscier DG, Young BJ. Autoimmunity in chronic lymphocytic leukaemia. J Clin Pathol. 1986;39(7):713–6.
60. Diehl LF, Ketchum LH. Autoimmune disease and chronic lymphocytic leukemia: autoimmune hemolytic anemia, pure red cell aplasia, and autoimmune thrombocytopenia. Semin Oncol. 1998;25(1):80–97.
61. Garratty G, Arndt PA. An update on drug-induced immune hemolytic anemia. Immunohematology. 2007;23(3):105–19.

62. LoBuglio AF, Jandl JH. The nature of the alpha-methyldopa red-cell antibody. N Engl J Med. 1967;276(12):658–65.
63. Worlledge SM, Carstairs KC, Dacie JV. Autoimmune haemolytic anaemia associated with alpha-methyldopa therapy. Lancet. 1966;2(7455):135–9.
64. Salama A, Santoso S, Mueller-Eckhardt C. Antigenic determinants responsible for the reactions of drug-dependent antibodies with blood cells. Br J Haematol. 1991;78(4):535–9.
65. Salama A, Mueller-Eckhardt C. On the mechanisms of sensitization and attachment of antibodies to RBC in drug-induced immune hemolytic anemia. Blood. 1987;69(4):1006–10.
66. Liesveld JL, Rowe JM, Lichtman MA. Variability of the erythropoietic response in autoimmune hemolytic anemia: analysis of 109 cases. Blood. 1987;69(3):820–6.
67. Dobryszycka W. Biological functions of haptoglobin—new pieces to an old puzzle. Eur J Clin Chem Clin Biochem. 1997;35(9):647–54.
68. Shih AW, McFarlane A, Verhovsek M. Haptoglobin testing in hemolysis: measurement and interpretation. Am J Hematol. 2014;89(4):443–7.
69. Marchand A, Galen RS, Van Lente F. The predictive value of serum haptoglobin in hemolytic disease. JAMA. 1980;243(19):1909–11.
70. Pollack W, Hager HJ, Reckel R, Toren DA, Singher H. A study of the forces involved in the second stage of Hemagglutination. Transfusion. 1965;5:158–83.
71. Kirschfink M, Knoblauch K, Roelcke D. Activation of complement by cold agglutinins. Infusionsther Transfusionsmed. 1994;21(6):405–9.
72. Jenkins WJ, Marsh WL, Noades J, Tippett P, Sanger R, Race RR. The I antigen and antibody. Vox Sang. 1960;5:97–121.
73. Marsh WL. Anti-i: a cold antibody defining the Ii relationship in human red cells. Br J Haematol. 1961;7:200–9.
74. Feizi T. Monotypic cold agglutinins in infection by mycoplasma pneumoniae. Nature. 1967;215(5100):540–2.
75. Deaton JG, Skaggs H Jr, Levin WC. Acute hemolytic anemia complicating infectious mononucleosis: the mechanism of hemolysis. Tex Rep Biol Med. 1967;25(3):309–17.
76. Rollof J, Eklund PO. Infectious mononucleosis complicated by severe immune hemolysis. Eur J Haematol. 1989;43(1):81–2.
77. Swiecicki PL, Hegerova LT, Gertz MA. Cold agglutinin disease. Blood. 2013;122(7):1114–21.
78. Sokol RJ, Hewitt S, Stamps BK, Hitchen PA. Autoimmune haemolysis in childhood and adolescence. Acta Haematol. 1984;72(4):245–57.
79. Gottsche B, Salama A, Mueller-Eckhardt C. Donath-Landsteiner autoimmune hemolytic anemia in children. A study of 22 cases. Vox Sang. 1990;58(4):281–6.
80. Heddle NM. Acute paroxysmal cold hemoglobinuria. Transfus Med Rev. 1989;3(3):219–29.
81. Qiao L, Chen J, Leng XM, Zhang W, Han B, Zhao Y, et al. Agranulocytosis and mixed-type autoimmune hemolytic anemia in primary sjogren's syndrome: a case report and review of the literature. Int J Rheum Dis. 2016;19(12):1351–3.

Chapter 6
Treatment of Autoimmune Hemolytic Anemia

Omar Niss and Russell E. Ware

Introduction

Autoimmune hemolytic anemia (AIHA) is a rare disorder that features red blood cell (RBC) destruction caused by self-recognizing immunoglobulin molecules (autoantibodies) directed against endogenous RBC antigens. AIHA is a rare condition, with an estimated incidence of 0.8–3 cases/100,000 adults annually and only 0.2–0.4 cases/100,000 per year for infants and children. It is a serious and often life-threatening disorder, however, with a mortality that reaches up to 11% in adults [1, 2].

Diagnosis and Classification

AIHA is most commonly diagnosed in the setting of characteristic laboratory features of hemolytic anemia (decreased hemoglobin concentration, reticulocytosis, indirect hyperbilirubinemia, elevated serum lactate dehydrogenase, low haptoglobin levels, and hemoglobinuria) plus the presence of anti-RBC antibodies that are detected by a positive direct antiglobulin test (DAT). AIHA can be classified in several ways, but the immunoglobulin class and optimal thermal binding of the autoantibodies provide a useful mechanistic description: warm AIHA, cold agglutinin disease (CAD), paroxysmal cold hemoglobinuria (PCH), and mixed forms (see Chapter on Pathophysiology, for further details).

O. Niss, MD · R. E. Ware, MD, PhD (✉)
Division of Hematology, Department of Pediatrics, Cincinnati Children's Hospital Medical Center and University of Cincinnati College of Medicine, Cincinnati, OH, USA
e-mail: russell.ware@cchmc.org

© Springer International Publishing AG, part of Springer Nature 2018   103
J. M. Despotovic (ed.), *Immune Hematology*,
https://doi.org/10.1007/978-3-319-73269-5_6

When the classical signs of hemolytic anemia are absent or difficult to interpret, and especially when the DAT is weakly positive or even negative, the diagnosis of AIHA can be challenging and often delayed. Reticulocytosis can be absent in 20% of adult cases and up to 39% of pediatric cases, especially early in the disease or when the autoantibodies also attack erythroid progenitors [3, 4]. The DAT can be negative in up to 10% of AIHA due to several possible mechanisms. First, the number of RBC-bound antibodies may be below the level of detection using visual agglutination; second, the causative autoantibodies may be "warm-reacting" IgM or IgA antibodies that are not detected by conventional anti-IgG reagents; and third, the RBC-bound antibodies may be lost during the DAT procedure due to low-affinity binding [5, 6]. If the suspicion for AIHA is high despite a negative DAT, alternative and enhanced DAT assays can be performed in reference laboratories in order to overcome the technical limitations of routine DAT testing, including the use of low ionic strength washing solutions, anti-IgA antisera, and more sensitive flow-based DAT assays [7]. Patients with "DAT-negative" AIHA appear to have a more severe course and higher mortality; [4] however, it is not clear if this is due to a delay in establishing the correct diagnosis and starting therapy or due to inherent characteristics of these cases.

Etiology

AIHA is idiopathic or primary in ~50% of adult and ~30% of pediatric cases. Lymphoproliferative diseases, autoimmune diseases, and malignancies are the most common causes of secondary AIHA in adults, while infections, autoimmune disorders, and immune dysregulation disorders are the most common underlying causes in pediatrics [1, 8]. As more disorders of immune dysregulation are recognized and explained at the genetic level, the proportion of secondary AIHA is expanding, especially in young patients and those with multilineage cytopenias such as Evans syndrome. Table 6.1 summarizes the most common causes of secondary AIHA, based on the characteristics of the autoantibodies and age of the patient.

A thorough personal and family history, coupled with a careful physical examination, should guide the investigations for an underlying cause of AIHA. Early identification of these secondary forms is prudent because secondary AIHA is frequently difficult to treat without treating the underlying cause. Drug-induced immune hemolytic anemia should also be considered early, since stopping exposure to the offending agent is often sufficient to ameliorate the problem [9, 10].

As discussed in detail in the previous chapter, several mechanisms involving multiple arms of the immune system are involved in the pathogenesis of AIHA, including autoantibody formation, autoreactive B and T lymphocytes, complement

Table 6.1 Causes of secondary autoimmune hemolytic anemia

Type of AIHA	Children	Adults
Warm AIHA	• Evans syndrome[a] • Infections[b] (EBV, parvovirus, mycoplasma, CMV) • Primary immune deficiencies and/or immune dysregulation syndromes (CVID, ALPS, DiGeorge syndrome, CTLA-4, LRBA, IPEX, STAT3-GOF, STAT1-GOF, WAS, CID, posttransplant) • Autoimmune diseases (SLE, hepatitis, thyroiditis, APS) • Infantile giant cell hepatitis	• Malignancies (CLL, NHL, HL) • Autoimmune disease (SLE, IBD, RA, APS) • Infections (hepatitis C, HIV, CMV, tuberculosis) • Primary immune deficiencies (CVID, ALPS)
Cold agglutinin disease	• Infections (mycoplasma, viral infections including EBV) • Posttransplantation	• MGUS • Lymphoproliferative disease • Macroglobulinemia • CLL • Solid tumors • Autoimmune disease • Posttransplant
Paroxysmal cold hemoglobinuria	• Infections (adenovirus, influenza A, syphilis, CMV, EBV, VZV, measles, mumps, mycoplasma, *E. coli*)	

The causes of AIHA in each category are listed in order of frequency
EBV Ebstein-Barr virus, *CMV* cytomegalovirus, *CVID* common variable immune deficiency, *ALPS* autoimmune lymphoproliferative syndrome, *CTLA-4* cytotoxic T-lymphocyte-associated protein 4 haploinsufficiency, *LRBA* lipopolysaccharide-responsive and beige-like anchor protein deficiency, *IPEX* immunodysregulation polyendocrinopathy enteropathy X-linked, *GOF* gain-of-function mutations, *WAS* Wiskott-Aldrich syndrome, *CID* combined immune deficiency, *SLE* systemic lupus erythematosus, *APS* antiphospholipid syndrome, *CLL* chronic lymphocytic leukemia, *NHL* non-Hodgkin lymphoma, *HL* Hodgkin lymphoma, *IBD* inflammatory bowel disease, *RA* rheumatoid arthritis, *MGUS* monoclonal gammopathy of undetermined significance
[a]The diagnosis of Evans syndrome may overlap with autoimmune diseases and primary immune deficiencies—see Chap. 7 for further details regarding Evans syndrome
[b]Infections can be a cause of AIHA by itself or a trigger for AIHA in other settings (e.g., autoimmune disease)

activation, macrophages, NK cells, regulatory T cells, and abnormal cytokines [11]. The contribution of each of these cells and mechanisms to AIHA underlies the heterogeneity in disease presentation, severity, and responses to treatment (Fig. 6.1). Further understanding of the specific mechanisms underlying different forms of AIHA in different patients may lead to "targeted" treatment approaches that are more precise and effective, while also being less toxic. Treatment of AIHA to date is mostly based on historical experience and a very limited number of randomized studies. The treatment of AIHA is guided by the type of AIHA and the acuity of presentation, rather than solid clinical evidence.

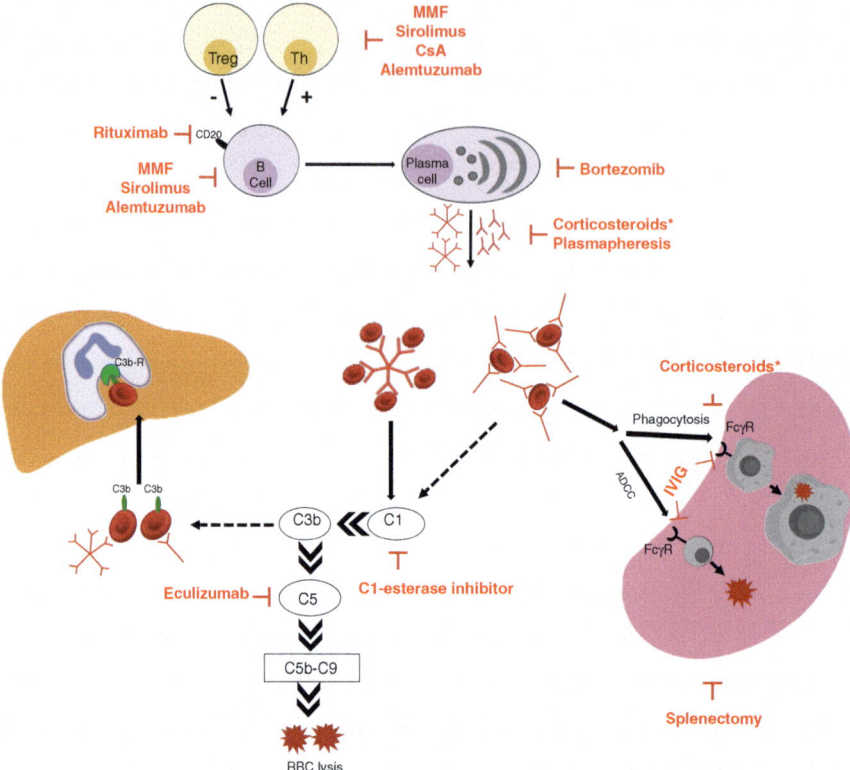

Fig. 6.1 Mechanisms and sites of action of AIHA therapies. Several immunosuppressive medications including MMF, sirolimus, and alemtuzumab inhibit both T and B lymphocytes. T cells regulate self-tolerance of B lymphocytes positively (helper T cells: Th1, Th2, and Th17) and negatively (regulatory T cells). Rituximab is a monoclonal antibody directed against CD20 that is expressed on immature, mature, and memory B cells but not on plasma cells. The proteasome inhibitor, bortezomib, preferentially targets the antibody-producing plasma cells. Antibodies can be temporarily removed from the circulation by plasmapheresis. IgG-coated erythrocytes in warm AIHA are destroyed primarily in the spleen by antibody-dependent cell-mediated cytotoxicity (ADCC) mediated by cytotoxic T cells and natural killer cells expressing receptors for the Fc portion of IgG, or phagocytosed by splenic macrophages carrying Fcγ receptors (FcγR). Corticosteroids decrease antibody production and inhibit extravascular hemolysis by inhibiting FcγR expression on splenic macrophages*, while IVIG directly blocks the uptake of antibody-coated red cells by FcγR. In cold AIHA, the pentameric IgM autoantibody has the ability to bind C1 and activate the complement system, culminating in the formation of the membrane attack complex (C5b-C9) causing intravascular hemolysis. A portion of the C3b-bound erythrocytes are also sequestered and destroyed in the liver. The complement system can also be activated by IgG molecules that have high affinity to complement or by high concentrations of IgG. Anticomplement agents, eculizumab and C1-esterase inhibitor, directly inhibit the complement cascade and decrease intravascular hemolysis in some cases of AIHA. *Corticosteroids exert their effect by different mechanisms that are not completely understood; only the main mechanisms are highlighted in this figure. Abbreviations: *ADCC* antibody-dependent cell-mediated cytotoxicity, *C3b-R* C3b receptor, *CsA* cyclosporin A, *FcγR* Fcγ receptor, *IVIG* intravenous immunoglobulins, *MMF* mycophenolate mofetil, *Th* helper T lymphocytes, *Treg* regulatory T lymphocytes

Frontline Treatment

The proper treatment of AIHA depends on the type of autoantibody, the clinical severity, additional or underlying conditions, and the age of the patient. Warm AIHA is the most common form and has a prolonged relapsing course in both children and adults. In the acute setting with a severe clinical presentation, blood transfusions should be utilized as a life-saving intervention, but are not generally recommended as an ongoing treatment option. Corticosteroids are the traditional first line of therapy for patients with warm AIHA.

Blood Transfusions

The onset of warm AIHA is typically abrupt and acute. Although most adult patients require inpatient management in the acute phase, some pediatric patients can be managed in the outpatient setting if their symptoms and anemia are not severe. The decision for blood transfusion is guided by the acuity of presentation and the presence of cardiovascular compromise or medical comorbidities, rather than the hemoglobin concentration alone. Because warm autoantibodies in AIHA are directed against RBC surface antigens and are usually pan-reactive, fully cross-matched blood is often not possible. However, transfusions should not be withheld from patients with severe, life-threatening anemia or those with severe hemolysis and a rapidly evolving presentation [12]. Transfusions can be life-saving for severe AIHA, and fear of transfusing incompatible erythrocytes should not prevent the procedure. Early communication between clinicians and the transfusion service is essential to minimize any delay in blood transfusion and to identify the optimal units of blood for transfusion.

Alloantibodies can form after exposure to transfused blood, but are masked by the presence of warm autoantibodies. Alloantibodies that complicate transfusions have been reported in 32% of AIHA, causing worsening hemolysis [13]. In urgent cases and when the presence of alloantibodies is unlikely (no history of prior transfusions, pregnancy, or organ transplantation), any ABO and RhD-compatible packed RBC unit can be administered safely [2]. In less emergent cases, ruling out the presence of alloantibodies by warm autoadsorption or allogeneic adsorption techniques, or when possible, transfusing phenotypically matched PRBCs, is advisable in order to minimize the risk of worsening hemolysis after transfusions [14].

When transfusion is given, packed RBC units should be leukocyte-depleted to decrease the risk of febrile reactions that result from anti-leukocyte antibodies. Blood should be transfused relatively slowly and the transfused volume is limited to the goal of ameliorating life-threatening anemia, manifested by neurological compromise or cardiovascular collapse, and not necessarily achieving a normal hemoglobin concentration [2]. Over-transfusing can be associated with increased hemolysis due to an increased RBC mass, which can be mistaken for alloimmunization. Some authors suggest "in vivo compatibility test" by infusing a small volume of 20 mL of packed RBC, followed by 20 min of observation for reactions before proceeding with the rest of the transfusion [8].

Corticosteroids

Despite the lack of systematic studies, there is general consensus that corticosteroids are the most effective "first-line" therapy for patients with warm AIHA. For severe clinical presentations, IV methylprednisolone should be administered at 1–4 mg/kg/day, divided every 6–8 h. Transitioning to oral prednisone or prednisolone is then accomplished at 1–2 mg/kg/day, usually divided into two or three doses, which is maintained for 2–3 weeks until a hemoglobin concentration of at least 10–11 g/dL is achieved without transfusion support. Additional labs should show a reduced reticulocytosis, but the DAT may still be positive. Higher doses of steroids, up to 1000 mg of methylprednisolone daily or 30 mg/kg/day in pediatrics for 3 days, have been used in several adult and pediatric case series, typically in the acute setting [1, 15]. For less severe clinical presentations, oral corticosteroids can be the initial treatment choice.

If a stable hemoglobin concentration can be maintained without transfusions, the oral corticosteroids can be tapered fairly rapidly in the first 1–2 months, aiming for a single daily dosing regimen that maintains stable counts followed by a slower tapering over several months. Despite high rates of initial response to steroids approaching 80% historically, relapse is very common during steroid tapering [4]. In a recent randomized trial ($N = 64$), 50% of newly diagnosed adults with AIHA treated with prednisolone alone achieved complete or partial response at 3 months, while only 36% remained in remission at 12 months [16]. A short duration of maintenance dosing and rapid tapering of corticosteroids are associated with increased risk of relapse, while the risk of recurrence is lower in patients receiving corticosteroids for longer than 6 months [17]. Therefore, subsequent tapering of corticosteroid dose after the first 1–2 months should occur more slowly over the following 4–6 months with close monitoring of hemoglobin concentration and reticulocyte count. Discontinuation of steroids should only be considered in patients who are stable on a low dose ($\leq$10 mg/day) after at least 4 months of corticosteroid treatment, and the final taper should be extended over at least 1–2 months.

Although there is no consensus on the definition of treatment responses among various studies, patients who fail to achieve any improvement in hemoglobin concentration after 3 weeks of corticosteroids or cannot discontinue transfusion support are generally considered refractory. Diagnostic reevaluation and additional therapies should be considered in these patients. In addition, patients who need high doses of corticosteroids to maintain remission or do not tolerate corticosteroids should be considered candidates for second-line treatment options due to the concerns about long-term medication effects, especially on growth and bone health. Among patients who respond to initial therapy, only ~50% of patients can be maintained in remission on an "acceptable" dose of steroid, defined as a prednisone dose <15 mg/day in adults or <0.1–0.2 mg/kg/day in pediatrics [8].

Second-Line Treatments

The decision to proceed to a second-line therapy for AIHA is determined by the balance between steroid efficacy and side effects. For patients who require high doses of steroids, experience significant side effects irrespective of the dose, or suffer frequent relapses requiring multiple dose escalations, a steroid-sparing strategy is needed. The two second-line therapies with proven short-term benefit are the anti-CD20 monoclonal antibody rituximab and splenectomy. There is controversy on the best order of these two therapies, with splenectomy used first for adults while rituximab is generally preferred before splenectomy in most pediatric centers [15]. Recently, promising results have also been achieved with the immunosuppressive medications mycophenolate mofetil (MMF) and sirolimus, which has prompted their addition to the list of second-line therapies.

Rituximab

This chimeric monoclonal antibody, developed for treatment of B-lymphocyte malignancies with specificity against the CD20 B-cell surface marker, is the preferred second-line therapy for children with AIHA, although this is not an FDA-approved clinical indication [1, 15]. Younger age and warm-type AIHA are the factors most predictive of response to rituximab [18]. Treatment is administered intravenously as per standard oncological indications, which is 375 mg/m^2 for four weekly doses. The overall short-term response rate with rituximab, based on the available small retrospective studies, ranges between 64 and 100%, with a complete response rate of 27–73% [19]. The median response duration is ~1 year, and 30% may have a sustained response up to 3 years; however, durable long-term responses are not confirmed [20]. In one of the few available phase III randomized trials in AIHA, the combination of rituximab and prednisolone was compared to prednisolone alone as a frontline therapy in adults with primary AIHA [16]. The combination therapy was associated with a higher rate of remission at 36 months compared to steroids alone (70% vs. 45%) without increased toxicity [16]. The time to response after rituximab is variable and ranges from a median of 1 month to several months in some patients [20]. A four-dose course of rituximab may be repeated in cases of relapse with good success. Although rituximab is an effective treatment for both primary and secondary warm AIHA, [2] the immunological background of the patient should be taken into consideration, as rituximab should be used with caution in primary immune deficiencies (discussed further below). Rituximab is generally well-tolerated with the exception of a few mild infusion-related side effects and rarely more severe anaphylactoid reactions [21]. Infectious complications following rituximab can occur in ~5% of patients, including hepatitis B reactivation and a rare progressive multifocal encephalopathy in immune-compromised patients. These encouraging data with rituximab have led some adult centers to adopt rituximab as the second-line therapy of choice, instead of the traditional splenectomy [4, 19]. In a recent study, a smaller dose of rituximab (100 mg/m²/dose weekly×4) had a similar efficacy rate to the standard dose; however, the relapse rate after low-dose rituximab was higher [22].

Splenectomy

Surgical total splenectomy has long been the main second-line therapy for AIHA in adults, after corticosteroids. Although splenectomy and rituximab have never been compared head to head, they both appear to have similar short-term efficacy rates [2]. Splenectomy is effective in ~67% of patients with primary warm AIHA, with an estimated cure rate of ~20% [2, 23]. Even those who do not have a complete response to splenectomy have decreased steroid requirements after splenectomy [8]. Unlike rituximab, splenectomy is less effective in secondary warm AIHA compared to primary cases (response rate of 19% compared to 82%) [24]. In patients with secondary AIHA or in patients with underlying medical conditions who are not candidates for splenectomy, rituximab may be the better option.

Although the complications of splenectomy have diminished over the years, some risks should be regarded when splenectomy is considered. Surgical advances and laparoscopic techniques have led to a reduction in perioperative complications, but the most feared complication remains the risk of postsplenectomy sepsis by encapsulated bacteria. Patients undergoing splenectomy should be vaccinated, prior to surgery, against encapsulated organisms like *S. pneumoniae* according to the recommended guidelines [25]. Splenectomy should be delayed in children younger than 5 years whenever possible, to allow development of the immune repertoire. Children who undergo splenectomy should receive postoperative antibiotic prophylaxis, typically penicillin, and should be instructed to seek immediate medical evaluation if they develop fever. The role of antibiotic prophylaxis in adults postsplenectomy is debatable, but our experience includes a case of fatal sepsis several decades after splenectomy. Patients with an underlying immune deficiency are at particularly high risk for postsplenectomy sepsis and death [26]. Therefore, an underlying immune disorder leading to secondary AIHA should be excluded before considering splenectomy. Finally, there is an increased risk of postsplenectomy thrombosis and a small risk of late-onset pulmonary hypertension, mainly in adults. The role of thromboprophylaxis in this setting is unclear; most adults who undergo splenectomy receive thromboprophylaxis postoperatively, while some receive it beyond hospital discharge [2].

Immunosuppressive Therapies

Although splenectomy and rituximab are the only established second-line therapies for warm AIHA, several immunosuppressive agents have been used with variable responses, especially before rituximab became available. Recently, MMF and sirolimus have emerged as possible steroid-sparing agents with promising results. MMF inhibits de novo purine synthesis by selectively inhibiting inosine monophosphate dehydrogenase present in proliferating T and B lymphocytes. MMF was initially developed as an antirejection medication but has also been useful in treating refractory cytopenias in children with autoimmune lymphoproliferative syndrome (ALPS) [27]. The effectiveness of MMF for AIHA is not fully elucidated, but the majority of treated adult and pediatric patients had refractory AIHA with heavy pretreatment including splenectomy, yet had a complete or good partial response [28–30]. MMF is generally well-tolerated but its long-term effects are not known. Although these encouraging results are based mostly on small observational studies, MMF is moving toward the front line in pediatric AIHA as a steroid-sparing agent and has also been included in the treatment arsenal for refractory AIHA in adults [1, 2, 29].

Sirolimus is a mammalian target of rapamycin (mTOR) inhibitor that inhibits cell proliferation and enhances apoptosis. Early case reports suggested a role for sirolimus in the treatment of immune cytopenia in posttransplant patients [31, 32]. In children, sirolimus can be an effective therapy even for refractory immune cytopenia, with complete response achieved in 75–100% of patients, including those who failed MMF [30, 33]. ALPS-related cytopenias also respond to sirolimus; however, sirolimus use has now been expanded to other cases of refractory primary and secondary cytopenia with comparable responses [34, 35]. Sirolimus is also well-tolerated with no reported infectious or metabolic complications in small studies, but its long-term side effects have not been determined. The most common reported side effect of sirolimus is mild stomatitis that resolves without intervention [34]. However, sirolimus is known to alter lipid metabolism so may have a different safety profile when other populations are treated, including older individuals with lipid abnormalities.

It is important to note that both MMF and sirolimus typically have a delayed response. Therefore, their use should be overlapped with a tapering course of corticosteroids over several weeks to months for initial control, until the desired blood levels (1–3.5 µg/mL for MMF and 4–12 ng/mL for sirolimus) and clinical effects of these medications are reached [1]. MMF and sirolimus can also serve as maintenance therapy after a rituximab response, to reduce the need for repeated rituximab dosing.

The available published evidence on these therapies in AIHA is limited which prompts cautious interpretation of these results and reduces the strength of the recommendations. Until stronger evidence is generated from larger studies and different second-line therapies are compared directly, the choice of a second-line treatment option is usually determined by the physician/institutional experience, patient preference, and an individualized benefit/risk balance in each patient. A treatment algorithm for warm AIHA is shown in Fig. 6.2.

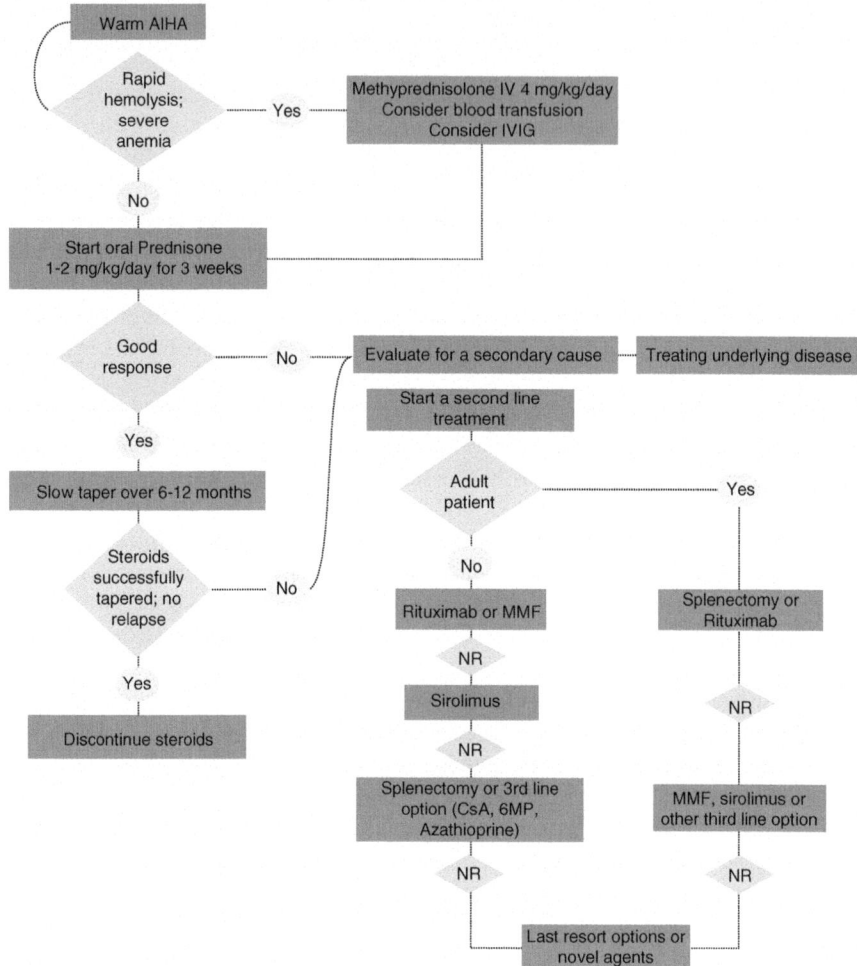

Fig. 6.2 Treatment algorithm for warm AIHA. *NR* no response, *IVIG* intravenous Immunoglobulin, *MMF* mycophenolate mofetil, *CsA* cyclosporin A, *6-MP* 6-mercaptopurine

Additional Treatment Options

The optimal treatment of AIHA in patients with severe or refractory disease, who fail to respond to the conventional therapies mentioned, is not known. Several agents have been used over the years with variable efficacy and toxicity results. Here, we present a brief overview of additional agents that have been used for the treatment of warm AIHA and their potential role.

Acute Temporizing Therapy

IVIG is much less effective for the treatment of AIHA than immune thrombocyto-penia (ITP). At best, IVIG is associated with a 40% short-term response rate in adults and up to 55% in children with AIHA [36]. IVIG use in AIHA is usually reserved for severe cases as a complementary agent or when ITP is present concur-rently with AIHA (see Chap. 7 for discussion of Evans syndrome). Plasmapheresis has been reported for a small number of severe cases as a temporizing measure dur-ing acute hemolysis, but with variable results [2]. Plasmapheresis is less effective in warm AIHA compared to cold AIHA, presumably because IgG-mediated hemolysis occurs outside of the intravascular space, and is therefore generally reserved for patients who fail several other therapies.

Third-Line Therapies

In the era before rituximab became available, several other immunosuppressive agents have been reported for refractory AIHA including azathioprine, cyclo-phosphamide, cyclosporin A, vincristine, and 6-mercaptopurine [2, 8, 15]. However, because of their limited effectiveness (<30% response rate) and much higher risk profile, these agents are now generally reserved for severe and life-threatening cases. Cyclosporin A has better results in combination with cortico-steroids or other immunosuppressive agents. Danazol, a synthetic anabolic steroid with mild androgenic effects, also can be used in combination with steroids, but its utility in the modern era is limited since more effective alternatives have become available [37].

"Last-Resort" Options

The humanized anti-CD52 antibody, alemtuzumab, which targets B and T lym-phocytes, has some effect in refractory AIHA cases in children and adults [23]. Also, high-dose cyclophosphamide (50 mg/kg/day for 4 days) has been used in refractory cases [38]. However, these therapies are reserved as last options because of their high toxicity. Very few data exist about the role of hematopoietic stem cell transplantation in AIHA, and it should probably be considered the last option for severe refractory cases. The overall complete remission rate is 50–60%, but with remission maintained in only 1/7 and 3/7 patients who underwent autolo-gous and allogeneic transplantation, respectively, with a transplant-related mortality of 15% [39, 40].

Emerging Novel Therapies

Recently the proteasome inhibitor, bortezomib, which targets the long-lived plasma cells that are not targeted by rituximab, has shown promise for treating refractory cytopenias in posttransplant patients who previously failed multiple therapies [41]. Additional novel alternative B-lymphocyte therapies include ofatumumab, a fully human monoclonal anti-CD20 antibody that has a superior complement-mediated cytotoxicity compared to rituximab. Ofatumumab was effective in treating two cases of warm AIHA associated with CLL and systemic lupus erythematosus that were refractory to multiple therapies including rituximab [42, 43]. Finally, the anti-C5 terminal complement inhibitor eculizumab was used to treat a case of refractory AIHA [44].

Treatment of Secondary AIHA

The immune mechanisms underlying secondary AIHA are heterogeneous and often mixed, which leads to a variable response to standard therapies. Treatment of the underlying disease is important to achieve disease control in secondary AIHA. The general treatment guidelines of primary AIHA are applicable in secondary AIHA; however, certain differences and considerations should be regarded. The following are examples of specific treatment considerations in selected secondary forms of AIHA.

Evans Syndrome

This eponymous disorder was identified over 60 years ago and has been historically defined by the presence of AIHA and ITP together without a known cause [45]. The definition has expanded over the years to include any immune-mediated cytopenia involving more than one cell lineage, and the cytopenias do not have to be concurrent. As new immune deficiencies and immune dysregulation disorders have been recognized and characterized, the proportion of patients with Evans syndrome (idiopathic cytopenia) has been shrinking. For example, almost half of patients diagnosed with Evans syndrome were found to have ALPS, after this disorder was characterized [46]. The diagnosis of Evans syndrome should only occur after a careful and thorough evaluation for an underlying immune deficiency or a broad autoimmune disease has been performed.

Although patients with Evans syndrome have similar initial response to corticosteroids, relapse and steroid dependency are common, and second-line therapies are often necessary [1]. Because most patients have ITP on presentation, IVIG is frequently given among the first-line therapies. The optimal dose and the efficacy rate of IVIG in this setting are not known, but the majority of patients who initially respond to IVIG will relapse and require additional therapies. IVIG is preferred over steroids in very young patients, due to steroid side effects on the growing child [47]. Rituximab, either alone or in combination with corticosteroids, has an efficacy rate approaching 75–82% in children and adults with Evans syndrome [48, 49]. In the setting of an underlying immune deficiency or immune dysregulation like ALPS, rituximab has lower efficacy and higher toxicity. Both MMF and sirolimus have also been successful; MMF was associated with complete response in 81% of patients with Evans syndrome or ALPS-related cytopenia, without toxicity [30, 50]. Similarly, the majority of patients treated with sirolimus had a complete or good partial response, although patients without ALPS had a slower response compared to those with ALPS [35, 51]. Splenectomy has lower efficacy in Evans syndrome compared to isolated AIHA, with reported short-term efficacy of only a few months [52]. Splenectomy should be reserved for patients who fail other therapies. Other immune suppressive agents similar to those used in primary AIHA have also been used with variable results [47].

ALPS

Autoimmune lymphoproliferative syndrome (ALPS) is a genetic disorder of defective lymphocyte apoptosis that is characterized by chronic nonmalignant lymphoproliferation, autoimmune diseases, and increased risk of malignancy. Abnormal $TCR\alpha\beta^+CD4^-CD8^-$ (double-negative) T lymphocytes are the signature of the disease, and their detection in peripheral blood is essential to establish the diagnosis [53]. Chronic, recurrent, multilineage cytopenia is the most common autoimmune manifestation of ALPS and the most common indication for treatment. Treatment of autoimmune cytopenia is needed in 59% of patients, but the need for treatment appears to decline with age [54]. ALPS-associated immune cytopenia is chronic, and a steroid-sparing agent should be considered early.

High-dose steroid pulses (5–10 mg/kg of intravenous methylprednisolone for 7–10 days) followed by a slow taper, with or without IVIG, is the recommended starting therapy [55]. MMF and sirolimus are the most studied steroid-sparing agents for ALPS. The majority of ALPS patients (60/64) treated with MMF for chronic cytopenia achieved an initial response lasting for at least 1 year, although one third (20 patients) relapsed and required other therapies [55]. Based on these results, MMF is considered the next treatment option after the acute presentation [55]. Sirolimus also led to a complete and durable response in 12 ALPS patients with cytopenia, including 7 patients who failed MMF [34]. Sirolimus is considered a secondary maintenance treatment for ALPS, especially in patients who fail MMF or have severe disease. Both MMF and sirolimus are well-tolerated in ALPS. Sirolimus has the unique benefit of directly targeting the double-negative T cells and lymphoproliferation in ALPS patients [34].

Second-line therapies for AIHA, namely, rituximab and splenectomy, should be avoided in ALPS. Rituximab is less effective in ALPS-related AIHA compared to primary AIHA and more toxic. In 12 ALPS patients treated with rituximab, 6/9 with ITP and 0/3 with AIHA had a clinical response. Importantly, three patients experienced prolonged hypogammaglobulinemia due to irreversible B-cell depletion which lasted several years [56]. Therefore, rituximab is not recommended for ALPS patients unless other treatment options are exhausted. Finally, splenectomy is associated with increased risk of mortality in ALPS. In a large cohort of ALPS patients, 40% underwent splenectomy, mostly before effective therapies or the diagnosis of ALPS were available. The likelihood of cytopenia relapse postsplenectomy was 30% by 4 years and >70% by 20 years. Importantly, 41% of splenectomized patients experienced at least one episode of sepsis and 9% died of overwhelming sepsis [54]. These poor results of splenectomy in ALPS, likely related to defective B-cell function, [26] indicate that splenectomy should be avoided in ALPS. Targeting T-cell pathology with MMF and sirolimus in ALPS, a primary disorder of T-cell dysregulation, is an example of a mechanism-based treatment approach that has proved to be more successful than conventional B-cell therapies, despite the apparent similarities between ALPS-related cytopenia and primary immune-mediated cytopenia [57].

Other Primary Immune Deficiencies

Similar to ALPS, cytopenias in primary immune deficiencies tend to be chronic and refractory, and a steroid-sparing strategy is often needed. AIHA can be the presenting feature of an underlying immune deficiency in 13% of patients [3]. Immune cytopenia can be the predominant feature of immune dysregulation or a first sign preceding other classic features. The presence of multilineage, refractory, or chronic cytopenias should prompt the clinician to investigate for an underlying primary immune deficiency. In addition, the presence of systemic autoimmune involvement, recurrent or opportunistic infections, and poor growth in children should raise the index of suspicion. The mechanisms of immune cytopenia are heterogeneous in this setting, but likely involve a failure to suppress autoreactive lymphocytes. Recently, a more targeted, mechanism-based second-line treatment approach has been used in this setting, resulting in better outcomes for this historically difficult-to-treat subgroup [57].

Common variable immune deficiency (CVID) is a heterogeneous group of disorders characterized by hypogammaglobulinemia, poor specific antibody titers, increased infections, and propensity to both autoimmune diseases and malignancy. Isolated AIHA can be diagnosed in 3–7% and Evans syndrome in 4% of CVID cases [57]. Notably, autoimmunity is diagnosed before the diagnosis of CVID is made in 49% of patients [58, 59]. Classical CVID is considered a primary B-cell disorder; however, true combined cases also exist. Rituximab provides a reasonable durable response in 59% of patients with resistant cytopenia. However, 24% of patients receiving rituximab developed severe bacterial infections, although most had previous splenectomy or were not receiving IVIG replacement therapy [60]. Patients with CVID or underlying immune deficiencies, who are considered for rituximab, should be counseled on the infectious risks, and immunoglobulin levels should be monitored routinely for possible replacement.

The cytotoxic T-lymphocyte antigen-4 haploinsufficiency (CTLA-4) and the lipopolysaccharide-responsive beige-like anchor (LRBA) deficiency are two recently described genetic immune deficiencies that cause regulatory T-cell defects leading to lymphoproliferation, variable immune deficiency, and immune cytopenia. AIHA is diagnosed in up to 28% and 57% of CTLA-4- and LRBA-deficient patients, respectively [61, 62]. Since immune dysregulation in both conditions is caused by CTLA-4 protein loss, the CTLA-4 agonist immunoglobulin abatacept has resulted in improvement of lymphoproliferation and autoimmune features in few patients who were resistant to several immunosuppressive therapies [63, 64]. An additional example of a successful targeted approach is the successful use of the JAK/STAT inhibitor ruxolitinib in controlling life-threatening autoimmune cytopenia in a patient with a STAT1-gain-of-function mutation [65].

Systemic Lupus Erythematosus

A diagnosis of systemic lupus erythematosus (SLE) underlies 4–10% of warm AIHA cases [66, 67]. A positive DAT is part of the diagnostic criteria for SLE, but does not always cause hemolytic anemia or require specific treatment for AIHA. When needed, corticosteroids are the preferred first-line therapy in SLE-related AIHA. Despite an excellent initial response, about one third of patients relapse, [68] so higher doses or prolonged courses of corticosteroids are commonly needed to treat SLE-related AIHA.

Second-line therapies used in primary AIHA have all been used in SLE. Rituximab was effective in treatment of refractory AIHA in childhood-onset SLE in two studies [69, 70]. Despite the risk of prolonged B-cell depletion, especially in patients with baseline hypogammaglobulinemia, the infection risk was low [70]. Splenectomy appears to have only short-term efficacy [68]. In a recent prospective study of sirolimus in refractory autoimmune cytopenia, two patients with SLE-related cytopenia had a durable complete response within 3 and 12 months of starting therapy [34]. MMF was also successful in treating SLE-related AIHA in case reports [71, 72].

Cold AIHA

Cold AIHA, characterized by the presence of RBC autoantibodies that bind preferentially at cold temperatures, is typically a secondary disease. The most common form, Cold Agglutinin Disease (CAD), is a chronic disease of adults caused by monoclonal IgM antibodies against erythrocyte carbohydrate antigens, most commonly associated with IgM monoclonal gammopathy of undetermined clinical significance (MGUS) or other lymphoproliferative diseases [73]. Other malignancies and autoimmune diseases have also been associated with CAD. In general, CAD is a long-term disease that affects the elderly (median age 72 years) and is often resistant to therapy. Conversely, CAD in children is caused by polyclonal IgM antibodies that are almost always post-infectious or para-infectious and spontaneously resolve, although treatment of the infection may speed resolution [3]. Mycoplasma and Epstein-Barr virus are the most common infections associated with CAD, but other bacteria and viruses have also been implicated.

Pharmacologic treatment of CAD is not always necessary. Supportive measures focused on avoiding cold exposure and pre-warming of blood products and fluids are the cornerstone of acute management to avoid exacerbation of hemolysis [73]. Blood transfusions can be given safely in CAD. Because of the nature of cold-reacting antibodies, blood compatibility should be performed strictly at 37 °C to exclude alloantibodies [14]. The use of in-line blood warmer may decrease autoantibody binding to the transfused erythrocytes.

Additional therapy is typically reserved for patients with symptomatic anemia who are transfusion-dependent or have circulatory compromise. In contrast to warm AIHA, CAD is not responsive to corticosteroids or splenectomy, since it is not IgG-mediated. Steroid use is discouraged in CAD [2]. Corticosteroids have a partial effect in 14–35% of cases; however, the need for unacceptably high doses of steroids to maintain remission in CAD has restricted their use [73, 74]. Because the clearance of complement-opsonized RBC occurs primarily in the liver, splenectomy is not effective and should not be performed in CAD. Eighty percent of patients who underwent splenectomy required further therapy [73]. Monotherapy with chlorambucil or cyclophosphamide has shown limited effect in small series [8, 74].

Rituximab has become the standard first-line therapy for adults with CAD. In this setting, targeting the pathogenic B-cell clone with rituximab is associated with a partial response rate of 45–80%, with a median duration of 11 months to 2 years [73, 75]. Although a large proportion eventually relapse, similar responses were observed when rituximab was repeated. In addition, the combination of rituximab with either fludarabine or bendamustine seems to have better and more durable response than rituximab alone. In 29 patients treated with fludarabine and rituximab, 76% responded including a complete response in 27%, with an estimated median response duration >66 months. Among 10 patients who failed rituximab monotherapy initially, this combination therapy was associated with a response rate of 70% [76]. Because of higher toxicity associated with this regimen, combination therapy is usually reserved for patients who fail multiple rounds of rituximab. Recently, the combination of rituximab and the antineoplastic bendamustine was reported to have a response rate of 71% in adults with CAD, including a 50% response rate in patients who were previously treated with fludarabine and rituximab [77].

Plasmapheresis has a salutary but limited effect in CAD management, primarily during acute hemolysis or during preoperative preparation in patients with high cold agglutinin titers, to minimize hypothermia-exacerbated hemolysis [2, 73]. Bortezomib led to transfusion independence in a severe case refractory to rituximab [78]. Finally, because of the role of complement activation in CAD, theoretically, targeting the complement system itself could be a successful strategy in management. Anticomplement agents eculizumab and C1-esterase inhibitor were successful in two cases of severe disease refractory to rituximab [79, 80].

Paroxysmal cold hemoglobinuria (PCH) is a rare form of AIHA that features cold-reactive IgG antibodies, typically against the erythrocyte P antigen, which fix complement avidly and lead to acute hemolytic anemia. PCH is frequently identified after a bacterial or viral infection and is usually self-limiting. Depending on the amount of intravascular hemolysis and degree of anemia, blood transfusion may be necessary at the time of clinical presentation. In severe PCH cases, corticosteroids may be additionally required, although their effectiveness has not been tested rigorously [2].

Conclusions

The treatment of AIHA is based primarily on historical clinical experience and few trials to provide evidence-based guidelines. Corticosteroids are the preferred first-line treatment in all forms of warm AIHA. Rituximab, splenectomy (in adults), and MMF/sirolimus (in children) are often used as second-line therapies (Fig. 6.2). Comparative studies are needed to establish the best second-line therapy. Diagnosing a primary immune deficiency in children with AIHA has significant therapeutic implications. Understanding the immune mechanisms underlying different forms of AIHA leads to better directed therapies that are more effective and less toxic. Cold AIHA in children is usually postinfectious and self-resolving. Rituximab is now the first-line therapy in adults with monoclonal cold agglutinin disease. Large-scale international studies are needed to generate evidence that changes the management of AIHA from opinion-based, currently, to evidence-based.

References

1. Miano M. How I manage Evans syndrome and AIHA cases in children. Br J Haematol. 2016;172(4):524–34.
2. Zanella A, Barcellini W. Treatment of autoimmune hemolytic anemias. Haematologica. 2014;99(10):1547–54.
3. Aladjidi N, Leverger G, Leblanc T, Picat MQ, Michel G, Bertrand Y, et al. New insights into childhood autoimmune hemolytic anemia: a French national observational study of 265 children. Haematologica. 2011;96(5):655–63.
4. Barcellini W, Fattizzo B, Zaninoni A, Radice T, Nichele I, Di Bona E, et al. Clinical heterogeneity and predictors of outcome in primary autoimmune hemolytic anemia: a GIMEMA study of 308 patients. Blood. 2014;124(19):2930–6.
5. Segel GB, Lichtman MA. Direct antiglobulin ("Coombs") test-negative autoimmune hemolytic anemia: a review. Blood Cells Mol Dis. 2014;52(4):152–60.

6. McGann PT, McDade J, Mortier NA, Combs MR, Ware RE. IgA-mediated autoimmune hemo-lytic anemia in an infant. Pediatr Blood Cancer. 2011;56(5):837–9.
7. Go RS, Winters JL, Kay NE. How I treat autoimmune hemolytic anemia. Blood. 2017;129(22):2971–9.
8. Lechner K, Jager U. How I treat autoimmune hemolytic anemias in adults. Blood. 2010;116(11):1831–8.
9. Garratty G. Drug-induced immune hemolytic anemia. Hematol Am Soc Hematol Educ Prog. 2009:73–9.
10. Borthakur G, O'Brien S, Wierda WG, Thomas DA, Cortes JE, Giles FJ, et al. Immune anae-mias in patients with chronic lymphocytic leukaemia treated with fludarabine, cyclophospha-mide and rituximab—incidence and predictors. Br J Haematol. 2007;136(6):800–5.
11. Barcellini W. New insights in the pathogenesis of autoimmune hemolytic anemia. Transfus Med Hemother. 2015;42(5):287–93.
12. Fattizzo B, Zaninoni A, Nesa F, Sciumbata VM, Zanella A, Cortelezzi A, et al. Lessons from very severe, refractory, and fatal primary autoimmune hemolytic anemias. Am J Hematol. 2015;90(8):E149–51.
13. Branch DR, Petz LD. Detecting alloantibodies in patients with autoantibodies. Transfusion. 1999;39(1):6–10.
14. Petz LD. A physician's guide to transfusion in autoimmune haemolytic anaemia. Br J Haematol. 2004;124(6):712–6.
15. Kalfa TA. Warm antibody autoimmune hemolytic anemia. Hematol Am Soc Hematol Educ Prog. 2016;2016(1):690–7.
16. Birgens H, Frederiksen H, Hasselbalch HC, Rasmussen IH, Nielsen OJ, Kjeldsen L, et al. A phase III randomized trial comparing glucocorticoid monotherapy versus glucocor-ticoid and rituximab in patients with autoimmune haemolytic anaemia. Br J Haematol. 2013;163(3):393–9.
17. Dussadee K, Taka O, Thedsawad A, Wanachiwanawin W. Incidence and risk factors of relapses in idiopathic autoimmune hemolytic anemia. J Med Assoc Thail. 2010;93(Suppl 1):S165–70.
18. Reynaud Q, Durieu I, Dutertre M, Ledochowski S, Durupt S, Michallet AS, et al. Efficacy and safety of rituximab in auto-immune hemolytic anemia: a meta-analysis of 21 studies. Autoimmun Rev. 2015;14(4):304–13.
19. Dierickx D, Kentos A, Delannoy A. The role of rituximab in adults with warm antibody auto-immune hemolytic anemia. Blood. 2015;125(21):3223–9.
20. Maung SW, Leahy M, O'Leary HM, Khan I, Cahill MR, Gilligan O, et al. A multi-centre ret-rospective study of rituximab use in the treatment of relapsed or resistant warm autoimmune haemolytic anaemia. Br J Haematol. 2013;163(1):118–22.
21. Zecca M, Nobili B, Ramenghi U, Perrotta S, Amendola G, Rosito P, et al. Rituximab for the treat-ment of refractory autoimmune hemolytic anemia in children. Blood. 2003;101(10):3857–61.
22. Barcellini W, Zaja F, Zaninoni A, Imperiali FG, Battista ML, Di Bona E, et al. Low-dose rituximab in adult patients with idiopathic autoimmune hemolytic anemia: clinical efficacy and biologic studies. Blood. 2012;119(16):3691–7.
23. Jaime-Perez JC, Rodriguez-Martinez M, Gomez-de-Leon A, Tarin-Arzaga L, Gomez-Almaguer D. Current approaches for the treatment of autoimmune hemolytic anemia. Arch Immunol Ther Exp. 2013;61(5):385–95.
24. Akpek G, McAneny D, Weintraub L. Comparative response to splenectomy in coombs-positive autoimmune hemolytic anemia with or without associated disease. Am J Hematol. 1999;61(2):98–102.
25. Centers for Disease Control and Prevention. Epidemiology and prevention of vaccine-preventable diseases. In: Hamborsky J, Kroger A, Wolfe S, editors, 13th ed. Washington, DC: Public Health Foundation; 2015.
26. Neven B, Bruneau J, Stolzenberg MC, Meyts I, Magerus-Chatinet A, Moens L, et al. Defective anti-polysaccharide response and splenic marginal zone disorganization in ALPS patients. Blood. 2014;124(10):1597–609.

27. Rao VK, Dugan F, Dale JK, Davis J, Tretler J, Hurley JK, et al. Use of mycophenolate mofetil for chronic, refractory immune cytopenias in children with autoimmune lymphoproliferative syndrome. Br J Haematol. 2005;129(4):534–8.
28. Howard J, Hoffbrand AV, Prentice HG, Mehta A. Mycophenolate mofetil for the treatment of refractory auto-immune haemolytic anaemia and auto-immune thrombocytopenia purpura. Br J Haematol. 2002;117(3):712–5.
29. Kotb R, Pinganaud C, Trichet C, Lambotte O, Dreyfus M, Delfraissy JF, et al. Efficacy of mycophenolate mofetil in adult refractory auto-immune cytopenias: a single center preliminary study. Eur J Haematol. 2005;75(1):60–4.
30. Miano M, Scalzone M, Perri K, Palmisani E, Caviglia I, Micalizzi C, et al. Mycophenolate mofetil and Sirolimus as second or further line treatment in children with chronic refractory primitive or secondary autoimmune cytopenias: a single centre experience. Br J Haematol. 2015.
31. Acquazzino MA, Fischer RT, Langnas A, Coulter DW. Refractory autoimmune hemolytic anemia after intestinal transplant responding to conversion from a calcineurin to mTOR inhibitor. Pediatr Transplant. 2013;17(5):466–71.
32. Valentini RP, Imam A, Warrier I, Ellis D, Ritchey AK, Ravindranath Y, et al. Sirolimus rescue for tacrolimus-associated post-transplant autoimmune hemolytic anemia. Pediatr Transplant. 2006;10(3):358–61.
33. Miano M, Calvillo M, Palmisani E, Fioredda F, Micalizzi C, Svahn J, et al. Sirolimus for the treatment of multi-resistant autoimmune haemolytic anaemia in children. Br J Haematol. 2014;167(4):571–4.
34. Bride KL, Vincent T, Smith-Whitley K, Lambert MP, Bleesing JJ, Seif AE, et al. Sirolimus is effective in relapsed/refractory autoimmune cytopenias: results of a prospective multi-institutional trial. Blood. 2016;127(1):17–28.
35. Teachey DT, Greiner R, Seif A, Attiyeh E, Bleesing J, Choi J, et al. Treatment with sirolimus results in complete responses in patients with autoimmune lymphoproliferative syndrome. Br J Haematol. 2009;145(1):101–6.
36. Flores G, Cunningham-Rundles C, Newland AC, Bussel JB. Efficacy of intravenous immunoglobulin in the treatment of autoimmune hemolytic anemia: results in 73 patients. Am J Hematol. 1993;44(4):237–42.
37. Pignon JM, Poirson E, Rochant H. Danazol in autoimmune haemolytic anaemia. Br J Haematol. 1993;83(2):343–5.
38. Moyo VM, Smith D, Brodsky I, Crilley P, Jones RJ, Brodsky RA. High-dose cyclophosphamide for refractory autoimmune hemolytic anemia. Blood. 2002;100(2):704–6.
39. Passweg JR, Rabusin M. Hematopoetic stem cell transplantation for immune thrombocytopenia and other refractory autoimmune cytopenias. Autoimmunity. 2008;41(8):660–5.
40. Snowden JA, Saccardi R, Allez M, Ardizzone S, Arnold R, Cervera R, et al. Haematopoietic SCT in severe autoimmune diseases: updated guidelines of the European Group for Blood and Marrow Transplantation. Bone Marrow Transplant. 2012;47(6):770–90.
41. Khandelwal P, Davies SM, Grimley MS, Jordan MB, Curtis BR, Jodele S, et al. Bortezomib for refractory autoimmunity in pediatrics. Biol Blood Marrow Transplant. 2014;20(10):1654–9.
42. Nader K, Patel M, Ferber A. Ofatumumab in rituximab-refractory autoimmune hemolytic anemia associated with chronic lymphocytic leukemia: a case report and review of literature. Clin Lymphoma Myeloma Leuk. 2013;13(4):511–3.
43. Karageorgas T, Zomas A, Kazakou P, Katsimbri P, Mantzourani M, Boumpas D. Successful treatment of life-threatening autoimmune haemolytic anaemia with ofatumumab in a patient with systemic lupus erythematosus. Rheumatology (Oxford). 2016;55(11):2085–7.
44. Ma K, Caplan S. Refractory IgG warm autoimmune hemolytic anemia treated with Eculizumab: a novel application of anticomplement therapy. Case Rep Hematol. 2016;2016:9181698.
45. Evans RS, Takahashi K, Duane RT, Payne R, Liu C. Primary thrombocytopenic purpura and acquired hemolytic anemia; evidence for a common etiology. AMA Arch Intern Med. 1951;87(1):48–65.

46. Teachey DT, Manno CS, Axsom KM, Andrews T, Choi JK, Greenbaum BH, et al. Unmasking Evans syndrome: T-cell phenotype and apoptotic response reveal autoimmune lymphoprolif-erative syndrome (ALPS). Blood. 2005;105(6):2443–8.
47. Norton A, Roberts I. Management of Evans syndrome. Br J Haematol. 2006;132(2):125–37.
48. Michel M, Chanet V, Dechartres A, Morin AS, Piette JC, Cirasino L, et al. The spectrum of Evans syndrome in adults: new insight into the disease based on the analysis of 68 cases. Blood. 2009;114(15):3167–72.
49. Bader-Meunier B, Aladjidi N, Bellmann F, Monpoux F, Nelken B, Robert A, et al. Rituximab therapy for childhood Evans syndrome. Haematologica. 2007;92(12):1691–4.
50. Miano M, Ramenghi U, Russo G, Rubert L, Barone A, Tucci F, et al. Mycophenolate mofetil for the treatment of children with immune thrombocytopenia and Evans syndrome. A retro-spective data review from the Italian association of paediatric haematology/oncology. Br J Haematol. 2016;175(3):490–5.
51. Jasinski S, Weinblatt ME, Glasser CL. Sirolimus as an effective agent in the treatment of immune thrombocytopenia (ITP) and Evans syndrome (ES): a single Institution's experience. J Pediatr Hematol Oncol. 2017;39(6):420–4.
52. Mathew P, Chen G, Wang W. Evans syndrome: results of a national survey. J Pediatr Hematol Oncol. 1997;19(5):433–7.
53. Oliveira JB, Bleesing JJ, Dianzani U, Fleisher TA, Jaffe ES, Lenardo MJ, et al. Revised diag-nostic criteria and classification for the autoimmune lymphoproliferative syndrome (ALPS): report from the 2009 NIH International Workshop. Blood. 2010;116(14):e35–40.
54. Price S, Shaw PA, Seitz A, Joshi G, Davis J, Niemela JE, et al. Natural history of auto-immune lymphoproliferative syndrome associated with FAS gene mutations. Blood. 2014;123(13):1989–99.
55. Rao VK, Oliveira JB. How I treat autoimmune lymphoproliferative syndrome. Blood. 2011;118(22):5741–51.
56. Rao VK, Price S, Perkins K, Aldridge P, Tretler J, Davis J, et al. Use of rituximab for refractory cytopenias associated with autoimmune lymphoproliferative syndrome (ALPS). Pediatr Blood Cancer. 2009;52(7):847–52.
57. Walter JE, Farmer JR, Foldvari Z, Torgerson TR, Cooper MA. Mechanism-based strategies for the management of autoimmunity and immune dysregulation in primary immunodeficiencies. J Allergy Clin Immunol Pract. 2016;4(6):1089–100.
58. Gathmann B, Mahlaoui N, Ceredih, Gérard L, Oksenhendler E, Warnatz K, et al. Clinical pic-ture and treatment of 2212 patients with common variable immunodeficiency. J Allergy Clin Immunol. 2014;134(1):116–26.
59. Heeney MM, Zimmerman SA, Ware RE. Childhood autoimmune cytopenia secondary to unsuspected common variable immunodeficiency. J Pediatr. 2003;143(5):662–5.
60. Gobert D, Bussel JB, Cunningham-Rundles C, Galicier L, Dechartres A, Berezne A, et al. Efficacy and safety of rituximab in common variable immunodeficiency-associated immune cytopenias: a retrospective multicentre study on 33 patients. Br J Haematol. 2011;155(4):498–508.
61. Gamez-Diaz L, August D, Stepensky P, Revel-Vilk S, Seidel MG, Noriko M, et al. The extended phenotype of LPS-responsive beige-like anchor protein (LRBA) deficiency. J Allergy Clin Immunol. 2016;137(1):223–30.
62. Schubert D, Bode C, Kenefeck R, Hou TZ, Wing JB, Kennedy A, et al. Autosomal domi-nant immune dysregulation syndrome in humans with CTLA4 mutations. Nat Med. 2014;20(12):1410–6.
63. Lee S, Moon JS, Lee CR, Kim HE, Baek SM, Hwang S, et al. Abatacept alleviates severe auto-immune symptoms in a patient carrying a de novo variant in CTLA-4. J Allergy Clin Immunol. 2016;137(1):327–30.
64. Lo B, Zhang K, Lu W, Zheng L, Zhang Q, Kanellopoulou C, et al. AUTOIMMUNE DISEASE. Patients with LRBA deficiency show CTLA4 loss and immune dysregulation responsive to abatacept therapy. Science. 2015;349(6246):436–40.

65. Weinacht KG, Charbonnier LM, Alroqi F, Plant A, Qiao Q, Wu H, et al. Ruxolitinib reverses dysregulated T helper cell responses and controls autoimmunity caused by a novel signal transducer and activator of transcription 1 (STAT1) gain-of-function mutation. J Allergy Clin Immunol. 2017;139(5):1629–40.
66. Bader-Meunier B, Armengaud JB, Haddad E, Salomon R, Deschênes G, Koné-Paut I, et al. Initial presentation of childhood-onset systemic lupus erythematosus: a French multicenter study. J Pediatr. 2005;146(5):648–53.
67. Roumier M, Loustau V, Guillaud C, Languille L, Mahevas M, Khellaf M, et al. Characteristics and outcome of warm autoimmune hemolytic anemia in adults: new insights based on a single-center experience with 60 patients. Am J Hematol. 2014;89(9):E150–5.
68. Gomard-Mennesson E, Ruivard M, Koenig M, Woods A, Magy N, Ninet J, et al. Treatment of isolated severe immune hemolytic anaemia associated with systemic lupus erythematosus: 26 cases. Lupus. 2006;15(4):223–31.
69. Kumar S, Benseler SM, Kirby-Allen M, Silverman ED. B-cell depletion for autoimmune thrombocytopenia and autoimmune hemolytic anemia in pediatric systemic lupus erythematosus. Pediatrics. 2009;123(1):e159–63.
70. Olfat M, Silverman ED, Levy DM. Rituximab therapy has a rapid and durable response for refractory cytopenia in childhood-onset systemic lupus erythematosus. Lupus. 2015;24(9):966–72.
71. Alba P, Karim MY, Hunt BJ. Mycophenolate mofetil as a treatment for autoimmune haemolytic anaemia in patients with systemic lupus erythematosus and antiphospholipid syndrome. Lupus. 2003;12(8):633–5.
72. Mak A, Mok CC. Mycophenolate mofetil for refractory haemolytic anemia in systemic lupus erythematosus. Lupus. 2005;14(10):856–8.
73. Swiecicki PL, Hegerova LT, Gertz MA. Cold agglutinin disease. Blood. 2013;122(7):1114–21.
74. Berentsen S, Ulvestad E, Langholm R, Beiske K, Hjorth-Hansen H, Ghanima W, et al. Primary chronic cold agglutinin disease: a population based clinical study of 86 patients. Haematologica. 2006;91(4):460–6.
75. Berentsen S, Ulvestad E, Gjertsen BT, Hjorth-Hansen H, Langholm R, Knutsen H, et al. Rituximab for primary chronic cold agglutinin disease: a prospective study of 37 courses of therapy in 27 patients. Blood. 2004;103(8):2925–8.
76. Berentsen S, Randen U, Vagan AM, Hjorth-Hansen H, Vik A, Dalgaard J, et al. High response rate and durable remissions following fludarabine and rituximab combination therapy for chronic cold agglutinin disease. Blood. 2010;116(17):3180–4.
77. Berentsen S, Randen U, Oksman M, Birgens H, Tvedt THA, Dalgaard J, et al. Bendamustine plus rituximab for chronic cold agglutinin disease: results of a Nordic prospective multicenter trial. Blood. 2017;130(4):537–41.
78. Carson KR, Beckwith LG, Mehta J. Successful treatment of IgM-mediated autoimmune hemolytic anemia with bortezomib. Blood. 2010;115(4):915.
79. Roth A, Huttmann A, Rother RP, Duhrsen U, Philipp T. Long-term efficacy of the complement inhibitor eculizumab in cold agglutinin disease. Blood. 2009;113(16):3885–6.
80. Wouters D, Stephan F, Strengers P, de Haas M, Brouwer C, Hagenbeeket A, et al. C1-esterase inhibitor concentrate rescues erythrocytes from complement-mediated destruction in autoimmune hemolytic anemia. Blood. 2013;121(7):1242–4.

Chapter 7
Evans Syndrome: Background, Clinical Presentation, Pathophysiology, and Management

Amanda B. Grimes

Introduction

Evans syndrome (ES) is defined as the presence of autoimmune cytopenias affecting two or more blood cell lines, either simultaneously or sequentially. Most often, this refers to the combination of autoimmune hemolytic anemia (AIHA) and immune thrombocytopenia (ITP) but can include autoimmune neutropenia (AIN) as well. The etiology of ES has historically been attributed to pathologic autoantibody production against the blood cells, with the true underlying cause remaining unknown. However, recent advances in our understanding of this complex disorder have revealed frequent association with more well-described underlying disorders of immune regulation. Nevertheless, "idiopathic" ES still precedes the diagnosis of an underlying autoimmune disorder or immunodeficiency in the majority of cases [1]. Improved insight into the pathology behind ES over the recent years highlights the importance of thorough investigation for underlying immune disorders when applying this "diagnosis of exclusion." This chapter will thoroughly review the background, clinical features, pathophysiology, and management of ES.

Background

History

Observations of leukopenia, thrombocytopenia, and hemolytic anemia co-occurring in the same patient were first reported in the 1940s [2–5], and most commonly noted are thrombocytopenia and hemolytic anemia [6]. However, it was

A. B. Grimes, MD
Baylor College of Medicine, Texas Children's Hospital, Houston, TX, USA
e-mail: abgrimes@txch.org

© Springer International Publishing AG, part of Springer Nature 2018   125
J. M. Despotovic (ed.), *Immune Hematology*,
https://doi.org/10.1007/978-3-319-73269-5_7

Evans and Duane who first discussed the implications of this finding in 1949 [6], postulating that the neutropenia and thrombocytopenia in these patients with acquired hemolytic anemia were "due to the presence of an immune body with a broader range of activity than the red cells or to a separate immune substance or substances more specific for platelet and white cell tissue." It was also at this time that the etiologies of "splenic neutropenia" and "classic thrombocytopenic purpura" were called into question, with Evans and Duane noting that "abnormal immune mechanisms could account for both excessive destruction...and deficient formation" [6]. Furthermore, in 1951, they suggested that the terms "hypersplenism and splenic panhematopenia should be supplanted, since it is evident that the spleen alone is not at fault in these diseases" [7]. In the subsequent years, the pathologic immune function driving both ITP (see Section "Platelet Autoantibodies" in Chap. 2) and AIHA (see Section "Historical Perspective" in Chap. 5) has been better elucidated; and unifying underlying disorders of immune regulation, such as common variable immunodeficiency (CVID) or autoimmune lymphoproliferative syndrome (ALPS), have been identified as drivers of ES more and more frequently [8].

Canale and Smith first described an ALPS-like phenotype in 1967, reporting five pediatric cases with a constellation of findings including generalized lymphadenopathy, hepatosplenomegaly, and immunological aberrations (autoimmune manifestations and/or abnormal immunoglobulin levels), causing them to postulate that the pathology driving these collection of symptoms was a "primary immunological disorder" [9]. Further studies of "Canale-Smith syndrome" throughout the following years led to the discovery of impaired lymphocyte apoptosis in the 1990s, specifically via defects in the Fas receptor, which transduces the intracellular signals necessary to initiate apoptosis [10], finally yielding an explanation for the autoimmunity and lymphoproliferation seen in this disease. With a unifying pathology and clinical phenotype, the syndrome was termed autoimmune lymphoproliferative syndrome (ALPS) moving forward; and subsequent investigations have identified several associated mutations in the *FAS* gene pathway, resulting in known genetic etiologies in >70% of patients with ALPS currently [11].

Definitions/Terminology

As noted previously, ES is a descriptive terminology, with classical definitions evolving over the years. Whereas the syndrome was previously defined strictly as a direct antiglobulin test (DAT)-positive hemolytic anemia plus ITP occurring simultaneously or in succession in the absence of a clear underlying diagnosis, it is now defined as autoimmune destruction of at least two hematologic cell lines, in which other diagnoses have been excluded [7, 12–15]. However, given that several years may elapse before underlying diagnoses are identified, the term "primary ES" refers to true idiopathic ES, and the term "secondary ES" refers to ES that is secondary to an identifiable well-defined disorder of immune regulation.

The changing definition of ES over the years affects the way in which studies can be compared, and the rarity of the disease and exclusionary nature of the diagnosis have made formal study of ES somewhat challenging. However, uniform definitions and inclusion criteria, as well as better understanding of the underlying pathology, have helped to make ongoing investigation in ES more productive.

Clinical Presentation

Epidemiology

The true incidence of ES in children and adults is unknown, given the relative rarity of this syndrome, as well as the varying and evolving definitions over the years. Recently, there are few larger series reported in children [16] and adults [17] with ES, but most of the literature is limited to case reports (<100 in the last 30 years) [16] and retrospective series, with inconsistent definitions and little long-term follow-up. However, the incidences of ITP and AIHA individually have been better established; and ES reported within the ITP and AIHA literature therefore allows for some estimation of ES incidence. ITP is diagnosed in 5–10 per 100,000 children per year [18–20] and ~3.5 per 100,000 adults per year [18, 21], while AIHA is diagnosed in 1–3 per 100,000 children and adults per year [22–24]. Most available data place the occurrence of ES among ITP patients at ~1%; [20, 21, 25] while the incidence of ES reported among those with AIHA is more variable, but consistently higher than in ITP, ranging from 13 to 73% [12–15, 26]. It should also be noted that the incidence of ES among chronic ITP patients is significantly higher than that among the generalized ITP population, cited at 6.7% in one large series of patients with chronic ITP [27]. Overall, most recent incidence data for ES [15, 16] remains consistent with older data from the 1960s to 1980s [28], reporting diagnosis of ES in 0.8 to 3.9% of all patients with either ITP or AIHA as the initial presentation. The average age at presentation among pediatric patients diagnosed with ES is around 5 years [1, 16]. No specific ethnic or gender predilection is noted among patients diagnosed with ES [12–14, 28], although there appears to be a tendency for male predominance in younger ES patients and female predominance in older ES patients [16, 17, 21].

Clinical Features

In both children and adults, the largest series of ES patients to date have shown AIHA and ITP to occur simultaneously upon initial presentation about half of the time (~48% of children and 55% of adults) [15–17]. However, many patients ultimately diagnosed with ES will present initially with only one autoimmune cytopenia—ITP first in ~29% and AIHA first in ~24% of children and 16% of adults [15–17]. AIN is present in 20% of children [16] and ~15% of adults with ES [17].

Clinically, patients with ES will present with symptoms related to the autoimmune cytopenia/s of which their syndrome is comprised (i.e., symptomatic anemia, jaundice, evidence of hemolysis in AIHA, or petechiae, bruising, and bleeding in ITP); and the clinical features of these entities are discussed in detail within their respective sections of this book. As opposed to the acutely presenting single lineage autoimmune cytopenias ITP, AIHA, and AIN, however, ES is often a chronic, relapsing, and treatment-refractory disease [13, 14, 16, 26]—especially ES which is determined to be secondary to an underlying disorder of immune regulation [16, 29]. Therefore, the diagnosis of ES should be considered even at the onset of a single lineage autoimmune cytopenia such as ITP or AIHA, as sequential autoimmune cytopenias occur an average of 2.4–4.2 years following diagnosis of the initial autoimmune cytopenia [15–17] but may still be more symptomatically severe at presentation [8, 16, 26].

Notably, mortality among patients with ES is reported to be as high as 10% in children [16] and as high as 24% in adults [17]—a mortality rate which is significantly increased above that seen among patients with ITP, AIHA, or AIN alone. For example, among a French cohort of 265 prospectively enrolled children diagnosed with AIHA from 2004 to 2007, overall mortality among children with AIHA was 4%, but among the subset of children with both AIHA and ITP (defined as ES), mortality was 10% [15]. Although the mortality is not clearly linked to cytopenia-related complications in all cases, it is notable that ES-related morbidity and mortality is consistently higher than that in any other autoimmune cytopenia alone.

Etiology

Although ES is traditionally known as an "idiopathic" condition, well-defined immune disorders are now being ultimately identified as the etiology of disease in ~50% of ES cases [1, 17]. The most commonly identified diseases driving ES are ALPS [30, 31], CVID [1, 15, 17, 32], and systemic autoimmune disease, most often systemic lupus erythematosus (SLE) [1, 16, 17]. With rapidly improving diagnostic capabilities, including increased access to genomic data, it is expected that inherited immunologic diseases responsible for driving the autoimmunity of ES will be increasingly identified [33]. Even as recently as 2015 though, the French reported that among a cohort of 156 children with Evans syndrome, a definitive underlying immune disorder was identified in only 10% of patients—2% with ALPS and 8% with SLE. However, 60% were noted to have more non-specific immune abnormalities such as lymphoproliferation, other autoimmune diseases, and hypogammaglobulinemia, which did not immediately meet diagnostic criteria for any formally recognized lymphoproliferative, autoimmune, or immunodeficiency syndrome, but for whom further immunologic investigation is ongoing [16]. Many similar cases are reported in the literature, with clear immunological aberrancies, including lymphadenopathy and/or hepatosplenomegaly, hypogammaglobulinemia, and autoimmune cytopenias, but still not meeting criteria for a unifying immune dysregulation diagnosis [34]. Importantly though, these unclassified cases appear to behave clinically similarly to secondary ES, requiring second-line therapies significantly more frequently (72%) than primary (or idiopathic) ES (55%) [16]. This highlights the importance of ongoing investigation in these cases with unclassified underlying immunopathology, as novel diagnostics and better defined immune disorders are continually emerging [33] and may uncover better targets for directed therapies.

The three most common etiologies underlying the clinical manifestations of ES—ALPS, CVID, and systemic autoimmune disease, most commonly SLE—will be further discussed here.

ALPS

Following the characterization of ALPS during the 1990s [10, 35–40], Teachey and colleagues first reported the association of ALPS with idiopathic ES, finding diagnostic evidence of underlying ALPS as defined by chronic nonmalignant lymphoproliferation, defective in vitro Fas-mediated lymphocyte apoptosis, and elevated TCRα/β$^+$CD3$^+$CD4$^-$CD8$^-$ double-negative T (DNT) cells in peripheral blood or lymphoid tissue, in 50% of idiopathic ES patients followed at their institution over a 5-year period [30]. A follow-up multi-institutional study in 2010 confirmed prior findings, with 21 of 45 pediatric ES patients (47%) meeting diagnostic criteria for ALPS [31]. Although the largest pediatric ES cohort recently published did not corroborate these findings, reporting a known diagnosis of ALPS in only 3 of the 156 children with ES, there were no ALPS-directed investigations deliberately conducted among this population, offering a likely explanation for this inconsistency; and further immunologic investigations are now ongoing among that cohort [16]. In another recent pediatric ES series including 23 patients, 30% were identified as having features of ALPS [1]. In order to streamline ongoing investigations within the field, revised diagnostic criteria and classification for ALPS were released following the NIH international workshop in 2009, with hopes of standardizing the diagnosis of ALPS and modernizing the classification to rely less heavily on outdated and cumbersome testing techniques such as Fas-mediated apoptosis assays and more heavily on the highly sensitive and specific DNT cell testing, as well as the newer mutation-specific variations of disease [41]. Regardless of these nuances, however, the strong association between ALPS and ES is clear and will likely be further clarified in the years ahead.

CVID

The prevalence of autoimmune cytopenias in CVID is ~10–20% [42–47], with one large series of 990 CVID patients specifically reporting ES in 3.8% of patients [47] and a smaller series of 326 CVID patients corroborating these findings, with a 3.4%

incidence of ES reported [42]. Importantly, the autoimmune cytopenias appear to precede the diagnosis of CVID more than 50% of the time [42, 48]; and the incidence of CVID among pediatric ES patients is reported at ~10% on average [1, 15], although some smaller series report CVID incidence up to 83% in pediatric ES patients [32]. The incidence of CVID among adults with ES is consistently lower than that seen in pediatric ES, reported at 6% in the largest adult ES cohort to date [17]. As a rule, ES is strongly and frequently associated with CVID, and all ES patients should be screened for this condition.

Systemic Autoimmunity

Autoimmune cytopenias may also be a presenting manifestation of systemic autoimmune disease; and systemic autoimmunity is in fact diagnosed in ~8% of pediatric ES patients [1, 16] and 21% of adult ES patients [17]. However, patients meeting diagnostic criteria for a systemic autoimmune disease such as SLE are no longer classified with the diagnosis of ES or secondary ES, as their autoimmune cytopenias are considered part of their primary autoimmune diagnosis and should be treated accordingly. As noted, SLE is the most common autoimmune disease diagnosed in patients with ES [16, 17], but other primary autoimmune diseases may be associated with ES as well, including Hashimoto's thyroiditis, type 1 diabetes [1], antiphospholipid antibody syndrome, and Sjögren syndrome [17]. At a minimum, however, ES patients should be screened for SLE [29].

Although significant advances have been made with regard to understanding the underlying pathogenesis of disease in ES, etiology remains unknown in ~50% of cases [1, 17]. However, "idiopathic" ES remains a diagnosis of exclusion, and thorough investigation for an underlying etiology should be completed in these cases. Given the above well-established associations, both children and adults should be screened for ALPS, CVID, and SLE, while screening in adults should also likely be expanded to include infectious etiologies such as human immunodeficiency virus (HIV) and hepatitis C virus (HCV), in addition to malignancies, as leukemias and lymphomas are reported in ~10% of adults with ES (compared to 0% in children with ES) [17, 29]. Beyond these routine recommendations, however, investigation should be conducted as clinically indicated, given the wide array of clinical entities capable of driving ES, including infections, drugs, vaccinations, immunodeficiencies (combined immunodeficiencies, DiGeorge syndrome, selective IgA deficiency), autoimmune diseases, lymphoproliferative diseases, hemophagocytic disorders, malignancies, and disorders of immune regulation, both well-established (immunodysregulation polyendocrinopathy enteropathy X-linked [IPEX] syndrome) and novel (cytotoxic T-lymphocyte antigen-4 [CTLA] deficiency, lipopolysaccharide-responsive beige-like anchor [LRBA] deficiency, activated phosphoinositide 3-kinase delta [PI3KD] syndrome, MonoMAC syndrome, and others) [26].

Pathophysiology

Evans Syndrome

The pathophysiology in ES is largely attributed to that of its individual components, ITP, AIHA, or AIN, which is described in detail within each respective section of this book. Traditionally, autoimmune cytopenias in ES have been ascribed to aberrant autoantibody production and the cascade of downstream events that follows, with more recent delineation of the role of cell-mediated immunity in the pathogenesis of disease as well. However, ES is unique in that a unifying underlying immune pathology has now been identified in ~50% of cases [1, 17], which allows for better understanding of the true mechanisms of pathogenesis in these cases of secondary ES.

The pathophysiology behind the most common underlying etiologies in ES, as well as some of the rarer and/or novel associated disorders of immune dysregulation, will be discussed briefly here.

ALPS

ALPS is a syndrome in which lymphocyte homeostasis is disrupted due to mutations affecting the *FAS* apoptotic pathway, resulting in aberrant lymphocyte survival, chronic lymphoproliferation, dysregulated immune tolerance, and autoimmunity [11, 29, 30, 49]. Fas expressed on the surface of activated B and T lymphocytes and Fas ligand expressed on activated T lymphocytes normally interact to trigger activation of the intracellular caspase cascade, leading to cellular apoptosis (Fig. 7.1) [29]. This apoptotic pathway typically functions to downregulate the immune response by eliminating excess activated and autoreactive lymphocytes but is rendered dysfunctional via mutations in *FAS* (60–70%), *FASL* (<1%), and *CASP10* genes (2–3%) in patients with ALPS [11]. This results in the persistence of TCRα/β$^+$CD3$^+$CD4$^-$CD8$^-$ double-negative T (DNT) cells characteristic of this condition, as well as the characteristic clinical phenotype of chronic lymphoproliferation and autoimmunity.

Although the result of defective Fas-mediated apoptosis is best described as a disruption in lymphocyte homeostasis, there are many other downstream disruptions of immunologic balance which account for both the cell-mediated and humoral autoimmunity seen in ALPS. There is a B and T cell lymphocytosis, comprised of abnormally persistent and abnormally activated lymphocyte populations, both in the peripheral blood and in the tissues. These appear to promote an immune milieu which downregulates T-helper 1 (Th1) responses and upregulates T-helper 2 (Th2) responses, as evidenced by the significantly increased levels of interleukin-10 (IL-10) seen in ALPS patients as compared to controls and other diseases states, and the decreased levels of Th1 cytokines [49]. The source of IL-10 production is not

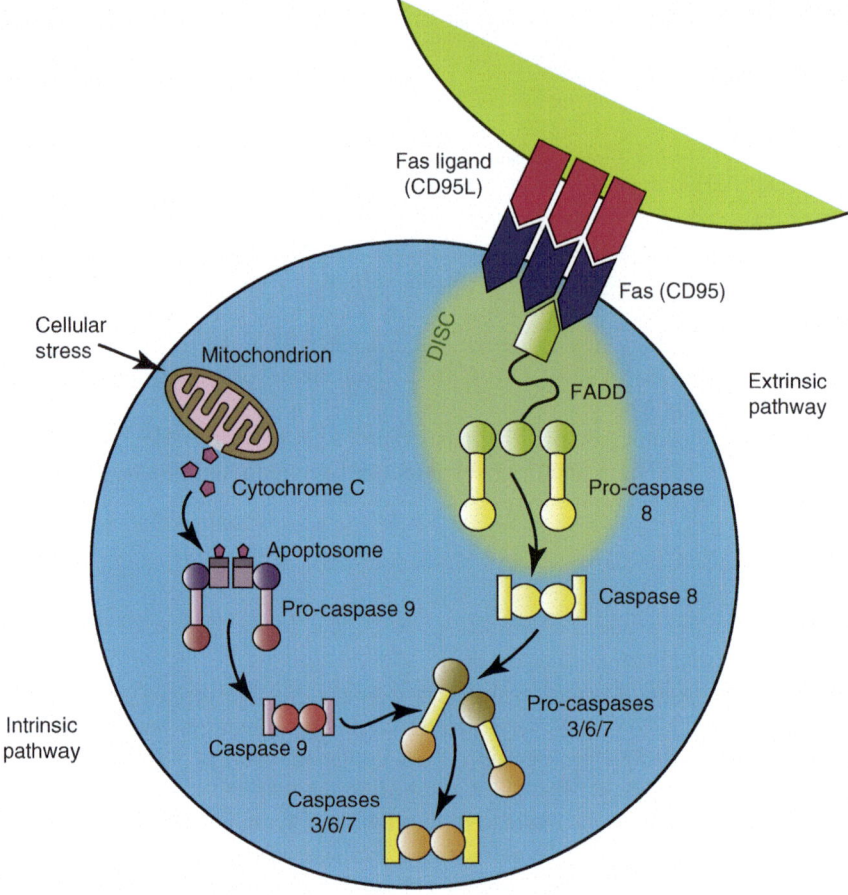

Fas ligand (CD95L)

Fas (CD95)

Cellular stress

Mitochondrion

DISC

FADD

Extrinsic pathway

Cytochrome C

Pro-caspase 8

Apoptosome

Pro-caspase 9

Caspase 8

Intrinsic pathway

Caspase 9

Pro-caspases 3/6/7

Caspases 3/6/7

Proteolysis, DNA degradation, apoptosis

Fig. 7.1 Cellular apoptosis Reprinted from Teachey DT, Lambert MP. Diagnosis and management of autoimmune cytopenias in childhood. Pediatr Clin North Am. 2013;60(6):1489–511 [29] with permission from Elsevier

entirely clear, though monocytes and macrophages from patients with ALPS have been demonstrated to produce ~5-fold more IL-10 than controls [49]; and evidence of potentially constitutive IL-10 expression by the DNT cell population in patients with ALPS has also been demonstrated [50]. IL-10 not only drives T cell differentiation toward a Th2 phenotype but also induces the anti-apoptotic protein Bcl-2 in both B cells and T cells, leading to further pathologic persistence and expansion of autoreactive lymphocytes. Th2 cytokines also stimulate T and B cell interactions necessary for autoantibody production, which could explain the excessive autoantibody production seen in ALPS [49].

Predictably, clinical and immunobiological phenotypes vary somewhat within ALPS, as explained by the variable genetics of the disease. Given our evolving understanding of the genetic pathogenesis, a gene-based classification system for ALPS was instituted following an international consensus conference at the NIH in 2009 [41]. The largest category, "ALPS-FAS," encompasses disease caused by germline mutations in *FAS*, which are generally inherited in an autosomal dominant fashion [51] and occur in 60–70% of patients affected by ALPS [11]. These are generally heterozygous, dominant negative mutations (i.e., producing a dominant or semidominant phenotype by acting antagonistically to the wild-type allele), which affect the intracellular domain of the fas-activating death domain [11]. However, ~30% of *FAS* mutations affect the extracellular domain of the fas-activating death domain and result in haploinsufficiency instead [52]. As opposed to dominant negative intracellular *FAS* mutations, which generally result in absence of fas activity and higher disease penetrance, these haploinsufficient extracellular mutations generally lead only to a decrease in Fas activity, which results in less disease penetrance [11, 52]. Somatic *FAS* mutations occur in ~10% of patients with ALPS and are categorized under "ALPS-sFAS" [11]. These somatic mutations are predominantly limited to the DNT cell compartment but produce a similar clinical phenotype to that of germline *FAS*-mutated patients, except that patients with germline mutations generally present with ALPS at a younger age [11]. Some crossover between the two categories of *FAS* mutations (ALPS-FAS and ALPS-sFAS) may still occur, as *FAS* mutations have variable penetrance, and some mutations require a second "hit" to result in clinically evident disease [11]. As an example, a small subset of ALPS patients with multiple *FAS* mutations have been identified, in whom a primary heterozygous germline *FAS* mutation results in no clinical evidence of disease but a somatic *FAS* mutation affecting the second allele produces clinical disease [53]. Furthermore, ALPS phenotypes have been described, in which both a *FAS* gene mutation and a second mutation in the *PRF1* (perforin) gene [54] or the *CASP10* gene [55] were identified, and family members carrying only one of the mutations had no clinical features of disease. The remaining categories used to classify ALPS are "ALPS-FASL," encompassing <1% of patients with germline *FASL* mutations; "ALPS-CASP10," encompassing 2–3% of patients with germline *CASP10* mutations; and "ALPS-U," which includes the remaining 20–30% of patients, in whom no mutation has yet been identified [11].

CVID

In contrast to ALPS, CVID is thought to be the result of multiple genetic, environmental, and immunologic factors, as no single causative mutation or pathway of mutations has been identified [56]. The defining features of the disease—hypogammaglobulinemia and impaired antibody responses [57]—provide clear rationale for the infectious complications common to this condition. However, as immunoglobulin replacement therapy has become standard practice, infectious complications have been surpassed by the autoimmune and lymphoproliferative complications of disease. Interestingly, the co-occurrence of autoimmune cytopenias, lymphoproliferation, and granulomatous disease is common within CVID [46, 58]. In a large cohort of 990 patients with CVID in the US Immunodeficiency Network, noninfectious CVID complications, such as lymphoproliferation, granulomatous disease, lymphoma, hepatic disease, enteropathy, and interstitial, granular, or nodular lung disease, occurred at a significantly increased rate among CVID patients with autoimmune cytopenias (69.4%) compared to those without autoimmune cytopenias (43.5%) [47]. This shared phenotype of autoimmunity and lymphoproliferative complications among this subset of CVID patients suggests a common underlying immunopathology.

While the immune dysregulation in CVID is classically thought to result from impaired B cell maturation [33], there are many complex immune mechanisms at play in the pathology of this diverse and multifaceted disease. For example, decreased levels of regulatory T cells have been noted in CVID complicated by autoimmunity [59, 60]. However, B-lymphocyte development certainly remains key to the pathology of disease, as impaired B cell maturation may result in altered B cell receptor signaling pathways, ultimately resulting in failure of central tolerance checkpoints. When central tolerance induction fails, autoreactive B cells normally selected for receptor editing or blocked development will evade detection and escape to the periphery unchecked [61, 62]. Decreased levels of isotype-switched memory B cells, suggesting defective germinal center development [58], and greater preservation of IgM production, suggesting potential defects in T cell involvement in immunoglobulin switching [43], have been associated with the development of autoimmunity in CVID as well. These associations have been further strengthened by the discovery of mutations in the *TNFRSF13B* gene encoding tumor necrosis factor receptor family member TACI (transmembrane activator and calcium-modulator and cyclophilin ligand receptor), which mediates isotype switching in B cells. These mutations are linked to the development of CVID, with a high association of autoimmune and lymphoproliferative complications [63, 64]. Furthermore, expansion of certain B cell populations have been identified in CVID-related autoimmunity, namely, CD19^{hi}CD21$^{lo/neg}$ B cells [65], which appear to express germline autoreactive antibodies [66].

Systemic Autoimmunity

Autoimmune cytopenias are a common feature of systemic autoimmune diseases and, as such, are included in the classification and diagnostic criteria for these diseases, rather than being considered as a "secondary" phenomenon of a separate underlying pathology. However, these autoimmune cytopenias may be an initial presentation of disease and therefore considered idiopathic until the underlying autoimmune disease is ultimately diagnosed. Among patients with SLE complicated by ES, for example, ~50% may be diagnosed with hematologic abnormalities (i.e., AIHA and/or ITP) months to years before developing full-blown clinical manifestations of SLE [67]. As expected, the pathophysiology of ES in the spectrum of these autoimmune diseases is quite diverse but also specific to the individual disease complex with which it is associated—a scope which is too broad to be covered here. However, one of the most prominent and unifying pathologic features of systemic autoimmunity is the failure to induce lymphocyte tolerance. Defective apoptosis in immature B cells, unbalanced pro-survival signals (i.e., as provided by BAFF [B cell activating factor]), and altered B cell receptor signaling are all cited as contributing to the failure of central and peripheral B cell tolerance induction in systemic autoimmunity [61, 62, 68]. Defective T cell tolerance may result from the failure to generate regulatory T cells or to anergize immature T cells which express autoreactive T cell receptors [62].

In SLE, humoral autoimmunity is largely implicated in the generation of autoimmune cytopenias, with immunological changes including increased plasma cell precursors [65], expansion of $CD19^{hi}CD21^{lo/neg}$ B cells [65] which appear to be anergic but express germline autoreactive antibodies [66], and several hematologic-specific autoantibodies identified. These include autoantibodies to the c-Mpl, or thrombopoietin receptor [69, 70], and antiplatelet glycoprotein antibodies (anti-GPIIb/IIIa) [70, 71] in patients with SLE-related ITP, as well as anti-CD40L autoantibodies, which have been identified in patients with both ITP and AIHA in the setting of SLE, but do not appear to be expressed in SLE without autoimmune cytopenias [71]. CD40L is expressed on the surface of activated $CD4^+$ T cells, as well as activated platelets, and these autoantibodies are thought to play a role in the dysregulation of lymphocyte tolerance and immune complex pathology, as well as potential augmentation of antiplatelet activity [71]. Additionally, the complement deficiency which is well-described in SLE [33], most notably involving C4, is significantly more pronounced in patients with ITP related to SLE [72] and ES related to SLE [67] as compared to patients with "primary" ITP or ES or SLE not complicated by autoimmune cytopenias [67].

Novel and Miscellaneous Disorders of Immune Dysregulation

In addition to these more well-defined entities, several ALPS-like syndromes and ALPS-CVID overlap syndromes have been described, in which clinical phenotypes including multilineage autoimmune cytopenias that may be initially identified as ES indicate similar underlying immune dysregulation. These syndromes are now being better defined and increasingly recognized among this population of patients. The most recently revised classification system for ALPS not only provides subclassifications for ALPS but also provides a classification system for ALPS-related disorders [41]. This includes RAS-associated autoimmune leukoproliferative disease (RALD), associated with somatic mutations in the *NRAS* or *KRAS* genes [41, 73, 74]; Dianzani autoimmune lymphoproliferative disease (DALD), in which an associated gene mutation has not yet been identified; and other classes in which lymphoproliferation and immunodeficiency, rather than autoimmunity, are more prominent features, including caspase 8 deficiency state (CEDS) [55, 75] and X-linked lymphoproliferative syndrome (XLP1) [41].

RALD is defined clinically by autoimmune cytopenias, monocytosis, and lymphoproliferation but may or may not fulfill all the diagnostic criteria for ALPS or exhibit typical elevation of IL-10, soluble FASL, or vitamin B12 levels, although the typical ALPS features such as elevated DNT cell population appear to be present more frequently in the *NRAS*-mutated variant [73, 76] than in the *KRAS*-mutated variant [74]. Importantly, there is no *FAS* pathway mutation, and the defective apoptosis noted in RALD is not Fas-mediated. RAS genes (including *NRAS* and *KRAS*) encode small GTP-binding intracellular signaling proteins which function in a variety of roles, including cell proliferation, growth, and apoptosis [77]. Germline activating mutations in *NRAS* augment RAF/MEK/ERK signaling, which decreases the pro-apoptotic protein Bcl-2-interacting mediator of cell death (BIM) and mitigates cytokine withdrawal-induced intrinsic apoptosis [73]. Similarly, activating *KRAS* mutations result in impaired intrinsic T cell apoptosis via the suppression of BIM and also appear to expedite cell proliferation via repression of the cell cycle inhibitor protein $p27^{kip1}$ [74]. DALD is also defined clinically by the autoimmunity and immunodeficiency typical of ALPS but distinct in that DNT cell populations are often not elevated, and despite evidence of defective Fas-mediated apoptosis, there are no identifiable *FAS* gene mutations. The defective apoptosis appears at least in part due to impaired ceramide-induced cell death, which indicates that DALD may be caused by downstream alterations in the Fas signaling pathway [55, 78, 79].

In today's genomic landscape, with next-generation and ever-advancing sequencing techniques, novel immune dysregulation disorders are being identified and better understood all the time. Some of the recently described ALPS-like syndromes with prominent autoimmune features are cytotoxic T-lymphocyte-associated protein 4 (CTLA-4) haploinsufficiency [80–82], lipopolysaccharide-responsive beige-like anchor (LRBA) protein deficiency [83–85], activated phosphoinositide 3-kinase δ (PI3KD) syndrome [86, 87], and signal transducer and activator of transcription (STAT) gain-of-function mutations [88], which will be described briefly here.

CTLA-4 is an important negative regulator of immune responses [80], and *CTLA-4* mutations which result in impaired ligand binding or CTLA-4 haploinsufficiency result in dysregulated $FoxP3^+$ regulatory T cells, hyperactivation of effector T cells, progressive loss of circulating B cells (with an increase of predominantly autoreactive $CD21^{lo/neg}$ B cells), both T- and B-lymphocytic infiltrations of organs, and generalized disruption of lymphocyte homeostasis [81]. Clinically, CTLA-4 haploinsufficiency is characterized by lymphoproliferation, lymphocytic infiltration of nonlymphoid organs, autoimmune cytopenias, hypogammaglobulinemia, and recurrent infections [80–82].

LRBA deficiency is characterized by a severe clinical phenotype, with early-onset hypogammaglobulinemia and autoimmunity—with AIHA and ITP in >50% of cases [84] and one report of a child with LRBA deficiency and Evans syndrome suffering fatal complications of ITP at 8.5 months of age [89]—and a strong association with inflammatory bowel disease as well [84, 85, 90]. Homozygous and compound heterozygous *LRBA* mutations result in clinically relevant disease, while heterozygous LRBA mutation carriers appear to remain clinically unaffected [83, 84]. Although the function of LRBA in immune function is not entirely clear, there is definite evidence of disrupted B cell development, with defects in B cell differentiation, defective autophagy, decreased switched memory B cells, decreased plasmablasts, impaired antibody responses, and hypogammaglobulinemia in LRBA deficiency [83, 84]; with some evidence of disrupted T cell homeostasis as well, given the decreased T regulatory cells also noted in these patients [84]. Recently, findings have led investigators to believe that LRBA may regulate the potent inhibitory immune regulator CTLA-4, which explains the similar immune phenotype of disease seen in CTLA-4 haploinsufficiency and LRBA deficiency [91]. Further investigations into the true pathogenesis underlying LRBA deficiency are ongoing, but the significant disruption in lymphocyte homeostasis and B cell development clearly drives a clinically severe disease, which should be suspected and diagnosed early in its course.

PI3KD syndrome results from dominant-activating germline gain-of-function mutations in the gene encoding the PI(3)K catalytic subunit p110δ. This catalytic subunit is selectively expressed in leukocytes; and again, although the understanding of its function in immune biology is not entirely clear, it is known to play an important role in adaptive immunity, at least in part via its role in mammalian target of rapamycin (mTOR) kinase activation [86]. In addition to activating mTOR, PI3K activates Akt (protein kinase B), which promotes translation of proteins including ribosomal s6 protein—all combining to promote differentiation of naïve T cells into effector T cells [86, 92–94]. The constitutively activated PI3K-Akt-mTOR pathway in PI3KD syndrome appears to result in a deficiency of naïve T cells and skewed differentiation of CD8$^+$ T cells to short-lived then senescent effector T cells, with severely impaired memory T- and B cell development [86]. The resultant immune dysregulation is clinically characterized most commonly by lymphoproliferative and infectious complications (including recurrent sinopulmonary infections and CMV and EBV viremia), but >1/3 of patients exhibit autoimmunity as well, including multilineage autoimmune cytopenias [87].

Gain-of-function mutations in signal transducer and activator of transcription (STAT) genes, in both STAT1 and STAT3, result in clinical phenotypes characterized by immunodeficiency, infectious susceptibility, and autoimmunity [88]. Sustained phosphorylation of STAT1 in STAT1 gain-of-function mutations results in impaired T_H17 cell differentiation and exaggerated responses to interferon stimulation [95]. These dysregulated T-helper cell responses generally result in a diverse phenotype of immune deficiency (including chronic mucocutaneous candidiasis) and autoimmunity [95, 96]. Similarly, STAT3 gain-of-function mutations (including both somatic and germline mutations) can produce diverse autoimmune and lymphoproliferative phenotypes [97–100], but germline mutations specifically result in an ALPS-like syndrome with lymphoproliferation, immunodeficiency, and autoimmunity—with hematologic autoimmunity as a major component [99, 101]. Notably, ALPS-like features including elevated DNT cell populations and defective Fas-mediated apoptosis have been identified in these disorders, with impairment of intrinsic apoptosis noted as well, likely via increased Bcl-2 anti-apoptotic proteins [101]. Upregulation of STAT3 transcriptional activity appears to produce other downstream signaling effects as well, with decreased phosphorylation of STAT1 and STAT5 in response to IFN-γ and IL-2, respectively, and decreased regulatory T cell populations [99].

Lastly, syndromes in which the features of ALPS and CVID overlap are now being increasingly identified [33, 55, 102]. While *hyper*gammaglobulinemia is reported in the majority of ALPS patients [103], as opposed to the hypogamma-globulinemia definitive of CVID, there are many overlapping immunopathological features occurring in these two syndromes. Namely, similar disturbances of B cell differentiation, most notably reduced levels of CD27$^+$ memory B cells, are seen in both syndromes [102–104]. More recently, the elevated DNT cell population and the defective Fas-mediated apoptosis that is typical of ALPS have been identified in several cases of CVID [55, 102, 105]; and there is clear evidence that Fas plays a significant role in proper B cell maturation [102]. At the same time, hypogamma-globulinemia much more typical of CVID has been identified in a subset of patients with ALPS, too [55, 102]. These "overlap" cases are complicated by autoimmune cytopenias, often multilineage, in >85% of cases [55]. Although few *FAS* gene mutations have been identified among these cases [102], the majority remain geneti-cally unclassified but clinically and immunophenotypically distinct, prompting the hypothesis that these ALPS-CVID overlap syndromes likely result from variable combinations of mutations involving two or more genes, albeit potentially Fas-mediated in some way [55].

Management

General Principles

ES is managed in accordance with the particular autoimmune cytopenias and accompanying symptoms with which a patient presents; and management of AIHA, ITP, and AIN are discussed in detail within their respective sections of this book. However, ES does tend to be a more refractory and chronic disease, often less responsive to frontline therapies used in the single lineage autoimmune cytopenias ITP, AIHA, and AIN [13, 14, 26, 29, 106, 107]. Furthermore, ES which is secondary to an underlying disorder of immune dysregulation such as ALPS warrants a man-agement strategy targeting the primary problem, as well as consideration of the other nuances of therapeutic options, i.e., toxicities or contraindications, in the con-text of the underlying disease. Additionally, as understanding of the pathophysiol-ogy of ES continues to improve, targeted immune therapies are replacing the more non-specific immune modulation strategies of the past.

Frontline management of ES does not differ from that of frontline ITP or AIHA management presenting alone, with the goal of controlling acute symptoms of bleeding or anemia, generally with corticosteroids or with intravenous immuno-globulin (IVIG) in the case of ITP. Children [26] and adults [17] with ES achieve at least partial response to corticosteroid therapy ~80% of the time. These response rates appear to be maintained with repeat steroid courses for relapsed autoimmune cytopenias; however, the chronic relapsing course of autoimmune cytopenias in ES, not to mention longer treatment duration requirements in ES, necessitates consideration of alternate treatment strategies in order to avoid prolonged corticosteroid therapy and accompanying side effects, both short- and long-term [108]. Similarly, the majority of ES patients who respond to frontline IVIG will have short-lived responses, may lose response to these therapies more quickly on repeat treatments [14], and will more than likely have persistent and/or relapsing disease, necessitating second-line therapies [26]. There are many "secondary" immunomodulating treatment options from which to choose, including azathioprine, cyclosporine, danazol, 6-thioguanine (6-TG), tacrolimus, vincristine, cyclophosphamide, splenectomy, alemtuzumab (anti-CD52 antibody), mycophenolate mofetil (MMF), rituximab (anti-CD20 antibody), and more recently rapamycin (sirolimus), and thrombopoietin receptor agonists (TPO-RAs) eltrombopag and romiplostim, among others [28, 109–111], but current advances in the understanding of ES have helped to narrow treatment strategies in the recent years.

Primary Evans Syndrome

For primary ES, with no apparent underlying disorder of immune dysregulation, the most well-studied and efficacious therapies include rituximab, MMF, and other immunomodulatory agents—with an aim toward targeting the global immune dysregulation of ES. Rituximab, an anti-CD20 antibody which causes rapid and targeted B cell depletion, results in a 75–80% initial response rate in children [112, 113] and adults [17] with ES, with a long-term relapse-free response rate ~60% in adults followed for 1–3.5 years [17] and a relapse-free response rate in children varying from 65% [112] down to 36% in those children followed for 6 years [113]. Interestingly, the complete response (CR) rate was significantly higher in children with AIHA alone treated with rituximab (74%) compared to those with ES treated with rituximab (46%); and a 6-year relapse-free survival for children with ES treated with rituximab was significantly lower (36%) than that for children with AIHA alone (53%) [113]. As with all monoclonal antibodies, rituximab carries a risk of infusion reaction. However, infusion reactions are generally mild, with grade 3 or 4 reactions occurring <1–9% of the time [114]. Other concerns related to the use of rituximab include prolonged hypogammaglobulinemia and infection risk following therapy. This is of particular concern in patients with known underlying ALPS, CVID, or other immunodeficiencies (see "Secondary Evans Syndrome" section) but should also be used with appropriate caution and counseling in all ES patients, given that some underlying disorders may take years to evolve.

MMF inactivates inosine monophosphate, a key enzyme in purine synthesis, inhibiting proliferation of T and B lymphocytes, and has been proven very effective in the treatment of ES, resulting in ~80% response rate in all patients with ES [115]. Importantly, the response seen with MMF is sustainable, allowing for the avoidance of less desirable treatment strategies or prolonged steroid exposure in many ES patients [106, 115, 116]. MMF is well-tolerated in general, although the most common treatment-limiting toxicities are cytopenias (leukopenia, neutropenia, anemia) and GI toxicities (diarrhea, abdominal pain, and transaminitis).

In the case of chronic or refractory ITP not controlled with systemic immunomodulation, TPO-RAs eltrombopag and romiplostim may be used, although ideal therapeutic options in the setting of ES are directed at the underlying immunopathology. Both eltrombopag [110, 117–120] and romiplostim [111, 121, 122] have shown excellent efficacy in the treatment of chronic and/or refractory ITP, with response rates ~80%, decreased bleeding events, improved health-related quality of life, and favorable adverse event profiles. However, patients receiving TPO-RA therapy should still be closely monitored for development of adverse events, including thrombosis (with both agents), transaminitis and potential cataract formation (with eltrombopag), and development of neutralizing antibodies (with romiplostim).

Secondary Evans Syndrome

Evans syndrome which is identified to be secondary to ALPS, an ALPS-related disorder, CVID, systemic autoimmune disease, or another disorder of immune dysregulation, requires careful strategization when considering treatment options. For example, while rituximab is generally an excellent treatment option for patients with refractory autoimmune cytopenias in ES, the response rate in patients with ALPS is 58%, as compared to a response rate of 76% in patients with primary ES [106, 112]. Furthermore, the risk of clinically significant hypogammaglobulinemia following rituximab therapy may be disproportionately high in patients with underlying immunodeficiency, including those with ALPS, given that a subset of ALPS patients are predisposed to develop CVID [51]. In one series, complications among ALPS patients treated with rituximab for refractory autoimmune cytopenias included prolonged hypogammaglobulinemia, prolonged impairment and/or absence of antibody responses, and prolonged neutropenia [106]. Therefore, rituximab therapy should generally be avoided in patients with ALPS. Similarly, splenectomy should be avoided in patients with ALPS, as responses in this population are generally short-lived and post-splenectomy toxicities are significantly more pronounced [106, 123–125]. More than 70% of patients with ES related to ALPS will ultimately relapse following splenectomy [125], with median time to relapse of ~1 month in one series but potentially occurring up to several years following splenectomy [14, 125]. More importantly, severe invasive bacterial infections are noted in up to 50% of splenectomized ALPS patients, with higher risk related to a younger age at the time of splenectomy, overall resulting in a bacteremia-related mortality rate ranging from 12–22% in splenectomized ALPS patients [123–125]. This increased susceptibility to invasive bacterial infection among splenectomized ALPS patients appears to correlate with lymphoproliferation and is thought to be caused by accumulation of DNT cells in the spleens of these patients, which interferes with correct localization of marginal zone B cells and results in an anti-polysaccharide IgM antibody production-specific defect [124].

On the other hand, responses to MMF are even better in patients with ALPS-related ES than those obtained in patients with primary ES [115], with 92% sustained response rate documented in ALPS patients treated with MMF for refractory autoimmune cytopenias [106, 116]. Additionally, Teachey and colleagues recently demonstrated that the mTOR inhibitor sirolimus is an effective and safe treatment for autoimmune cytopenias in highly refractory ES patients. Moreover, this medication is effective when used alone, thereby sparing the effects of additional steroid therapy. Significantly, the treatment effect was better among ES patients treated with sirolimus than among those with single lineage autoimmune cytopenias, with particularly excellent activity in ALPS [107]. The cohort of ALPS patients had rapid response in autoimmune cytopenias, durable CR, improvement in lymphoproliferative symptoms, and disappearance of DNT cell populations (with sparing of other lymphocyte populations) as well [107, 109]. The most common adverse effects associated with sirolimus therapy were grade 1–2 mucositis and elevations of triglyceride and cholesterol levels, with rarer events including hypertension, headache, acne, sun sensitivity, and exacerbation of gastroesophageal reflux; but with an overall good safety and tolerability profile [107]. Given these findings, sirolimus is now considered as an earlier treatment option in ALPS patients who require chronic therapy [107].

Even as ES therapies are evolving toward more mechanistically driven approaches (i.e., targeting lymphocyte dysregulation with MMF and sirolimus in ALPS) and away from the broader empiric immunosuppressive approaches, work remains ongoing toward further honing more targeted approaches to therapy. Some of the genetically novel ALPS-related disorders now being described provide good examples for targeted therapeutic possibilities. For example, in the ALPS-like syndrome driven by *NRAS* mutations (RALD), RAS-inactivating drugs such as farnesyltransferase inhibitors [73] or other therapeutics directed at blocking ERK or RAS which are currently under development could be useful in the future [74]. For CTLA-4 haploinsufficiency, the immunoglobulin-CTLA-4 fusion protein abatacept is available for use in restoring the immunosuppressive activity of CTLA-4. This drug has been reported to improve autoimmune manifestations and restore regulatory T cell function, as evidenced by an increase in FoxP3 expression in one case of CTLA-4 haploinsufficiency [126]. Furthermore, Lo et al. recently reported excellent clinical response to abatacept in LRBA-deficient patients, corroborating the hypothesis that LRBA is necessary to regulate the potent inhibitory immune regulator CTLA-4, and highlighting the potential for CTLA-4 restorative therapy in both of these conditions [91]. Another excellent example for the potential use of targeted therapies is PI3KD syndrome, given that hyperactivation of the PI3K-Akt-mTOR pathway is implicated in the pathology of this disease, and there is a readily available and safe medication which targets mTOR inhibition—rapamycin or sirolimus. When trialed in vivo, rapamycin was not only shown to decrease ribosomal protein s6 phosphorylation [127] but was also shown to restore naïve T cell percentages, decrease CD8$^+$ T cell levels, and restore normal proliferative responses of the T cells, essentially

restoring a more normal balance of naïve, effector, and memory $CD8^+$ T cell populations [86]. Additionally, clinical improvement as demonstrated by amelioration of
lymphoproliferative symptoms was demonstrated in these patients [86]. Furthermore,
in vitro studies utilizing the newer selective PI3Kδ inhibitor leniolisib, or CDZ173,
resulted in decreased Akt and s6 phosphorylation [127]; and early clinical trials
have shown similarly encouraging results, demonstrating a dose-dependent suppression of PI3Kδ pathway hyperactivation as measured by decreased phosphorylation of Akt and s6 in patient cells, along with improvement in immunophenotypical
and clinical features among patients with PI3KD syndrome [128]. Theoretically,
STAT1 gain-of-function mutations and resultant excess STAT1 activation could be
reduced by blocking the upstream IFN-γ receptor-associated JAK1 and JAK2; and
in actuality, use of the JAK1/2 inhibitor ruxolitinib did in fact decrease hyperre-
sponsiveness to IFN, normalize T_H1 and follicular T-helper cell responses, improve
T_H17 differentiation, and ultimately result in resolution of clinical mucocutaneous
candidiasis and life-threatening autoimmune cytopenias in a patient with STAT1
gain-of-function mutation [96]. In a patient with STAT3 gain-of-function mutation,
the use of a small molecule Bcl-2 inhibitor, ABT-737, which targets the Bcl-2
homology 3 (BH3) domain of Bcl-2, resulted in restoration of apoptosis in patient
cells with constitutively activated STAT3 [101]. Meanwhile, given the IL-6 elevation in STAT3 gain-of-function mutations, which prolongs STAT3 phosphorylation,
the anti-IL-6 antibody tocilizumab was also trialed in a similar patient, resulting in
T_H17 cell normalization and clinical improvement in the patient's RA and AIHA
[99]. These are a collection of examples in which targeted therapies may result in
improved outcomes for these secondary ES patients in the future.

An ancillary consideration in secondary ES pertains to the increased risk for
secondary malignancy and the need for careful surveillance in this population of
patients. Although the increased risk for lymphoma in ALPS is not definitively
established [11], most data suggest ~5–10% risk for secondary lymphomas in ALPS
patients [29]. These lymphomas are most common in patients with *FAS* mutations
[29], especially dominant negative intracellular mutations [52], with a lifetime risk
of developing non-Hodgkin lymphoma cited at 14 times greater than that expected
in the general population and for Hodgkin lymphoma, 51 times greater than that
expected in the general population among patients with germline *FAS* mutations
[129]. Additionally, CVID patients carry a higher risk of developing lymphomas as
well [56], particularly when CVID is complicated by lymphoproliferation [43].
CVID-associated lymphomas are most commonly non-Hodgkin's B cell lymphomas [43]; and the risk is higher when TACI mutations are involved [64].

ES therapy must be individualized, as some patients may need chronic therapy
for recalcitrant symptomatic disease, while some patients may require only intermittent therapy for occasional symptomatic disease flares [28, 29]. For example,
patients with CVID receiving replacement doses of IVIG may respond to treatment
doses of IVIG when complications related to autoimmune cytopenias arise [29].
Meanwhile, patients with systemic autoimmune disease are not expected to respond
like either the primary or secondary ES populations described here, as their autoimmune cytopenias fall within the constellation of findings related to their systemic

disease, and treatment should be aimed toward the driving disease pathology, following which autoimmune cytopenias will generally respond alongside the other autoimmune manifestations of disease. In general, invasive therapies such as splenectomy, and certainly hematopoietic stem cell transplant, should be reserved for multi-treatment-refractory and severely symptomatic ES patients.

Conclusion

ES is a descriptive diagnosis, defining a condition in which two or more autoimmune cytopenias occur in one patient, either simultaneously or sequentially. Disease course is generally more chronic, severe, and treatment-refractory in ES than in isolated autoimmune cytopenias, likely due to the complex underlying immune dysregulation. Immunopathology in ES can generally be ascribed to a disturbance in lymphocyte development or function, such that the immune balance is tipped toward autoreactivity; and the genetic and biological drivers of immune dysregulation are now being identified in ~50% of ES cases. At this time, however, ES remains a diagnosis of exclusion, and a thorough investigation for underlying etiologies should be completed prior to making this diagnosis, especially given that treatment strategies may differ significantly for secondary ES.

References

1. Al Ghaithi I, Wright NAM, Breakey VR, Cox K, Warias A, Wong T, et al. Combined autoimmune cytopenias presenting in childhood. Pediatr Blood Cancer. 2016;63:292–8.
2. Wiseman BK, Doan CA. Primary splenic neutropenia; a newly recognized syndrome closely related to congenital hemolytic icterus and essential thrombocytopenic purpura. Ann Intern Med. 1942;16:1097.
3. Rogers MH, Hall BE. Primary splenic neutropenia. Arch Intern Med. 1945;75:192.
4. Fisher JA. The cryptogenic acquired hemolytic anemias. Quart J Med. 1947;16:245.
5. Dameshek W, Estren S. Spleen and hypersplenism. New York: Grune & Stratton; 1948.
6. Evans RS, Duane RT. Acquired hemolytic anemia; the relation of erythrocyte antibody production to activity of the disease; the significance of thrombocytopenia and leukopenia. Blood. 1949;4(11):1196–213.
7. Evans RS, Takahashi K, Duane RT, Payne R, Liu C. Primary thrombocytopenic purpura and acquired hemolytic anemia; evidence for a common etiology. AMA Arch Intern Med. 1951;87(1):48–65.
8. Ghosh S, Seidel MG. Editorial: current challenges in immune and other acquired cytopenias of childhood. Front Pediatr. 2016;4:3.
9. Canale VC, Smith CH. Chronic lymphadenopathy simulating malignant lymphoma. J Pediatr. 1967;70(6):891–9.
10. Drappa J, Vaishnaw AK, Sullivan KE, Chu JL, Elkon KB. Fas gene mutations in the Canale-Smith syndrome, an inherited lymphoproliferative disorder associated with autoimmunity. N Engl J Med. 1996;335(22):1643–9.
11. Teachey D. New advances in the diagnosis and treatment of autoimmune lymphoproliferative syndrome. Curr Opin Pediatr. 2012;24:1–8.

12. Pui CH, Wilimas J, Wang W. Evans syndrome in childhood. J Pediatr. 1980;97(5):754–8.
13. Wang WC. Evans syndrome in childhood: pathophysiology, clinical course, and treatment. Am J Pediatr Hematol Oncol. 1988;10(4):330–8.
14. Mathew P, Chen G, Wang W. Evans syndrome: results of a national survey. J Pediatr Hematol Oncol. 1997;19(5):433–7.
15. Aladjidi N, Leverger G, Leblanc T, Quitterie Picat M, Michel G, Bertrand Y, et al. New insights into childhood autoimmune hemolytic anemia: a French national observational study of 265 children. Haematologica. 2011;96(5):655–63.
16. Aladjidi N, Fernandes H, Leblanc T, Vareliette A, Rieux-Laucat F, Bertrand Y, et al. Evans syndrome in children: long-term outcome in a prospective French national observational cohort. Front Pediatr. 2015;3:79.
17. Michel M, Chanet V, Dechartres A, Morin AS, Piette JC, Cirasino L, et al. The spectrum of Evans syndrome in adults: new insight into the disease based on the analysis of 68 cases. Blood. 2009;114(15):3167–72.
18. Terrell DR, Beebe LA, Vesely SK, Neas BR, Segal JB, George JN. The incidence of immune thrombocytopenic purpura in children and adults: a critical review of published reports. Am J Hematol. 2010;85(3):174.
19. Yong M, Schoonen WM, Li L, Kanas G, Coalson J, Mowat F, et al. Epidemiology of paediatric immune thrombocytopenia in the General Practice Research Database. Br J Haematol. 2010;149(6):855–64.
20. Segal JB, Powe NR. Prevalence of immune thrombocytopenia: analyses of administrative data. J Thromb Haemost. 2006;4(11):2377–83.
21. Schoonen WM, Kucera G, Coalson J, Li L, Rutstein M, Mowat F, et al. Epidemiology of immune thrombocytopenic purpura in the General Practice Research Database. Br J Haematol. 2009;145(2):235–44.
22. Aladjidi N, Jutand MA, Beaubois C, Fernandes H, Jeanpetit J, Coureau G, et al. Reliable assessment of the incidence of childhood autoimmune hemolytic anemia. Pediatr Blood Cancer. 2017;64:e26683.
23. Gehrs BC, Friedberg RC. Autoimmune haemolytic anemia. Am J Hematol. 2002;69(4):258–71.
24. Roumier M, Loustau V, Guillaud C, Languille L, Mahevas M, Khellaf M, et al. Characteristics and outcome of warm autoimmune hemolytic anemia in adults: new insights based on a single-center experience with 60 patients. Am J Hematol. 2014;89(9):150–5.
25. Cines DB, McMillan R. Management of adult idiopathic thrombocytopenic purpura. Annu Rev Med. 2005;56:425–42.
26. Miano M. How I manage Evans syndrome and AIHA cases in children. Br J Haematol. 2016;172:524–34.
27. Sipurzynski J, Fahrner B, Kerbl R, Crazzolara R, Jones N, Ebetsberger G, et al. Management of chronic immune thrombocytopenia in children and adolescents: lessons from an Austrian national cross-sectional study of 81 patients. Semin Hematol. 2016;53(S1):S43–7.
28. Norton A, Roberts I. Management of Evans syndrome. Br J Haematol. 2005;132:125–37.
29. Teachey DT, Lambert MP. Diagnosis and management of autoimmune cytopenias in childhood. Pediatr Clin N Am. 2013;60(6):1489–511.
30. Teachey DT, Manno CS, Axsom KM, Andrews T, Choi JK, Greenbaum BH, et al. Unmasking Evans syndrome: T-cell phenotype and apoptotic response reveal autoimmune lymphoproliferative syndrome (ALPS). Blood. 2005;105(6):2443–8.
31. Seif AE, Manno CS, Sheen C, Grupp SA, Teachey DT. Identifying autoimmune lymphoproliferative syndrome in children with Evans syndrome: a multi-institutional study. Blood. 2010;115(11):2142–5.
32. Savaşan S, Warrier I, Buck S, Kaplan J, Ravindranath Y. Increased lymphocyte Fas expression and high incidence of common variable immunodeficiency disorder in childhood Evans' syndrome. Clin Immunol. 2007;125(3):224–9.
33. Seidel MG. Autoimmune and other cytopenias in primary immunodeficiencies: pathomechanisms, novel differential diagnoses, and treatment. Blood. 2014;124(15):2337–44.

34. Li E, Grimes AB, Rider NL, Mahoney DH, Fleisher TA, Shearer WT. Diagnostic dilemma: ALPS versus Evans syndrome. Clin Immunol. 2017;183:247–8.
35. Watanabe-Fukunaga R, Brannan CI, Copeland NG, Jenkins NA, Nagata S. Lymphoproliferative disorder in mice explained by defects in Fas antigen that mediates apoptosis. Nature. 1992;356(6367):314–7.
36. Sneller MC, Straus SE, Jaffe ES, Jaffe JS, Fleisher TA, Stetler-Stevenson M, et al. A novel lymphoproliferative/autoimmune syndrome resembling murine lpr/gld disease. J Clin Invest. 1992;90(2):334–41.
37. Takahashi T, Tanaka M, Brannan CI, Jenkins NA, Copeland NG, Suda T, et al. Generalized lymphoproliferative disease in mice, caused by a point mutation in the Fas ligand. Cell. 1994;76(6):969–76.
38. Rieux-Laucat F, Le Deist F, Hivroz C, Roberts IA, Debatin KM, Fischer A, et al. Mutations in Fas associated with human lymphoproliferative syndrome and autoimmunity. Science. 1995;268(5215):1347–9.
39. Fisher GH, Rosenberg FJ, Straus SE, Dale JK, Middleton LA, Lin AY, et al. Dominant interfering Fas gene mutations impair apoptosis in a human autoimmune lymphoproliferative syndrome. Cell. 1995;81(6):935–46.
40. Sneller MC, Wang J, Dale JK, Strober W, Middleton LA, Choi Y, et al. Clinical, immunologic, and genetic features of an autoimmune lymphoproliferative syndrome associated with abnormal lymphocyte apoptosis. Blood. 1997;89(4):1341–8.
41. Oliveira JB, Bleesing JJ, Dianzani U, Fleisher TA, Jaffe ES, Lenardo MJ, et al. Revised diagnostic criteria and classification for the autoimmune lymphoproliferative syndrome (ALPS): report from the 2009 NIH International Workshop. Blood. 2010;116(14):e35–40.
42. Wang J, Cunningham-Rundles C. Treatment and outcome of autoimmune hematologic disease in common variable immunodeficiency (CVID). J Autoimmun. 2005;25(1):57–62.
43. Chapel H, Lucas M, Lee M, Bjorkander J, Webster D, Grimbacher B, et al. Common variable immunodeficiency disorders: division into distinct clinical phenotypes. Blood. 2008;112(2):277–86.
44. Boileau J, Mouillot G, Gerard L, Carmagnat M, Rabian C, Oksenhendler E, et al. Autoimmunity in common variable immunodeficiency: correlation with lymphocyte phenotype in the French DEFI study. J Autoimmun. 2011;36:25–32.
45. Resnick ES, Moshier EL, Godbold JH, Cunningham-Rundles C. Morbidity and mortality in common variable immune deficiency over 4 decades. Blood. 2012;119(7):1650.
46. Gathmann B, Mahlaoui N, Ceredih L, Gerard E, Oksenhendler K, Warnatz I, et al. European Society for Immunodeficiencies Registry Working. Clinical picture and treatment of 2212 patients with common variable immunodeficiency. J Allergy Clin Immunol. 2014;134:116–26.
47. Feuille EJ, Anooshiravani N, Sullivan KE, Fuleihan RL, Cunningham-Rundles C. Autoimmune cytopenias and associated conditions in CVID: a report from the USIDNET Registry. J Clin Immunol. 2017;38(1):28–34. https://doi.org/10.1007/s10875-017-0456-9. [Epub ahead of print].
48. Michel M, Chanet V, Galicier L, Ruivard M, Levy Y, Hermine O, et al. Autoimmune thrombocytopenia purpura and common variable immunodeficiency: analysis of 21 cases and review of the literature. Medicine (Baltimore). 2004;83(4):254–63.
49. Straus SE, Sneller M, Lenardo MJ, Puck JM, Strober W. An inherited disorder of lymphocyte apoptosis: the autoimmune lymphoproliferative syndrome. Ann Intern Med. 1999;130:591–601.
50. Ohga S, Nomura A, Takahata Y, Ihara K, Takada H, Wakiguchi H, et al. Dominant expression of interleukin 10 but not interferon gamma in CD4(-)CD8(-)alphabeta T cells of autoimmune lymphoproliferative syndrome. Br J Haematol. 2002;119(2):535–8.
51. Teachey DT, Seif AE, Grupp SA. Advances in the management and understanding of autoimmune lymphoproliferative syndrome (ALPS). Br J Haematol. 2010;148:205–16.
52. Kuehn HS, Caminha I, Niemela JE, Rao VK, Davis J, Fleisher TA, et al. FAS haploinsufficiency is a common disease mechanism in the human autoimmune lymphoproliferative syndrome. J Immunol. 2011;186(10):6035–43.

53. Magerus-Chatinet A, Neven B, Stolzenberg MC, Daussy C, Arkwright PD, Lanzarotti N, et al. Onset of autoimmune lymphoproliferative syndrome (ALPS) in humans as a consequence of genetic defect accumulation. J Clin Invest. 2011;121(1):106–12.
54. Clementi R, Dagna L, Dianzani U, Dupré L, Dianzani I, Ponzoni M, et al. Inherited perforin and Fas mutations in a patient with autoimmune lymphoproliferative syndrome and lymphoma. N Engl J Med. 2004;351(14):1419–24.
55. Campagnoli MF, Garbarini L, Quarello P, Garelli E, Carando A, Baravalle V, et al. The broad spectrum of autoimmune lymphoproliferative disease: molecular bases, clinical features and long-term follow-up in 31 patients. Haematologica. 2006;91(4):538–41.
56. Maglione PJ. Autoimmune and lymphoproliferative complications of common variable immunodeficiency. Curr Allergy Asthma Rep. 2016;16(3):19.
57. Ameratunga R, Brewerton M, Slade C, Jordan A, Gillis D, Steele R, et al. Comparison of diagnostic criteria for common variable immunodeficiency disorder. Front Immunol. 2014;5:415.
58. Wehr C, Kivioja T, Schmitt C, Ferry B, Witte T, Eren E, et al. The EUROclass trial: defining subgroups in common variable immunodeficiency. Blood. 2008;111(1):77–85.
59. Carter CR, Aravind G, Smalle NL, Cole JY, Savic S, Wood PM. CVID patients with autoimmunity have elevated T cell expression of granzyme B and HLA-DR and reduced levels of Treg cells. J Clin Pathol. 2013;66(2):146–50.
60. Genre J, Errante PR, Kokron CM, Toldeo-Barros M, Camara NO, Rizzo LV. Reduced frequency of CD4(+)CD25(HIGH)FOXP3(+) cells and diminished FOXP3 expression in patients with common variable immunodeficiency: a link to autoimmunity? Clin Immunol. 2009;132(2):215–21.
61. Meffre E. The establishment of early B cell tolerance in humans: lessons from primary immunodeficiency diseases. Ann N Y Acad Sci. 2011;1246:1–10.
62. von Boehmer H, Melchers F. Checkpoints in lymphocyte development and autoimmune disease. Nat Immunol. 2010;11(1):14–20.
63. Salzer U, Chapel HM, Webster AD, Pan-Hammarström Q, Schmitt-Graeff A, Schlesier M, et al. Mutations in TNFRSF13B encoding TACI are associated with common variable immunodeficiency in humans. Nat Genet. 2005;37(8):820–8.
64. Castigli E, Wilson SA, Garibyan L, Rachid R, Bonilla F, Schneider L, et al. TACI is mutant in common variable immunodeficiency and IgA deficiency. Nat Genet. 2005;37(8):829–34.
65. Warnatz K, Wehr C, Dräger R, Schmidt S, Eibel H, Schlesier M, et al. Expansion of CD19(hi) CD21(lo/neg) B cells in common variable immunodeficiency (CVID) patients with autoimmune cytopenia. Immunobiology. 2002;206(5):502–13.
66. Isnardi I, Ng YS, Menard L, Meyers G, Saadoun D, Srdanovic I, et al. Complement receptor 2/CD21- human naïve B cells contain mostly autoreactive unresponsive clones. Blood. 2010;115(24):5026–36.
67. Zhang L, Wu X, Wang L, Li J, Chen H, Zhao Y, et al. Clinical features of systemic lupus erythematosus patients complicated with Evans syndrome: a case-control, single center study. Medicine (Baltimore). 2016;95(15):e3279.
68. Newman K, Owlia MB, El-Hemaidi I, Akhtari M. Management of immune cytopenias in patients with systemic lupus erythematosus—old and new. Autoimmun Rev. 2013;12(7):784–91.
69. Kuwana M, Okazaki Y, Kajihara M, Kaburaki J, Miyazaki H, Kawakami Y, et al. Autoantibody to c-Mpl (thrombopoietin receptor) in systemic lupus erythematosus: relationship to thrombocytopenia with megakaryocytic hypoplasia. Arthritis Rheum. 2002;46:2148–59.
70. Cines DB, Liebman H, Stasi R. Pathobiology of secondary immune thrombocytopenia. Semin Hematol. 2009;46(1 Suppl 2):S2–14.
71. Nakamura M, Tanaka Y, Satoh T, Kawai M, Hirakata M, Kaburaki J, et al. Autoantibody to CD40 ligand in systemic lupus erythematosus: association with thrombocytopenia but not thromboembolism. Rheumatology (Oxford). 2006;45(2):150–6.
72. Liu Y, Chen S, Sun Y, Lin Q, Liao X, Zhang J, et al. Clinical characteristics of immune thrombocytopenia associated with autoimmune disease: a retrospective study. Medicine (Baltimore). 2016;95(50):e5565.

73. Oliveira JB, Bidère N, Niemela JE, Zheng L, Sakai K, Nix CP, et al. NRAS mutation causes a human autoimmune lymphoproliferative syndrome. Proc Natl Acad Sci U S A. 2007;104(21):8953–8.
74. Niemela J, Lu L, Fleisher TA, Davis J, Caminha I, Natter M, et al. Somatic *KRAS* mutations associated with a human nonmalignant syndrome of autoimmunity and abnormal leukocyte homeostasis. Blood. 2011;117:2883–6.
75. Chun HJ, Zheng I, Ahmad M, Wang J, Speirs CK, Siegel RM, et al. Pleiotropic defects in lymphocyte activation caused by caspase-8 mutations lead to human immunodeficiency. Nature. 2002;419(6905):395–9.
76. Shiota M, Yang X, Kubokawa M, Morishima T, Tanaka K, Mikami M, et al. Somatic mosaicism for a NRAS mutation associates with disparate clinical features in RAS-associated leukoproliferative disease: a report of two cases. J Clin Immunol. 2015;35(5):454–8.
77. Malumbres M, Barbacid M. RAS oncogenes: the first 30 years. Nat Rev Cancer. 2003;3(6):459–65.
78. Dianzani U, Bragardo M, DiFranco D, Alliaudi C, Scagni P, Buonfiglio D, et al. Deficiency of the Fas apoptosis pathway without Fas gene mutations in pediatric patients with autoimmunity/lymphoproliferation. Blood. 1997;89(8):2871–9.
79. Ramenghi U, Bonissoni S, Migliaretti G, DeFranco S, Bottarel F, Gambaruto C, et al. Deficiency of the Fas apoptosis pathway without Fas gene mutations is a familial trait predisposing to development of autoimmune diseases and cancer. Blood. 2000;95(10):3176–82.
80. Schubert D, Bode C, Kenefeck B, Hou TZ, Wing JB, Kennedy A, et al. Autosomal dominant immune dysregulation syndrome in humans with CTLA4 mutations. Nat Med. 2014;20(12):1410–6.
81. Kuehn HS, Ouyang W, Lo B, Deenick EK, Niemela JE, Avery DT, et al. Immune dysregulation in human subjects with heterozygous germline mutations in CTLA4. Science. 2014;345(6204):1623–7.
82. Kucuk ZY, Charbonnier LM, McMasters RL, Chatila T, Bleesing JJ. CTLA-4 haploinsufficiency in a patient with an autoimmune lymphoproliferative disorder. J Allergy Clin Immunol. 2017;140(3):862–4.
83. Lopez-Herrera G, Tampella G, Pan-Hammarström Q, Herholz P, Trujillo-Vargas CM, Phadwal K, et al. Deleterious mutations in LRBA are associated with a syndrome of immune deficiency and autoimmunity. Am J Hum Genet. 2012;90(6):986–1001.
84. Gámez-Díaz L, August D, Stepensky P, Revel-Vilk S, Seidel MG, Noriko M, et al. The extended phenotype of LPS-responsive beige-like anchor protein (LRBA) deficiency. J Allergy Clin Immunol. 2016;137(1):223–30.
85. Kostel Bal S, Haskologlu S, Serwas NK, Islamoglu C, Aytekin C, Kendirli T, et al. Multiple presentations of LRBA deficiency: a single-center experience. J Clin Immunol. 2017;37(8):790–800.
86. Lucas CL, Kuehn HS, Zhao F, Niemela JE, Deenick EK, Palendira U, et al. Dominant-activating germline mutations in the gene encoding the PI(3)K catalytic subunit p110δ result in T cell senescence and human immunodeficiency. Nat Immunol. 2014;15(1):88–97.
87. Coulter TI, Chandra A, Bacon CM, Babar J, Curtis J, Screaton N, et al. Clinical spectrum and features of activated phosphoinositide 3-kinase δ syndrome: a large patient cohort study. J Allergy Clin Immunol. 2017;139(2):597–606.
88. Consonni F, Dotta L, Todaro F, Vairo D, Badolato R. Signal transducer and activator of transcription gain-of-function primary immunodeficiency/immunodysregulation disorders. Curr Opin Pediatr. 2017;29(6):711–7.
89. Lévy E, Stolzenberg MC, Bruneau J, Breton S, Neven B, Sauvion S, et al. LRBA deficiency with autoimmunity and early onset chronic erosive polyarthritis. Clin Immunol. 2016;168: 88–93.
90. Revel-Vilk S, Fischer U, Keller B, Nabhani S, Gámez-Díaz L, Rensing-Ehl A, et al. Autoimmune lymphoproliferative syndrome-like disease in patients with LRBA mutation. Clin Immunol. 2015;159(1):84–92.

91. Lo B, Zhang K, Lu W, Zheng L, Zhang Q, Kanellopoulou C, et al. Autoimmune disease. Patients with LRBA deficiency show CTLA4 loss and immune dysregulation responsive to abatacept therapy. Science. 2015;349(6246):436–40.
92. Kaech SM, Cui W. Transcriptional control of effector and memory CD8+ T cell differentiation. Nat Rev Immunol. 2012;12(11):749–61.
93. Xu X, Ye L, Araki K, Ahmed R. mTOR, linking metabolism and immunity. Semin Immunol. 2012;24(6):429–35.
94. Alessi DR, James SR, Downes CP, Holmes AB, Gaffney PR, Reese CB, et al. Characterization of a 3-phosphoinositide-dependent protein kinase which phosphorylates and activates protein kinase Balpha. Curr Biol. 1997;7(4):261–9.
95. Liu L, Okada S, Kong XF, Kreins AY, Cypowyj S, Abhyankar A, et al. Gain-of-function human STAT1 mutations impair IL-17 immunity and underlie chronic mucocutaneous candidiasis. J Exp Med. 2011;208(8):1635–48.
96. Weinacht KG, Charbonnier LM, Alrogi F, Plant A, Qiao Q, Wu H, et al. Ruxolitinib reverses dysregulated T helper cell responses and controls autoimmunity caused by a novel signal transducer and activator of transcription 1 (STAT1) gain-of-function mutation. J Allergy Clin Immunol. 2017;139(5):1629–40.
97. Flanagan SE, Haapaniemi E, Russell MA, Caswell R, Allen HL, De Franco E, et al. Activating germline mutations in STAT3 cause early-onset multi-organ autoimmune disease. Nat Genet. 2014;46(8):812–4.
98. Haapaniemi EM, Kaustio M, Rajala HL, van Adrichem AJ, Kainulainen L, Glumoff V, et al. Autoimmunity, hypogammaglobulinemia, lymphoproliferation, and mycobacterial disease in patients with activating mutations in STAT3. Blood. 2015;125(4):639–48.
99. Milner JD, Vogel TP, Forbes L, Ma CA, Stray-Pederson A, Niemela JE, et al. Early-onset lymphoproliferation and autoimmunity caused by germline STAT3 gain-of-function mutations. Blood. 2015;125(4):591–999.
100. Forbes LR, Milner J, Haddad E. Signal transducer and activator of transcription 3: a year in review. Curr Opin Hematol. 2016;23(1):23–7.
101. Nabhani S, Schipp C, Miskin H, Levin C, Postovsky S, Dujovny T, et al. STAT3 gain-of-function mutations associated with autoimmune lymphoproliferative syndrome like disease deregulate lymphocyte apoptosis and can be targeted by BH3 mimetic compounds. Clin Immunol. 2017;181:32–42.
102. Rensing-Ehl A, Warnatz K, Fuchs S, Schlesier M, Salzer U, Draeger R, et al. Clinical and immunological overlap between autoimmune lymphoproliferative syndrome and common variable immunodeficiency. Clin Immunol. 2010;137(3):357–65.
103. Bleesing JJ, Brown MR, Straus SE, Dale JK, Siegel RM, Johnson M, et al. Immunophenotypic profiles in families with autoimmune lymphoproliferative syndrome. Blood. 2001;98(8):2466–73.
104. Caminha I, Fleisher TA, Hornung RL, Dale JK, Niemela JE, Price S, et al. Using biomarkers to predict the presence of FAS mutations in patients with features of the autoimmune lymphoproliferative syndrome. J Allergy Clin Immunol. 2010;125(4):946–9.
105. Iglesias J, Matamoros N, Raga S, Ferrer JM, Mila J. CD95 expression and function on lymphocyte subpopulations in common variable immunodeficiency (CVID); related to increased apoptosis. Clin Exp Immunol. 1999;117(1):138–46.
106. Rao VK, Oliveira JB. How I treat autoimmune lymphoproliferative syndrome. Blood. 2011;118(22):5741–51.
107. Bride KL, Vincent T, Smith-Whitley K, Lambert MP, Bleesing JJ, Seif AE, et al. Sirolimus is effective in relapsed/refractory autoimmune cytopenias: results of a prospective multi-institutional trial. Blood. 2016;127(1):17–28.
108. Fan J, He H, Zhao W, Wang Y, Lu J, Li J, et al. Clinical features and treatment outcomes of childhood autoimmune hemolytic anemia: a retrospective analysis of 68 cases. J Pediatr Hematol Oncol. 2016;38(2):e50–5.

109. Teachey DT, Greiner R, Seif A, Attiyeh E, Bleesing J, Choi J, et al. Treatment with sirolimus results in complete responses in patients with autoimmune lymphoproliferative syndrome. Br J Haematol. 2009;145(1):101–6.
110. Bussel JB, Cheng G, Saleh MN, Psaila B, Kovaleva L, Meddeb B, et al. Eltrombopag for the treatment of chronic idiopathic thrombocytopenic purpura. N Engl J Med. 2007;357: 2237–47.
111. Kuter DJ, Bussel JB, Lyons RM, Pullarkat V, Gernsheimer TB, Senecal FM, et al. Efficacy of romiplostim in patients with chronic immune thrombocytopenic purpura: a double-blind randomised controlled trial. Lancet. 2008;371:395–403.
112. Bader-Meunier B, Aladjidi N, Bellmann F, Monpoux F, Nelken B, Robert A, et al. Rituximab therapy for childhood Evans syndrome. Haematologica. 2007;92(12):1691–4.
113. Ducassou S, Leverger G, Fernandes H, Chambost H, Bertrand Y, Armari-Alla C, et al. Benefits of rituximab as a second-line treatment for autoimmune haemolytic anaemia in children: a prospective French cohort study. Br J Haematol. 2017;177(5):751–8.
114. Rituxan (rituximab) package insert. South San Francisco, CA: Genentech; 2013.
115. Miano M, Ramenghi U, Russo G, Rubert L, Barone A, Tucci F, et al. Mycophenolate mofetil for the treatment of children with immune thrombocytopenia and Evans syndrome. A retrospective data review from the Italian association of paediatric haematology/oncology. Br J Haematol. 2016;175(3):490–5.
116. Rao VK, Dugan F, Dale JK, Davis J, Tretler J, Hurley JK, et al. Use of mycophenolate mofetil for chronic, refractory immune cytopenias in children with autoimmune lymphoproliferative syndrome. Br J Haematol. 2005;129(4):534–8.
117. Bussel JB, Provan D, Shamsi T, Cheng G, Psaila B, Kovaleva L, et al. Effect of Eltrombopag on platelet counts and bleeding during treatment of chronic idiopathic thrombocytopenic purpura: a randomised, double-blind, placebo-controlled trial. Lancet. 2009;373:641–8.
118. Cheng G, Saleh MN, Marcher C, Vasey S, Mayer B, Aivado M, et al. Eltrombopag for management of chronic immune thrombocytopenia (RAISE): a 6-month, randomised, phase 3 study. Lancet. 2011;377:393–402.
119. Bussel JB, Saleh MN, Vasey SY, Mayer B, Arning M, Stone NL. Repeated short-term use of eltrombopag in patients with chronic immune thrombocytopenia (ITP). Br J Haematol. 2013;160:538–46.
120. Saleh MN, Bussel JB, Cheng G, Meyer O, Bailey CK, Arning M, et al. Safety and efficacy of eltrombopag for treatment of chronic immune thrombocytopenia: results of the long-term, open-label EXTEND study. Blood. 2013;121:537–45.
121. Kuter DJ, Rummel M, Boccia R, Macik G, Pabinger I, Selleslag D, et al. Romiplostim or standard of care in patients with immune thrombocytopenia. N Engl J Med. 2010;363(20): 1889–99.
122. Rodeghiero F, Stasi R, Giagounidis A, Viallard JF, Godeau B, Pabinger I, et al. Long-term safety and tolerability of romiplostim in patients with primary immune thrombocytopenia: a pooled analysis of 13 clinical trials. Eur J Haematol. 2013;91:423–36.
123. Neven B, Magerus-Chatinet A, Florkin B, Gobert D, Lambotte O, De Somer L, et al. A survey of 90 patients with autoimmune lymphoproliferative syndrome related to *TNFRSF6* mutation. Blood. 2011;118(18):4798–807.
124. Neven B, Bruneau J, Stolzenberg MC, Meyts I, Magerus-Chatinet A, Moens L, et al. Defective anti-polysaccharide response and splenic marginal zone disorganization in ALPS patients. Blood. 2014;124(10):1597–609.
125. Price S, Shaw PA, Seitz A, Joshi G, Davis J, Niemela JE, et al. Natural history of autoimmune lymphoproliferative syndrome associated with FAS gene mutations. Blood. 2014;123(13):1989–99.
126. Lee S, Moon JS, Lee CR, Kim HE, Baek SM, Hwang S, et al. Abatacept alleviates severe autoimmune symptoms in a patient carrying a de novo variant in CTLA-4. J Allergy Clin Immunol. 2016;137(1):327–30.

127. Notarangelo LD, Fleisher TA. Targeted strategies directed at the molecular defect: toward precision medicine for select primary immunodeficiency disorders. J Allergy Clin Immunol. 2017;139(3):715–23.
128. Rao VK, Webster S, Dalm VASH, Sedivá A, van Hagen PM, Holland S, et al. Effective 'Activated PI3Kδ Syndrome'-targeted therapy with the PI3Kδ inhibitor leniolisib. Blood. 2017;130(21):2307–16. https://doi.org/10.1182/blood-2017-08-801191. [Epub ahead of print].
129. Straus SE, Jaffe ES, Puck JM, Dale JK, Elkon KB, Rösen-Wolff A, et al. The development of lymphomas in families with autoimmune lymphoproliferative syndrome with germline Fas mutations and defective lymphocyte apoptosis. Blood. 2001;98(1):194–200.

Part III
Thrombotic Thrombocytopenic
Purpura (TTP)

Chapter 8
Background and Presentation of Thrombotic Thrombocytopenic Purpura

Clay Cohen

Historical Perspective

The first case of TTP was described in 1924 by Eli Moschcowitz in a 16-year-old female who presented with upper extremity weakness, fever, and pallor. She eventually succumbed to heart failure; and autopsy revealed platelet-rich thrombi in the terminal arterioles and capillaries of various organs [1]. Prior to universal acceptance of the term TTP, the disease process had many different names, including Moschcowitz's disease, thrombocytic acro-angiothrombosis, and platelet thrombosis syndrome. A 1950 review described a rapidly progressive fatal syndrome characterized clinically by vague non-localizing symptoms, fever, purpura, and anemia, with prominent neurological changes. Histologically, widespread occlusive platelet-rich thrombi in arterioles and capillaries with endothelial proliferation were noted as common features [2]. A review of the 271-then reported cases of TTP in 1966 documented the natural history of TTP, including the characteristic pentad of TTP (thrombocytopenic purpura, hemolytic anemia, fever, neurologic manifestations, and renal disease) [3].

A platelet-aggregating factor was inferred in 1979 by Lian et al. as the cause of TTP after noting decreased platelet-aggregating activity when plasma of patients with TTP was incubated with plasma of normal patients [4, 5]. This factor was discovered and described by Moake and associates in 1982 as "unusually large" complexes containing factor VIII (FVIII) and von Willebrand factor (VWF) multimers accumulating in the plasma of patients with chronic relapsing forms of TTP capable of aggregating circulating platelets in a shear-induced manner [6, 7]. Currently referred to as ultra-large (UL)VWF, these endothelial cell secreted multimers were correctly hypothesized to have defective processing resulting in increased platelet

C. Cohen, MD
Department of Pediatric Hematology and Oncology, Baylor College of Medicine,
Houston, TX, USA
e-mail: ctcohen@texaschildrens.org

© Springer International Publishing AG, part of Springer Nature 2018   153
J. M. Despotovic (ed.), *Immune Hematology*,
https://doi.org/10.1007/978-3-319-73269-5_8

agglutination with subsequent vascular ischemia and tissue damage. Moake and colleagues also hypothesized that the defective processing was possibly due to "missing large VIII-vWF depolymerase activity" during clinical relapses. Proteolysis of the VWF polypeptide was later found to be induced when the complexes were exposed to normal plasma in a shear-dependent manner [8]. The protease responsible for processing the large VWF polymers into smaller VWF multimers was discovered in 1996 by two groups and was described as a novel metalloprotease [9, 10]. Nonfamilial TTP was found to be due to an inhibitor of the VWF-cleaving protease by the same two groups in 1998 [11, 12]. A genome-wide analysis performed on four pedigrees affected by familial TTP mapped the genetic locus of this protease to chromosome 9q34, representing the 13th member of the ADAMTS (a disintegrin and metalloproteinase with thrombospondin-1 motifs) family of zinc metalloproteinase genes [13], explaining the enzyme name of ADAMTS13.

Decreased activity of ADAMTS13 can be caused by either a congenital absence or acquired inhibition of the protease. The congenital deficiency of ADAMTS13, referred to as Upshaw-Schulman syndrome (USS) (OMIM #274150), was described by Upshaw and Schulman in two individuals with recurrent episodes of microangiopathic hemolysis and thrombocytopenia that were reversed by the administration of normal plasma [14, 15]. Acquired antibodies that inhibit ADAMTS13 were suspected in cases of TTP in which remission was achieved by immunosuppressive therapy [16, 17].

Prior to the development of therapy, TTP was universally fatal. As understanding of the disease has evolved over time, so has treatment. In 1959, when the majority of patients with TTP were dying within 8 weeks of disease onset and survival beyond 1 year was exceedingly rare, prolonged remission was first achieved by using high-dose corticosteroids [18]. Later in that same year, a case of remission achieved following fresh whole blood transfusion was published [19]. Plasma was identified as the beneficial component of whole blood in 1977 after relapses in chronic TTP were able to be reversed or prevented by fresh frozen plasma transfusions [20]. Plasma exchange was also found to be beneficial in that same year [21]. A randomized controlled trial comparing plasma infusion and plasma exchange, published in 1991, demonstrated a higher and more prolonged survival in the group that received plasma exchange [22].

Incidence

The annual incidence of acquired TTP is greater in adults compared to children under 18 years of age. In adults, TTP with severe, acquired ADAMTS13 deficiency (<10% activity) occurs in 2.17 per 100,000 people per year. Studies have found a sevenfold increased incidence of TTP in black patients compared to non-blacks and a two- to threefold higher incidence in women compared to men [23]. Thrombotic thrombocytopenic purpura is seen in all ages throughout adulthood, with the highest incidence occurring in patients 18–49 years of age. In children under 18 years, the incidence is 0.09 per 100,000 children per year [23]. The age and gender distribution in children is difficult to assess due to the small number of reported cases. There does, however, appear to be a similar gender pattern as seen in adults, with females being affected more than males. In an epidemiologic study, while death from the initial TTP episode was less in children, other characteristics between children and adults were similar, including incidence of TTP relapse following the acute episode (33% of children compared to 36% of adult patients) [23].

The hereditary TTP registry estimates 0.5 to 4 cases of USS per million people in Europe [24]. In patients with a severe constitutional ADAMTS13 deficiency, the age of first acute TTP episode varies. Approximately half of USS patients will have an episode in the first 5 years of their life, considered early onset. The other half may remain asymptomatic until adulthood [25], often with their first TTP event being triggered by pregnancy [26, 27]. Pregnancy is also a risk factor for acquired TTP in addition to unmasking the hereditary form. A cross-sectional analysis of the French national registry for thrombotic microangiopathy evaluated 772 patients with TMA episodes and ADAMTS13 activity less than 10%. Of these patients, 21 (3%) were determined to have the inherited form of TTP, and 565 (73%) were anti-ADAMTS13 IgG positive and determined to have autoimmune acquired TTP. In the 186 remaining patients, no antibody was detected although ADAMTS13 increased to detectable levels in remission, indicating an autoimmune cause of their TTP episodes as opposed to a congenital absence of the protease [28]. The congenital form of TTP is inherited in an autosomal dominant manner with over 75 ADAMTS13 mutations currently reported [29].

Differential Diagnosis

Thrombotic thrombocytopenic purpura (both acquired and hereditary) is a TMA syndrome, a term used to describe a group of disorders characterized by small vessel occlusion by platelet- and fibrin-rich thrombi, resulting in thrombocytopenia, microangiopathic hemolytic anemia, and elevated serum levels of lactate dehydrogenase. The anemia is a result of erythrocyte fragmentation within the microcirculation by partially occlusive platelet aggregates, while the elevated serum lactate dehydrogenase is due to the resulting tissue ischemia and necrosis [30]. The discussion of the differential diagnosis for TTP begins with a description of other syndromes of TMA (Table 8.1).

Shiga Toxin-Mediated Hemolytic-Uremic Syndrome

The hemolytic-uremic syndrome (HUS) is often used to describe two separate syndromes, the Shiga toxin-mediated hemolytic-uremic syndrome (ST-HUS) and complement-mediated TMA (often referred to as "atypical HUS"); and these two

Table 8.1 Differential diagnosis of thrombotic thrombocytopenic purpura

Syndromes of thrombotic microangiopathy (TMA)
– Shiga toxin-mediated hemolytic-uremic syndrome (HUS)
– Complement-mediated TMA (atypical HUS)
– Drug-mediated TMA
– Coagulation-mediated TMA
• Diacylglycerol kinase ε (DGKE) deficiency
• Thrombomodulin dysfunction
Disseminated intravascular coagulation (DIC)
Severe hypertension
Systemic rheumatologic disorders
– Systemic lupus erythematosus
– Antiphospholipid syndrome
– Systemic sclerosis
Evans syndrome
Pregnancy-related conditions
– Preeclampsia/eclampsia
– Hemolysis, elevated liver enzymes, and low platelet (HELLP) syndrome

disorders will be discussed separately. *Escherichia coli* O157 is the most common member of the Shiga toxin-producing organisms, associated with ST-HUS in Europe and the Americas [31]. The term enterohemorrhagic *E. coli* (EHEC) refers to the ability of the organism to induce bloody diarrhea, with or without the development of HUS. Invasive *Streptococcus pneumoniae* infections may also lead to HUS, and *Shigella dysenteriae* type 1 remains a cause of ST-HUS in other countries [32]. The main source of *E. coli* O157 is cattle [33] although other animals including sheep and pigs [34] have been found to act as carriers of the organism as well.

Shiga toxin-producing *E. coli* (STEC) adhere to the mucosal surfaces of colonic epithelial cells, damaging underlying tissue and vasculature via the Shiga exotoxin, leading to bloody diarrhea [30]. Further pro-inflammatory and pro-thrombotic action by Shiga toxin includes inducing VWF secretion from endothelial cells [35]. This promotes platelet adhesion and aggregation to the large VWF multimers, ultimately leading to platelet consumption and thrombocytopenia. Anemia is marked and develops rapidly secondary to intravascular hemolysis. Unlike TTP, ST-HUS is not associated with reduction of plasma ADAMTS13 activity. After entering the intestinal circulation, Shiga toxins attach to glomerular capillary endothelial cells, mesangial cells, and tubular epithelial cells, initiating a sequence of events leading to fibrin thrombi [36–39]. The result is renal injury and often acute renal failure.

The most common age of presentation of ST-HUS in Europe and North America is between ages 1 and 5 years. The time from exposure, often from contaminated foods, water, vegetables, or other food sources, to the onset of bloody diarrhea (which occurs in about 90% of cases) is less than 1 week, frequently 3–4 days. While massive HUS outbreaks have occurred [40], most cases occur sporadically or in small clusters [41]. When HUS develops, the mean length of time from the onset of diarrhea is 4 days, with a range of 1–10 days [32]. In children affected by the

EHEC-associated gastroenteritis, characterized by abdominal pain, fever, and vomiting, in addition to bloody diarrhea, about 85% will have spontaneous resolution without the development of HUS [41].

Management of ST-HUS is mainly supportive. As azotemia develops, maintaining renal perfusion while avoiding fluid overload and electrolyte disturbances is crucial. Hypertension is common, with vasodilators being the preferred agents of treatment due to the potential development of oliguria or anuria with HUS [41]. Dialysis is often indicated due to complications of acute renal failure. While neurological manifestations are part of the clinical pentad of TTP, CNS complications are also key contributors to morbidity and mortality of ST-HUS, as up to 20% of children with STEC-induced HUS may have CNS involvement [42]. Cerebral microvascular thrombi may cause tissue ischemia, with manifestations ranging from confusion and irritability to seizures and coma [43]. Moreover, the combination of thrombocytopenia, hypertension, and azotemia may predispose to intracranial bleeding.

Complement-Mediated TMA

Complement-mediated TMA, also referred to as atypical HUS, is a result of uncontrolled activation of the alternative complement pathway. The cause is defective regulation of the complement system from inhibition of regulatory proteins and complement components including factor H (CFH), factor I (CFI), or membrane cofactor protein (MCP; CD46) due to inherited defects or acquired antibodies [44–48]. Gain-of-function mutations in the genes coding C3 and factor B produce similar effects [46, 49]. The result is enhanced formation of the C3 convertase (C3bBb), increasing the formation of the C5b-9 terminal complement complex (or membrane attack complex). The effect of complement activation is uncontrolled platelet and neutrophil activation, endothelial cell injury, and the development of glomerular capillary and arteriole thrombi. The damage to renal microcirculation and glomerular endothelial cells leads to acute kidney injury [50, 51].

Unlike TTP, there is no specific laboratory test that can diagnose complement-mediated TMA at this time, as normal plasma levels of complement factors H, B, I, C3, and C4 do not exclude the diagnosis [52]. Genetic mutations in complement-regulating factors are found in 40–60% of patients with complement-mediated TMA [53, 54]. Genetic variations, when found, may be clinically relevant as patients with MCP mutations have a better prognosis and outcome with kidney transplantation in comparison to patients with CFH and CFI mutations [55]. Many of the complement mutations causing TMA are heterozygous, having variable penetrance as many affected family members are asymptomatic. Point mutations in the gene coding complement CFH occur in 25–30% of complement-mediated TMA with over 80 different mutations identified [56]. These mutations may result in rapid progression to renal failure with a high risk of relapse after renal transplant [57]. Autoantibodies to CFH occur in 6–10% of atypical HUS cases, often presenting before 16 years of age with a clinical course characterized by clinical relapses [56, 58].

Acute kidney injury and hypertension are the prominent clinical manifestations of complement-mediated TMA. The clinical characteristics used in a prospective phase 2 trial evaluating the C5 monoclonal antibody eculizumab in patients with atypical hemolytic-uremic syndrome included thrombocytopenia, impaired renal function (elevated creatinine), ADAMTS13 activity >5%, and evidence of hemolysis (elevated LDH, decreased haptoglobin, or schistocytes), excluding those patients with evidence of a Shiga toxin-producing *E. coli* infection [59]. Morbidity and mortality of complement-mediated TMA are high, with a 25% mortality rate during the acute phase and up to 50% progressing to end-stage renal failure [55].

Previously the approach to treatment of TMA included plasma exchange. Those patients with complement-mediated TMA, as opposed to TTP, respond poorly to this treatment, frequently progressing to end-stage renal failure (although there may be efficacy in FH deficiency) [60, 61]. Currently treatment is centered on eculizumab, a humanized monoclonal antibody that binds to C5, preventing the formation of C5a and C5b, thereby decreasing the production of the membrane attack complex, C5b-9 [59, 60]. Those with genetic variants in C5 may not respond to eculizumab [62]. Widespread use of this therapy is currently limited due to high cost, and moreover, pretreatment meningococcal vaccination is important due to the increased risk of infection with eculizumab [63].

Drug-Mediated TMA

Drugs can cause a picture of TMA via immunologic reactions or in a toxic dose-related manner [52]. The first drug to be associated with TMA was quinine, initially described in 1980 [64]. Quinine was found to induce TMA through the development of platelet-reactive antibodies, red blood cell and granulocyte antibodies were also found [65]. These antibodies are thought to cause TMA through endothelial cell activation, capable of causing clinical relapses upon reexposure to the drug [66, 67]. The US Food and Drug Administration issued a ban on over-the-counter use for quinine, previously commonly used for treatment or prevention of nocturnal leg cramps, in 1994. Quetiapine [68] and gemcitabine [69] have also been demonstrated to cause TMA with repeated exposure. The antiplatelet drugs ticlopidine [70] and clopidogrel [71] have both been connected to the development of TTP. The majority of episodes of TTP developed within 2 weeks of clopidogrel initiation, while events with ticlopidine were delayed in comparison. In kidney transplant patients, use of sirolimus, in association with decreased vascular endothelial growth factor, is causative of TMA [72]. Other medications that have been implicated in episodes of TMA include mitomycin; pre-bone marrow therapy conditioning regimens including combinations of cyclosporine, etoposide, teniposide, cytarabine, and carmustine; and total body irradiation [73, 74]. Episodes of TMA have been demonstrated after solid-organ and small-bowel transplantation as well [75, 76]. Recently intravenous use of the oral long-acting opioid oxymorphone hydrochloride has been associated with episodes of microangiopathic hemolytic anemia and acute kidney injury [77–79].

Disorders of Vitamin B$_{12}$ Metabolism

Cobalamin (Cb1) , also known as vitamin B$_{12}$, is an essential water-soluble compound [80]. The most common disorder of vitamin B$_{12}$ metabolism is methylmalonic aciduria and homocystinuria, cobalamin C (Cb1C) complementation type (MMACHC) disease, accounting for about 80% of cases [52, 80]. Cobalamin is a cofactor for two enzymes: methionine synthase (converting homocysteine to methionine) and methylmalonyl-CoA mutase (converting methylmalonyl-CoA to succinyl-CoA) [81]. Cobalamin C disease results in elevated homocysteine and methylmalonic acid, with a decrease in methionine. Elevated homocysteine levels lead to endothelial cell injury, increased platelet activation and consumption, and coagulation via increased expression of tissue factor, coagulation factors V and XII, with decreased expression of thrombomodulin and antithrombin III [82]. Renal TMA may be seen as a result. A review of 36 patients with Cb1C defects and renal disease revealed common features of intravascular hemolysis, hematuria, and proteinuria; biopsies when available were consistent with TMA (demonstrating endothelial damage and glomerular fibrin thrombi). The age of presentation varied, although infantile onset occurred in 44% of patients. Neurological and neurocognitive manifestations are commonly seen, including failure to thrive, developmental delay, and hypotonia. Treatment with parenteral hydroxycobalamin has been demonstrated to improve renal function [83], although chronic kidney disease with hypertension and proteinuria is seen [80].

Coagulation-Mediated TMA

Autosomal recessive mutations in the gene coding for diacylglycerol kinase ε (DGKE) have been linked to episodes of TMA [84, 85]. Unlike cases of complement-mediated TMA, DGKE encodes an intracellular enzyme with no known effect on the complement system. Rather, it is involved in the activation of protein kinase C (PKC), which has roles in production of both pro- and anti-thrombotic factors in endothelial cells [86–91]. Activation of PKC also leads to the downregulation of the VEGF receptor in podocytes, which has been associated with TMA [92, 93]. DGKE has been located in endothelial cells, platelets, and podocytes; and loss of function results in a pro-thrombotic state due to increased production of VWF, plasminogen activator inhibitor-1, platelet-activating factor, and tissue factor [84]. Patients commonly presented within the first year of life with microangiopathic hemolytic anemia, thrombocytopenia, and acute renal failure. Biopsies were consistent with chronic TMA. Complement-regulatory treatments are ineffective, and renal transplantation may be an option for affected patients [94].

Defects in the thrombomodulin gene (*THBD*) have been found to cause atypical hemolytic-uremic syndrome. Thrombomodulin is a ubiquitous transmembrane endothelial cell glycoprotein that accelerates the activation of protein C, which suppresses thrombin generation [95, 96]. Thrombomodulin also acts as a negative regulator of the complement system via CFI-mediated inactivation of C3b and through accelerated C3a and C5a inactivation. One study identified mutations in the gene encoding thrombomodulin in approximately 5% of 152 studied cases of atypical hemolytic-uremic syndrome [95].

Other non-TMA disorders share characteristics and therefore may be confused with TTP. Specifically, the combination of thrombocytopenia and microangiopathic hemolytic anemia (evidence of hemolysis with schistocytosis) can be seen in disseminated intravascular coagulation (DIC), the pregnancy complications of pre-eclampsia/eclampsia and HELLP syndrome (*h*emolysis, *e*levated *l*iver enzymes, and *l*ow *p*latelets), severe hypertension, systemic rheumatologic disorders (including systemic lupus erythematosus, antiphospholipid syndrome, systemic sclerosis), and Evans syndrome (combination of autoimmune thrombocytopenia and autoimmune hemolysis).

Clinical Presentation

Thrombotic thrombocytopenic purpura has classically been defined by a pentad of clinical signs and symptoms: thrombocytopenia, microangiopathic hemolytic anemia, neurologic abnormalities, renal failure, and fever. In reality, however, TTP does not often manifest with the "classic pentad," as only 5% of the Oklahoma TTP-HUS registry presented in this way [97]. The laboratory triad of thrombocytopenia, schistocytosis, and elevated lactate dehydrogenase is enough to suggest TTP [22, 30, 98]. The thrombocytopenia may be severe, frequently below 20,000 cells/μL, and may parallel the reduction in ADAMTS13 activity at the time of presentation, as ADAMTS13 activity <10% is often associated with a lower platelet count [99]. Plasma ADAMTS13 activity in healthy adults typically ranges from 50 to 178% of normal [30]. Intravascular erythrocyte fragmentation is a result of the inability of erythrocytes to traverse through the platelet-adhering ULVWF strings in microcirculation. This fragmentation is represented by schistocytes on the peripheral blood smear. Reticulocytosis and nucleated red blood cells are also frequently seen in the peripheral blood as the bone marrow responds to the brisk hemolysis. The elevation of serum lactate dehydrogenase is largely the result of subsequent ischemic or necrotic tissue rather than erythrocyte lysis, and 64% of patients have evidence of organ ischemia at the time of diagnosis [30, 100]. Coagulation studies are typically normal at acute presentation, although may become abnormal with increased tissue necrosis, tissue factor exposure, and DIC development [30]. In the neonatal period, patients with congenital TTP may present with severe hyperbilirubinemia [101].

In addition to the Oklahoma TTP-HUS registry, the French national registry for thrombotic microangiopathy [100] has added to the understanding of the natural history of TTP. Between the two patient cohorts, features of the initial TTP episode included fever in 23–36%, neurological abnormalities (including headache, confusion, coma, seizures, stroke, or transient neurological defects) in 40–66%, gastrointestinal symptoms in 69%, impaired renal function in 42%, and cardiac disorder in 7%. Many of the symptoms of acute TTP are likely secondary to tissue ischemia. Patients who do not present with neurological changes at the time of diagnosis may go on to develop new symptoms during the course of their treatment. In rare cases, TTP may initially manifest as thrombotic episodes such as cardiac thrombosis or cerebral vascular accident prior to the development of hematological manifestations [102]. Acute pancreatitis has been reported as a precipitating event for episodes of TTP, implicating the marked inflammation caused by pancreatitis as a triggering event for TTP [103]. The thrombocytopenia of TTP results in bleeding symptoms in about half of acute cases [97]. The risk of tissue ischemia and damage as a result of microthrombi, however, are far greater than the risk of hemorrhagic complications. Jaundice may develop as a result of the microangiopathic hemolytic anemia.

Cardiac consequences of TTP may be under-reported. One retrospective review of 41 patients with TTP found 22 patients with troponin- T levels above 0.05 µg/L, indicating myocardial necrosis associated with microvascular thrombi. Only 12 of the 22 patients reported cardiac symptoms, while 8 complained of chest pain [104]. Microvascular occlusions affecting the cardiac conducting system may result in rhythm abnormalities and sudden death [105–107]. One autopsy study revealed that the most common immediate cause of death in TTP was cardiac in origin, due to a combination of myocardial ischemia, infarction, or microvascular occlusion [108]. The 2001–2010 Nationwide Inpatient Sample database of adult patients ($\geq$18 years) revealed an in-hospital mortality rate of 11.1%, with a 5.7% acute myocardial infarction rate [109]. Pulmonary involvement in acute TTP has been rarely described and, if present, may suggest an alternative diagnosis [110].

Both congenital and acquired TTP may present with the initial episode during pregnancy, with an incidence of 1 in every 25,000 pregnancies [111]. The UK Thrombotic Thrombocytopenic Purpura Registry described the largest cohort of women with congenital and acquired TTP relating to pregnancy [112]. In this group of patients, 66% of women that presented with TTP during pregnancy or immediately postpartum had previously undiagnosed congenital TTP. The majority of presentations were after 30 weeks gestational age, differing from previous data suggesting that the second trimester was the most common time period for presentation [113]. The outcome of pregnancy in women presenting with either congenital or acquired TTP is dependent on the gestational age at presentation, with pregnancy loss occurring more often in the second trimester compared to the third [112]. The most common symptoms in pregnancy-associated congenital TTP were proteinuria, elevated blood pressure, headache, transient ischemic attacks, and blurred vision. In acquired episodes, acute collapse, pulmonary embolism, and abdominal and chest pain were additional presenting symptoms. The presentation of TTP during pregnancy may lead to a delay in diagnosis and treatment due to the overlap in symptoms seen in TTP, preeclampsia, and HELLP syndrome [111].

Initial Evaluation/Workup

Due to the high morbidity and mortality of TTP, early recognition of the disorder is critical for patient outcome. Patients presenting with their first acute episode of TTP are often previously healthy and may complain of nonspecific systemic symptoms as previously discussed. In cases of thrombocytopenia with anemia, evaluation of the peripheral smear is essential. With evidence of microangiopathic hemolytic anemia, specifically schistocytosis (having at least one fragmented red blood cell per high powered field) [56], TTP should be at the top of the differential diagnosis. In a study of six patients with TTP, the mean schistocyte count was 8.3% of red blood cells with a range of 1.0–18.4% of red cells [114]. The median platelet count is typically 10,000–30,000 cells/μL, although mild to severe cases may present with platelet levels from 80,000 to 1,000 cells/μL, respectively. Median hemoglobin levels at presentation are typically 8–10 g/dL [56, 98]. Beyond the complete blood count (CBC), laboratory evaluation (Table 8.2) should include reticulocyte count, coagulation studies, including D-dimers, fibrin degradation products, prothrombin time (PT), partial thromboplastin time (PTT), and fibrinogen levels to differentiate TTP from DIC. Acute TTP should have a normal coagulation profile, which will be markedly abnormal in DIC. Direct antiglobulin, or Coombs, testing is typically negative. Decreased serum haptoglobin along with an elevated reticulocyte count and bilirubin in the setting of anemia is also consistent with the intravascular hemolysis of TTP. Lactate dehydrogenase levels will be elevated representing ischemic or necrotic tissue cells.

While determining the ADAMTS13 level is an important step in confirming the diagnosis, initiation of treatment for presumed TTP should not wait on the laboratory result, as results of ADAMTS13 activity assays are often not readily available. Inhibitors to ADAMTS13 may be detected by mixing the patient plasma with normal plasma and determining the resultant ADAMTS13 activity [115]. ADAMTS13

Table 8.2 Laboratory workup and findings in acute TTP

Complete blood count (CBC)	Thrombocytopenia and anemia
ADAMTS13 activity	Decreased (often below 10% of normal)
Lactate dehydrogenase	Elevated
Serum creatinine	Normal to elevated
Coagulation studies (PT, PTT, fibrinogen, D-dimers, fibrin degradation products)	Normal (may be abnormal with development of secondary DIC)
Peripheral blood smear	Schistocytosis, reticulocytosis, nucleated red blood cells, helmet cells
Haptoglobin	Decreased
Bilirubin	Elevated (specifically indirect bilirubin)

activity assays are reported as the protease percent activity compared to normal individuals. Severe deficiency is defined as an ADAMTS13 activity of <10% and is typically confirmatory of the diagnosis [116]. Normal levels of ADAMTS13 activity are ≥50%; levels between 10 and 50% are considered low and may occur in systemic inflammatory disorders (such as malignancy [117, 118], sepsis [119, 120], or HELLP syndrome [121]). Levels above 10% may be possible for patients with TTP who have been transfused plasma containing blood products, which contain ADAMTS13. One study that used ADAMTS13 activity >11% as criteria to either not initiate or to discontinue plasma exchange did not demonstrate a difference in mortality between the two groups [122]. This is consistent with the previous observations that platelet consumption does not occur when ADAMTS13 activity is greater than 10% in TTP [123].

Head imaging, computed tomography (CT) or magnetic resonance imaging (MRI), may be warranted as patients are at an increased risk for intracranial hemorrhage and infarction. The most common abnormality in a series of TTP patients who underwent brain imaging was posterior reversible encephalopathy syndrome (PRES), with many of the brain imaging findings being reversible with treatment of TTP [124]. Obtaining serum chemistries and creatinine is important as acute kidney injury is common, although progression to anuria and acute renal failure is rare compared to other TMA syndromes [52]. An infectious workup, including blood cultures, is warranted in patients exhibiting signs of a systemic infection. Similarly, in patients with diarrhea, especially bloody diarrhea, stool cultures and testing for Shiga toxin and Shiga toxin-producing organisms are important to rule out HUS. Serologic testing for systemic lupus erythematosus and other autoimmune disease may be indicated in certain cases (i.e., acquired TTP), especially prior to the initiation of plasma exchange.

Conclusion

As our understanding of TTP has improved, so have treatments and patient outcomes. It remains critical for physicians to have a high index of suspicion for TTP in cases of thrombocytopenia and hemolytic anemia even without the presence of the clinical pentad of TTP. If TTP is high on the differential diagnosis, efforts should be made toward initiating therapy in order to avoid devastating consequences of delayed treatment.

References

1. Moschcowitz E. Hyaline thrombosis of the terminal arterioles and capillaries: a hitherto undescribed disease. Proc N Y Pathol Soc. 1924;24:21–4.
2. Gore I. Disseminated arteriolar and capillary platelet thrombosis; a morphologic study of its histogenesis. Am J Pathol. 1950;26(1):155–75, incl 4 pl

3. Amorosi E, Ultmann J. Thrombotic thrombocytopenic purpura: report of 16 cases and review of the literature. Medicine. 1966;45(2):139–60.
4. Lian EC, Harkness DR, Byrnes JJ, Wallach H, Nunez R. Presence of a platelet aggregating factor in the plasma of patients with thrombotic thrombocytopenic purpura (TTP) and its inhibition by normal plasma. Blood. 1979;53(2):333–8.
5. Lian EC. The role of increased platelet aggregation in TTP. Semin Thromb Hemost. 1980;6(4):401–15.
6. Moake JL, Rudy CK, Troll JH, Weinstein MJ, Colannino NM, Azocar J, et al. Unusually large plasma factor VIII:von Willebrand factor multimers in chronic relapsing thrombotic thrombocytopenic purpura. N Engl J Med. 1982;307(23):1432–5.
7. Moake JL, Turner NA, Stathopoulos NA, Nolasco LH, Hellums JD. Involvement of large plasma von Willebrand factor (vWF) multimers and unusually large vWF forms derived from endothelial cells in shear stress-induced platelet aggregation. J Clin Invest. 1986;78(6):1456–61.
8. Tsai HM, Sussman II, Nagel RL. Shear stress enhances the proteolysis of von Willebrand factor in normal plasma. Blood. 1994;83(8):2171–9.
9. Furlan M, Robles R, Lammle B. Partial purification and characterization of a protease from human plasma cleaving von Willebrand factor to fragments produced by in vivo proteolysis. Blood. 1996;87(10):4223–34.
10. Tsai HM. Physiologic cleavage of von Willebrand factor by a plasma protease is dependent on its conformation and requires calcium ion. Blood. 1996;87(10):4235–44.
11. Furlan M, Robles R, Galbusera M, Remuzzi G, Kyrle PA, Brenner B, et al. von Willebrand factor-cleaving protease in thrombotic thrombocytopenic purpura and the hemolytic-uremic syndrome. N Engl J Med. 1998;339(22):1578–84.
12. Tsai HM, Lian EC. Antibodies to von Willebrand factor-cleaving protease in acute thrombotic thrombocytopenic purpura. N Engl J Med. 1998;339(22):1585–94.
13. Levy GG, Nichols WC, Lian EC, Foroud T, McClintick JN, McGee BM, et al. Mutations in a member of the ADAMTS gene family cause thrombotic thrombocytopenic purpura. Nature. 2001;413(6855):488–94.
14. Upshaw JD Jr. Congenital deficiency of a factor in normal plasma that reverses microangiopathic hemolysis and thrombocytopenia. N Engl J Med. 1978;298(24):1350–2.
15. Schulman I, Pierce M, Lukens A, Currimbhoy Z. Studies on thrombopoiesis. I. A factor in normal human plasma required for platelet production; chronic thrombocytopenia due to its deficiency. Blood. 1960;16:943–57.
16. Furlan M, Robles R, Solenthaler M, Lammle B. Acquired deficiency of von Willebrand factor-cleaving protease in a patient with thrombotic thrombocytopenic purpura. Blood. 1998;91(8):2839–46.
17. Moake JL, Rudy CK, Troll JH, Schafer AI, Weinstein MJ, Colannino NM, et al. Therapy of chronic relapsing thrombotic thrombocytopenic purpura with prednisone and azathioprine. Am J Hematol. 1985;20(1):73–9.
18. Burke HA Jr, Hartmann RC. Thrombotic thrombocytopenic purpura two patients with remission associated with the use of large amounts of steroids. AMA Arch Intern Med. 1959;103(1):105–12.
19. Rubinstein MA, Kagan BM, Macgillviray MH, Merliss R, Sacks H. Unusual remission in a case of thrombotic thrombocytopenic purpura syndrome following fresh blood exchange transfusions. Ann Intern Med. 1959;51:1409–19.
20. Byrnes JJ, Khurana M. Treatment of thrombotic thrombocytopenic purpura with plasma. N Engl J Med. 1977;297(25):1386–9.
21. Bukowski RM, King JW, Hewlett JS. Plasmapheresis in the treatment of thrombotic thrombocytopenic purpura. Blood. 1977;50(3):413–7.
22. Rock GA, Shumak KH, Buskard NA, Blanchette VS, Kelton JG, Nair RC, et al. Comparison of plasma exchange with plasma infusion in the treatment of thrombotic thrombocytopenic purpura. Canadian Apheresis Study Group. N Engl J Med. 1991;325(6):393–7.

23. Reese JA, Muthurajah DS, Kremer Hovinga JA, Vesely SK, Terrell DR, George JN. Children and adults with thrombotic thrombocytopenic purpura associated with severe, acquired Adamts13 deficiency: comparison of incidence, demographic and clinical features. Pediatr Blood Cancer. 2013;60(10):1676–82.
24. Mansouri Taleghani M, von Krogh AS, Fujimura Y, George JN, Hrachovinova I, Knobl PN, et al. Hereditary thrombotic thrombocytopenic purpura and the hereditary TTP registry. Hamostaseologie. 2013;33(2):138–43.
25. Furlan M, Lammle B. Aetiology and pathogenesis of thrombotic thrombocytopenic purpura and haemolytic uraemic syndrome: the role of von Willebrand factor-cleaving protease. Best Pract Res Clin Haematol. 2001;14(2):437–54.
26. Moatti-Cohen M, Garrec C, Wolf M, Boisseau P, Galicier L, Azoulay E, et al. Unexpected frequency of Upshaw-Schulman syndrome in pregnancy-onset thrombotic thrombocytopenic purpura. Blood. 2012;119(24):5888–97.
27. von Auer C, von Krogh AS, Kremer Hovinga JA, Lammle B. Current insights into thrombotic microangiopathies: thrombotic thrombocytopenic purpura and pregnancy. Thromb Res. 2015;135(Suppl 1):S30–3.
28. Mariotte E, Azoulay E, Galicier L, Rondeau E, Zouiti F, Boisseau P, et al. Epidemiology and pathophysiology of adulthood-onset thrombotic microangiopathy with severe ADAMTS13 deficiency (thrombotic thrombocytopenic purpura): a cross-sectional analysis of the French national registry for thrombotic microangiopathy. Lancet Haematol. 2016;3(5):e237–45.
29. Lotta LA, Garagiola I, Palla R, Cairo A, Peyvandi F. ADAMTS13 mutations and polymorphisms in congenital thrombotic thrombocytopenic purpura. Hum Mutat. 2010;31(1):11–9.
30. Moake JL. Thrombotic microangiopathies. N Engl J Med. 2002;347(8):589–600.
31. Pennington H. Escherichia coli O157. Lancet. 2010;376(9750):1428–35.
32. Mark TC. Enterohaemorrhagic Escherichia coli and Shigella dysenteriae type 1-induced haemolytic uraemic syndrome. Pediatr Nephrol. 2008;23(9):1425–31.
33. Hussein HS, Bollinger LM. Prevalence of Shiga toxin-producing Escherichia coli in beef cattle. J Food Prot. 2005;68(10):2224–41.
34. Milnes AS, Stewart I, Clifton-Hadley FA, Davies RH, Newell DG, Sayers AR, et al. Intestinal carriage of verocytotoxigenic Escherichia coli O157, Salmonella, thermophilic Campylobacter and Yersinia enterocolitica, in cattle, sheep and pigs at slaughter in Great Britain during 2003. Epidemiol Infect. 2008;136(6):739–51.
35. Huang J, Motto DG, Bundle DR, Sadler JE. Shiga toxin B subunits induce VWF secretion by human endothelial cells and thrombotic microangiopathy in ADAMTS13-deficient mice. Blood. 2010;116(18):3653–9.
36. Chandler WL, Jelacic S, Boster DR, Ciol MA, Williams GD, Watkins SL, et al. Prothrombotic coagulation abnormalities preceding the hemolytic-uremic syndrome. N Engl J Med. 2002;346(1):23–32.
37. Robinson LA, Hurley RM, Lingwood C, Matsell DG. *Escherichia coli* verotoxin binding to human paediatric glomerular mesangial cells. Pediatr Nephrol. 1995;9(6):700–4.
38. Lingwood CA. Verotoxin-binding in human renal sections. Nephron. 1994;66(1):21–8.
39. Hughes AK, Stricklett PK, Kohan DE. Shiga toxin-1 regulation of cytokine production by human glomerular epithelial cells. Nephron. 2001;88(1):14–23.
40. Bell BP, Goldoft M, Griffin PM, Davis MA, Gordon DC, Tarr PI, et al. A multistate outbreak of *Escherichia coli* O157:H7-associated bloody diarrhea and hemolytic uremic syndrome from hamburgers. The Washington experience. JAMA. 1994;272(17):1349–53.
41. Tarr PI, Gordon CA, Chandler WL. Shiga-toxin-producing *Escherichia coli* and haemolytic uraemic syndrome. Lancet. 2005;365(9464):1073–86.
42. Fakhouri F, Zuber J, Fremeaux-Bacchi V, Loirat C. Haemolytic uraemic syndrome. Lancet. 2017;390(10095):681–96.
43. Bale JF Jr, Brasher C, Siegler RL. CNS manifestations of the hemolytic-uremic syndrome. Relationship to metabolic alterations and prognosis. Am J Dis Child. 1980;134(9):869–72.

44. Fremeaux-Bacchi V, Dragon-Durey MA, Blouin J, Vigneau C, Kuypers D, Boudailliez B, et al. Complement factor I: a susceptibility gene for atypical haemolytic uraemic syndrome. J Med Genet. 2004;41(6):e84.
45. Richards A, Kemp EJ, Liszewski MK, Goodship JA, Lampe AK, Decorte R, et al. Mutations in human complement regulator, membrane cofactor protein (CD46), predispose to development of familial hemolytic uremic syndrome. Proc Natl Acad Sci U S A. 2003;100(22):12966–71.
46. Goicoechea de Jorge E, Harris CL, Esparza-Gordillo J, Carreras L, Arranz EA, Garrido CA, et al. Gain-of-function mutations in complement factor B are associated with atypical hemolytic uremic syndrome. Proc Natl Acad Sci U S A. 2007;104(1):240–5.
47. Ying L, Katz Y, Schlesinger M, Carmi R, Shalev H, Haider N, et al. Complement factor H gene mutation associated with autosomal recessive atypical hemolytic uremic syndrome. Am J Hum Genet. 1999;65(6):1538–46.
48. Dragon-Durey MA, Loirat C, Cloarec S, Macher MA, Blouin J, Nivet H, et al. Anti-factor H autoantibodies associated with atypical hemolytic uremic syndrome. J Am Soc Nephrol. 2005;16(2):555–63.
49. Fremeaux-Bacchi V, Miller EC, Liszewski MK, Strain L, Blouin J, Brown AL, et al. Mutations in complement C3 predispose to development of atypical hemolytic uremic syndrome. Blood. 2008;112(13):4948–52.
50. Sperati CJ, Moliterno AR. Thrombotic microangiopathy: focus on atypical hemolytic uremic syndrome. Hematol Oncol Clin North Am. 2015;29(3):541–59.
51. Greenbaum LA. Atypical hemolytic uremic syndrome. Adv Pediatr. 2014;61(1):335–56.
52. George JN, Nester CM. Syndromes of thrombotic microangiopathy. N Engl J Med. 2014;371(7):654–66.
53. Bresin E, Rurali E, Caprioli J, Sanchez-Corral P, Fremeaux-Bacchi V, Rodriguez de Cordoba S, et al. Combined complement gene mutations in atypical hemolytic uremic syndrome influence clinical phenotype. J Am Soc Nephrol. 2013;24(3):475–86.
54. Nayer A, Asif A. Atypical hemolytic-uremic syndrome: a clinical review. Am J Ther. 2016;23(1):e151–8.
55. Caprioli J, Noris M, Brioschi S, Pianetti G, Castelletti F, Bettinaglio P, et al. Genetics of HUS: the impact of MCP, CFH, and IF mutations on clinical presentation, response to treatment, and outcome. Blood. 2006;108(4):1267–79.
56. Shatzel JJ, Taylor JA. Syndromes of thrombotic microangiopathy. Med Clin North Am. 2017;101(2):395–415.
57. Loirat C, Niaudet P. The risk of recurrence of hemolytic uremic syndrome after renal transplantation in children. Pediatr Nephrol. 2003;18(11):1095–101.
58. Skerka C, Jozsi M, Zipfel PF, Dragon-Durey MA, Fremeaux-Bacchi V. Autoantibodies in haemolytic uraemic syndrome (HUS). Thromb Haemost. 2009;101(2):227–32.
59. Legendre CM, Licht C, Muus P, Greenbaum LA, Babu S, Bedrosian C, et al. Terminal complement inhibitor eculizumab in atypical hemolytic-uremic syndrome. N Engl J Med. 2013;368(23):2169–81.
60. Mannucci PM, Cugno M. The complex differential diagnosis between thrombotic thrombocytopenic purpura and the atypical hemolytic uremic syndrome: laboratory weapons and their impact on treatment choice and monitoring. Thromb Res. 2015;136(5):851–4.
61. Licht C, Weyersberg A, Heinen S, Stapenhorst L, Devenge J, Beck B, et al. Successful plasma therapy for atypical hemolytic uremic syndrome caused by factor H deficiency owing to a novel mutation in the complement cofactor protein domain 15. Am J kidney Dis. 2005;45(2): 415–21.
62. Nishimura J, Yamamoto M, Hayashi S, Ohyashiki K, Ando K, Brodsky AL, et al. Genetic variants in C5 and poor response to eculizumab. N Engl J Med. 2014;370(7):632–9.
63. Benamu E, Montoya JG. Infections associated with the use of eculizumab: recommendations for prevention and prophylaxis. Curr Opin Infect Dis. 2016;29(4):319–29.
64. Webb RF, Ramirez AM, Hocken AG, Pettit JE. Acute intravascular haemolysis due to quinine. N Z Med J. 1980;91(651):14–6.

65. Gottschall JL, Neahring B, McFarland JG, Wu GG, Weitekamp LA, Aster RH. Quinine-induced immune thrombocytopenia with hemolytic uremic syndrome: clinical and serological findings in nine patients and review of literature. Am J Hematol. 1994;47(4):283–9.
66. Glynne P, Salama A, Chaudhry A, Swirsky D, Lightstone L. Quinine-induced immune thrombocytopenic purpura followed by hemolytic uremic syndrome. Am J Kidney Dis. 1999;33(1):133–7.
67. Kojouri K, Vesely SK, George JN. Quinine-associated thrombotic thrombocytopenic purpura-hemolytic uremic syndrome: frequency, clinical features, and long-term outcomes. Ann Intern Med. 2001;135(12):1047–51.
68. Huynh M, Chee K, Lau DH. Thrombotic thrombocytopenic purpura associated with quetiapine. Ann Pharmacother. 2005;39(7–8):1346–8.
69. Saif MW, Xyla V, Makrilia N, Bliziotis I, Syrigos K. Thrombotic microangiopathy associated with gemcitabine: rare but real. Expert Opin Drug Saf. 2009;8(3):257–60.
70. Bennett CL, Weinberg PD, Rozenberg-Ben-Dror K, Yarnold PR, Kwaan HC, Green D. Thrombotic thrombocytopenic purpura associated with ticlopidine. A review of 60 cases. Ann Intern Med. 1998;128(7):541–4.
71. Bennett CL, Connors JM, Carwile JM, Moake JL, Bell WR, Tarantolo SR, et al. Thrombotic thrombocytopenic purpura associated with clopidogrel. N Engl J Med. 2000;342(24):1773–7.
72. Sartelet H, Toupance O, Lorenzato M, Fadel F, Noel LH, Lagonotte E, et al. Sirolimus-induced thrombotic microangiopathy is associated with decreased expression of vascular endothelial growth factor in kidneys. Am J Transpl. 2005;5(10):2441–7.
73. Rabadi SJ, Khandekar JD, Miller HJ. Mitomycin-induced hemolytic uremic syndrome: case presentation and review of literature. Cancer Treat Rep. 1982;66(5):1244–7.
74. Moake JL, Byrnes JJ. Thrombotic microangiopathies associated with drugs and bone marrow transplantation. Hematol Oncol Clin North Am. 1996;10(2):485–97.
75. Singh N, Gayowski T, Marino IR. Hemolytic uremic syndrome in solid-organ transplant recipients. Transpl Int. 1996;9(1):68–75.
76. Humar A, Jessurun J, Sharp HL, Gruessner RW. Hemolytic uremic syndrome in small-bowel transplant recipients: the first two case reports. Transpl Int. 1999;12(5):387–90.
77. Ambruzs JM, Serrell PB, Rahim N, Larsen CP. Thrombotic microangiopathy and acute kidney injury associated with intravenous abuse of an oral extended-release formulation of oxymorphone hydrochloride: kidney biopsy findings and report of 3 cases. Am J Kidney Dis. 2014;63(6):1022–6.
78. Centers for Disease Control and Prevention (CDC). Thrombotic thrombocytopenic purpura (TTP)-like illness associated with intravenous Opana ER abuse—Tennessee, 2012. MMWR Morb Mortal Wkly Rep. 2013;62(1):1–4.
79. Lammle B. Opana ER-induced thrombotic microangiopathy. Blood. 2017;129(7):808–9.
80. Beck BB, van Spronsen F, Diepstra A, Berger RM, Komhoff M. Renal thrombotic microangiopathy in patients with cblC defect: review of an under-recognized entity. Pediatr Nephrol. 2016;32(5):733–41.
81. Koenig JC, Rutsch F, Bockmeyer C, Baumgartner M, Beck BB, Kranz B, et al. Nephrotic syndrome and thrombotic microangiopathy caused by cobalamin C deficiency. Pediatr Nephrol. 2015;30(7):1203–6.
82. Coppola A, Davi G, De Stefano V, Mancini FP, Cerbone AM, Di Minno G. Homocysteine, coagulation, platelet function, and thrombosis. Semin Thromb Hemost. 2000;26(3):243–54.
83. Brunelli SM, Meyers KE, Guttenberg M, Kaplan P, Kaplan BS. Cobalamin C deficiency complicated by an atypical glomerulopathy. Pediatr Nephrol. 2002;17(10):800–3.
84. Lemaire M, Fremeaux-Bacchi V, Schaefer F, Choi M, Tang WH, Le Quintrec M, et al. Recessive mutations in DGKE cause atypical hemolytic-uremic syndrome. Nat Genet. 2013;45(5):531–6.
85. Ozaltin F, Li B, Rauhauser A, An SW, Soylemezoglu O, Gonul II, et al. DGKE variants cause a glomerular microangiopathy that mimics membranoproliferative GN. J Am Soc Nephrol. 2013;24(3):377–84.

86. Pettitt TR, Martin A, Horton T, Liossis C, Lord JM, Wakelam MJ. Diacylglycerol and phosphatidate generated by phospholipases C and D, respectively, have distinct fatty acid compositions and functions. Phospholipase D-derived diacylglycerol does not activate protein kinase C in porcine aortic endothelial cells. J Biol Chem. 1997;272(28):17354–9.
87. Carew MA, Paleolog EM, Pearson JD. The roles of protein kinase C and intracellular Ca2+ in the secretion of von Willebrand factor from human vascular endothelial cells. Biochem J. 1992;286(Pt 2):631–5.
88. Ren S, Shatadal S, Shen GX. Protein kinase C-beta mediates lipoprotein-induced generation of PAI-1 from vascular endothelial cells. Am J Physiol Endocrinol Metab. 2000;278(4):E656–62.
89. Whatley RE, Nelson P, Zimmerman GA, Stevens DL, Parker CJ, McIntyre TM, et al. The regulation of platelet-activating factor production in endothelial cells. The role of calcium and protein kinase C. J Biol Chem. 1989;264(11):6325–33.
90. Herbert JM, Savi P, Laplace MC, Dumas A, Dol F. Chelerythrine, a selective protein kinase C inhibitor, counteracts pyrogen-induced expression of tissue factor without effect on thrombomodulin down-regulation in endothelial cells. Thromb Res. 1993;71(6):487–93.
91. Levin EG, Marotti KR, Santell L. Protein kinase C and the stimulation of tissue plasminogen activator release from human endothelial cells. Dependence on the elevation of messenger RNA. J Biol Chem. 1989;264(27):16030–6.
92. Eremina V, Jefferson JA, Kowalewska J, Hochster H, Haas M, Weisstuch J, et al. VEGF inhibition and renal thrombotic microangiopathy. N Engl J Med. 2008;358(11):1129–36.
93. Hoshi S, Nomoto K, Kuromitsu J, Tomari S, Nagata M. High glucose induced VEGF expression via PKC and ERK in glomerular podocytes. Biochem Biophys Res Commun. 2002;290(1):177–84.
94. Quaggin SE. DGKE and atypical HUS. Nat Genet. 2013;45(5):475–6.
95. Delvaeye M, Noris M, De Vriese A, Esmon CT, Esmon NL, Ferrell G, et al. Thrombomodulin mutations in atypical hemolytic-uremic syndrome. N Engl J Med. 2009;361(4):345–57.
96. Esmon C. Do-all receptor takes on coagulation, inflammation. Nat Med. 2005;11(5):475–7.
97. George JN. How I treat patients with thrombotic thrombocytopenic purpura: 2010. Blood. 2010;116(20):4060–9.
98. Scully M, Hunt BJ, Benjamin S, Liesner R, Rose P, Peyvandi F, et al. Guidelines on the diagnosis and management of thrombotic thrombocytopenic purpura and other thrombotic microangiopathies. Br J Haematol. 2012;158(3):323–35.
99. Kremer Hovinga JA, Vesely SK, Terrell DR, Lammle B, George JN. Survival and relapse in patients with thrombotic thrombocytopenic purpura. Blood. 2010;115(8):1500–11; quiz 662
100. Joly BS, Stepanian A, Leblanc T, Hajage D, Chambost H, Harambat J, et al. Child-onset and adolescent-onset acquired thrombotic thrombocytopenic purpura with severe ADAMTS13 deficiency: a cohort study of the French national registry for thrombotic microangiopathy. Lancet Haematol. 2016;3(11):e537–e46.
101. Schiff DE, Roberts WD, Willert J, Tsai HM. Thrombocytopenia and severe hyperbilirubinemia in the neonatal period secondary to congenital thrombotic thrombocytopenic purpura and ADAMTS13 deficiency. J Pediatr Hematol Oncol. 2004;26(8):535–8.
102. Kalish Y, Rottenstreich A, Rund D, Hochberg-Klein S. Atypical presentations of thrombotic thrombocytopenic purpura: a diagnostic role for ADAMTS13. J Thromb Thrombolysis. 2016;42(2):155–60.
103. Swisher KK, Doan JT, Vesely SK, Kwaan HC, Kim B, Lammle B, et al. Pancreatitis preceding acute episodes of thrombotic thrombocytopenic purpura-hemolytic uremic syndrome: report of five patients with a systematic review of published reports. Haematologica. 2007;92(7):936–43.
104. Hughes C, McEwan JR, Longair I, Hughes S, Cohen H, Machin S, et al. Cardiac involvement in acute thrombotic thrombocytopenic purpura: association with troponin T and IgG antibodies to ADAMTS 13. J Thromb Haemost. 2009;7(4):529–36.

105. James TN, Monto RW. Pathology of the cardiac conduction system in thrombotic thrombo-cytopenic purpura. Ann Intern Med. 1966;65(1):37–43.
106. Ridolfi RL, Hutchins GM, Bell WR. The heart and cardiac conduction system in thrombotic thrombocytopenic purpura. A clinicopathologic study of 17 autopsied patients. Ann Intern Med. 1979;91(3):357–63.
107. Bell MD, Barnhart JS Jr, Martin JM. Thrombotic thrombocytopenic purpura causing sudden, unexpected death—a series of eight patients. J Forensic Sci. 1990;35(3):601–13.
108. Nichols L, Berg A, Rollins-Raval MA, Raval JS. Cardiac injury is a common postmortem finding in thrombotic thrombocytopenic purpura patients: is empiric cardiac monitoring and protection needed? Ther Apher Dial. 2015;19(1):87–92.
109. Balasubramaniyam N, Kolte D, Palaniswamy C, Yalamanchili K, Aronow WS, McClung JA, et al. Predictors of in-hospital mortality and acute myocardial infarction in thrombotic thrombocytopenic purpura. Am J Med. 2013;126(11):1016.e1–7.
110. Nokes T, George JN, Vesely SK, Awab A. Pulmonary involvement in patients with thrombotic thrombocytopenic purpura. Eur J Haematol. 2014;92(2):156–63.
111. Gasparri ML, Bellati F, Brunelli R, Perrone G, Pecorini F, Papadia A, et al. Thrombotic thrombocytopenic purpura during pregnancy versus imitator of preeclampsia. Transfusion. 2015;55(10):2516–8.
112. Scully M, Thomas M, Underwood M, Watson H, Langley K, Camilleri RS, et al. Thrombotic thrombocytopenic purpura and pregnancy: presentation, management, and subsequent pregnancy outcomes. Blood. 2014;124(2):211–9.
113. Martin JN Jr, Bailey AP, Rehberg JF, Owens MT, Keiser SD, May WL. Thrombotic thrombocytopenic purpura in 166 pregnancies: 1955-2006. Am J Obstet Gynecol. 2008;199(2):98–104.
114. Burns ER, Lou Y, Pathak A. Morphologic diagnosis of thrombotic thrombocytopenic purpura. Am J Hematol. 2004;75(1):18–21.
115. Horton TM, Stone JD, Yee D, Dreyer Z, Moake JL, Mahoney DH. Case series of thrombotic thrombocytopenic purpura in children and adolescents. J Pediatr Hematol Oncol. 2003;25(4):336–9.
116. George JN. Measuring ADAMTS13 activity in patients with suspected thrombotic thrombocytopenic purpura: when, how, and why? Transfusion. 2015;55(1):11–3.
117. Mannucci PM, Karimi M, Mosalaei A, Canciani MT, Peyvandi F. Patients with localized and disseminated tumors have reduced but measurable levels of ADAMTS-13 (von Willebrand factor cleaving protease). Haematologica. 2003;88(4):454–8.
118. Bohm M, Gerlach R, Beecken WD, Scheuer T, Stier-Bruck I, Scharrer I. ADAMTS-13 activity in patients with brain and prostate tumors is mildly reduced, but not correlated to stage of malignancy and metastasis. Thromb Res. 2003;111(1–2):33–7.
119. Nguyen TC, Liu A, Liu L, Ball C, Choi H, May WS, et al. Acquired ADAMTS-13 deficiency in pediatric patients with severe sepsis. Haematologica. 2007;92(1):121–4.
120. Ono T, Mimuro J, Madoiwa S, Soejima K, Kashiwakura Y, Ishiwata A, et al. Severe secondary deficiency of von Willebrand factor-cleaving protease (ADAMTS13) in patients with sepsis-induced disseminated intravascular coagulation: its correlation with development of renal failure. Blood. 2006;107(2):528–34.
121. Lattuada A, Rossi E, Calzarossa C, Candolfi R, Mannucci PM. Mild to moderate reduction of a von Willebrand factor cleaving protease (ADAMTS-13) in pregnant women with HELLP microangiopathic syndrome. Haematologica. 2003;88(9):1029–34.
122. Shah N, Rutherford C, Matevosyan K, Shen YM, Sarode R. Role of ADAMTS13 in the management of thrombotic microangiopathies including thrombotic thrombocytopenic purpura (TTP). Br J Haematol. 2013;163(4):514–9.
123. Tsai HM. Untying the knot of thrombotic thrombocytopenic purpura and atypical hemolytic uremic syndrome. Am J Med. 2013;126(3):200–9.
124. Burrus TM, Wijdicks EF, Rabinstein AA. Brain lesions are most often reversible in acute thrombotic thrombocytopenic purpura. Neurology. 2009;73(1):66–70.

Chapter 9
Pathophysiology of Thrombotic Thrombocytopenic Purpura

Sarah E. Sartain

Introduction

The pathophysiologic abnormalities observed in thrombotic thrombocytopenic purpura (TTP) are the result of decreased concentrations of the von Willebrand factor (VWF)-cleaving protease ADAMTS13 (a disintegrin and metalloproteinase with a thrombospondin type 1 motif, member 13) [1–3]. Deficiencies of ADAMTS 13 are secondary to congenital production defects or are acquired secondary to development of an inhibitor antibody directed against the protease [2] and result in microvascular thrombosis and endothelial injury, microangiopathic hemolytic anemia (MAHA), thrombocytopenia, and end-organ damage. This chapter will review the normal function of VWF and ADAMTS13, focus on the mechanisms of TTP pathogenesis, and conclude with review of new concepts in immune-mediated TTP pathophysiology.

Normal Pathophysiology of VWF and ADAMTS13

VWF

VWF is synthesized and stored in endothelial cells and platelets [4–6]. Within the endothelial cell, VWF is packaged into secretory granules, known as Weibel-Palade bodies (WPBs) [7], as multimeric forms called ultra-large VWF (ULVWF); within the platelet, ULVWF is packaged into alpha granules [8]. These multimers are secreted from endothelial cells and platelets in response to a variety of physiologic agonists, including epinephrine, histamine, thrombin, inflammatory cytokines, and

S. E. Sartain, MD
Baylor College of Medicine, Texas Children's Hospital, Houston, TX, USA
e-mail: sesartai@txch.org

© Springer International Publishing AG, part of Springer Nature 2018   171
J. M. Despotovic (ed.), *Immune Hematology*,
https://doi.org/10.1007/978-3-319-73269-5_9

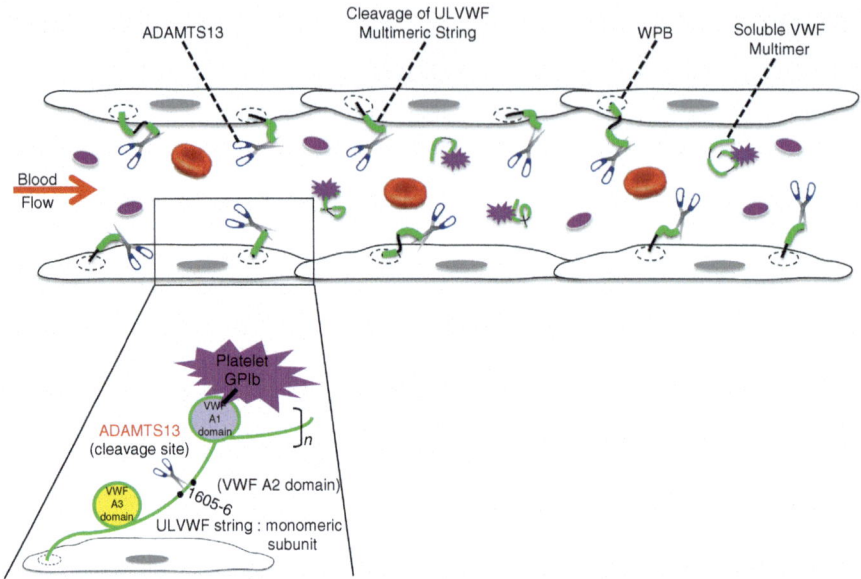

Fig. 9.1 Normal proteolysis of ULVWF multimers by ADAMTS13 in a microvessel (arteriole-capillary). At the site of vascular injury, ULVWF multimers are secreted from WPBs and become anchored to microvascular endothelial cells. Platelets bind to the A1 domain of ULVWF via the GPIb component of the GP Ib/IX/V receptor (see insert). Upon binding, the platelets become activated, leading to platelet aggregation. In normal individuals, periods of shear stress lead to the partial unfolding of endothelial cell-anchored ULVWF multimers, allowing ADAMTS13 cleavage at the Tyr-Met (1605–1606) bond in the A2 domain of VWF, resulting in the release of varying sizes of soluble VWF into the plasma. ADAMTS13: a disintegrin and metalloproteinase with a thrombospondin type 1 motif, member 13; *ULVWF:* ultra-large von Willebrand factor; *WPB:* Weibel-Palade body; *n:* number of VWF multimers. Platelets (purple): round = not activated, spiny = activated. Figure provided by Nancy A. Turner, used with permission.

hormones [9–15]. The VWF protein is composed of several repetitive domains, each with different functional properties [16–18] and containing the binding sites for FVIII, platelet glycoproteins, heparin, collagen, and ristocetin [19–23], as well as the cleavage site for ADAMTS13 [1].

At the site of vascular injury, ULVWF multimers are secreted from WPBs, become anchored to the endothelial cell surface, and bind platelets [24], thereby initiating primary hemostasis (Fig. 9.1). Platelets bind more efficiently to ULVWF multimers than to smaller circulating VWF forms, likely because the binding sites for platelets are more effectively exposed on ULVWF during high shear stress [25–27]. Platelets bind to the first A-domain (A1) of ULVWF [21, 22, 28] via the glycoprotein (GP) Ib component of the GP Ib/IX/V receptor (Fig. 9.1) [25, 29]. Upon binding, the platelets become activated and expose their GP IIb/IIIa complex, leading to platelet aggregation on the multimeric strings and the subendothelium [30].

In circulation, VWF plays an indirect role in secondary hemostasis as a carrier for the factor VIII (FVIII) coagulation protein [31]. It prolongs FVIII half-life by protecting it from proteolytic inactivation by activated protein C and protein S [32–34]. FVIII is synthesized in endothelial cells and packaged within the WPBs along with VWF [35]; it travels in the circulation bound to VWF at the D'D3 domain [20]. FVIII becomes activated (FVIIIa) upon cleavage by thrombin, wherein it is released from VWF and becomes a fully functional cofactor in thrombin generation [33].

ADAMTS13

ADAMTS13 is produced and secreted by endothelial cells, megakaryocytes, and hepatic stellate cells [36–39] and is responsible for cleaving ULVWF multimers anchored to the endothelium. Periods of shear stress lead to the partial unfolding of endothelial cell-anchored ULVWF multimers, allowing ADAMTS13 cleavage at the Tyr-Met (tyrosine 1605–1606 methionine) bond in the second A-domain (A2) of VWF [1, 3, 40, 41], resulting in the release of varying sizes of VWF into the circulation (Fig. 9.1). Soluble VWF coils into a conformation that buries the A2 domain, thereby preventing further VWF cleavage by ADAMTS13 [42, 43].

After secretion from endothelial cells, ADAMTS13 cleaves newly secreted ULVWF multimers within seconds to minutes [44]; however, ULVWF proteolysis is dependent upon the amount of ULVWF and ADAMTS13 secreted by endothelial cells and the processing capacity of ADAMTS13, and alterations in this balance can lead to excessive bleeding or clotting [9].

Pathogenesis of TTP

Endothelial Injury, Microvascular Thrombosis, and Organ Dysfunction

Severe ADAMTS13 deficiency is caused by congenital homozygous or double-heterozygous *ADAMTS13* gene mutations [45] or by acquired production of poly-clonal autoantibodies directed against the metalloprotease [2, 46, 47]. With deficiencies in ADAMTS13 to less than 10% of normal plasma levels [2, 46–48], ULVWF multimers are not cleaved sufficiently, leading to their accumulation on the endothelium [44, 49]. Endothelial cell injury in the microcirculation of patients with TTP is well described. Tissue biopsy from TTP patients reveals endothelial proliferation, endothelial swelling and detachment, and subendothelial hyaline deposits [50, 51]. Early *in vitro* studies demonstrated that addition of plasma from TTP patients to human umbilical vein endothelial cells (HUVECs) in culture resulted in progressive cytoplasmic and nuclear degeneration [50]. More recent studies have found that during acute TTP episodes, markers of endothelial damage such as thrombomodulin, tissue plasminogen activator (TPA), intracellular adhesion molecule-1 (ICAM-1), vascular adhesion molecule-1 (VCAM-1), and endothelial microparticles (EMPs) are released [52–54]. The pathophysiologic mechanisms of this endothelial injury have been difficult to elucidate, and there is continued debate as to whether microthrombi formation is a result or the cause of endothelial injury. Investigators have suggested multiple other mechanisms for the etiology of endothelial damage, including direct endothelial injury by antibodies against endothelial cells [55–58], nitric oxide [59], oxidative stress [60], neutrophil activation [59, 61], and activation of the Fas pathway leading to endothelial cell apoptosis [62, 63].

Disruption of the endothelium secondary to injury results in a high shear stress environment, as well as release of ULVWF multimers from endothelial cell WPBs. ULVWF is more active than normal plasma VWF in promoting platelet adhesion and aggregation secondary to high shear stress [64, 65]. With the excess ULVWF multimeric forms present in TTP, pathologic platelet aggregation occurs (Fig. 9.2). Due to their small size, the microvessels have higher shear stress than larger size vessels, and therefore platelet-VWF microthrombi have a propensity to form in the smaller arterioles and capillaries [66]. While fibrin may be present in small amounts, the microvascular thromboses characteristic of TTP are composed primarily of platelets and VWF [44, 67, 68].

Endothelial injury and microvascular thrombosis lead to impaired organ perfusion and can result in multi-organ failure, likely the most devastating consequence of TTP. The organs most commonly involved are the central nervous system [49, 69–73], kidney [49, 70, 74, 75], heart [76–82], and gastrointestinal tract [69], although autopsies of deceased TTP patients demonstrate microvascular thrombi in almost all organs [69].

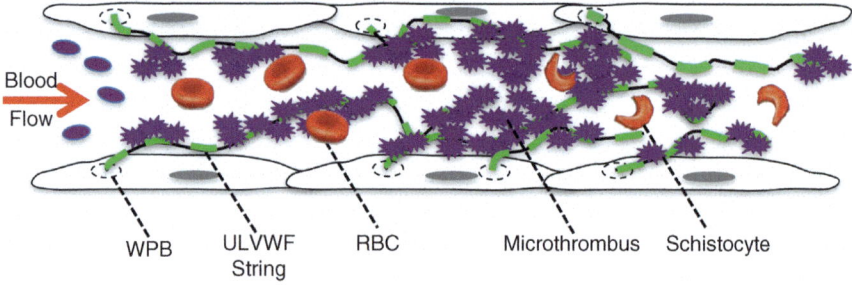

Fig. 9.2 Pathogenesis of TTP in a microvessel. When ADAMTS13 levels are below ~10% of normal in hereditary or autoantibody-mediated TTP, microvascular endothelial cell-anchored ULVWF string cleavage is severely reduced. This results in excessive platelet adherence, activation, and aggregation on the ULVWF multimeric strings, ultimately resulting in formation of platelet-VWF microthrombi. The RBCs are sheared as they flow through the microvessels partially occluded by platelet clumps, producing schistocytes and hemolysis *WPB:* Weibel-Palade body; *ULVWF:* ultra-large von Willebrand factor; RBC: red blood cell. Platelets (purple): round = not activated, spiny = activated. Figure provided by Nancy A Turner, used with permission

Hematologic Findings

The development of systemic microvascular thrombosis leads to MAHA and thrombocytopenia. The proposed mechanism of MAHA is mechanical fragmentation as the red blood cells (RBCs) cross the platelet thrombi (Fig. 9.2) [83]. The presence and degree of MAHA can be assessed by review of the peripheral blood smear, which will demonstrate schistocytes—fragmented RBCs that are irregularly shaped or jagged—reflecting intravascular destruction. Thrombocytopenia is thought to be secondary to platelet activation and consumption by systemic microthrombi formation on ULVWF multimers (Fig. 9.2) .

Antibodies in Acquired TTP

In many cases, the etiology for inhibitory antibody production against ADAMTS13 is unknown. In some patients, infections may trigger autoantibody development, while in others, immune system dysregulation may be the cause [84]. Many autoimmune disorders have been associated with TTP, including systemic lupus erythematosus (SLE), antiphospholipid antibody syndrome, autoimmune vasculitides, Sjogren syndrome, connective tissue disorders, scleroderma, type 1 diabetes mellitus, inflammatory bowel disease, Raynaud syndrome, sarcoidosis, psoriasis, multiple sclerosis, autoimmune hemolytic anemia, autoimmune thyroiditis, primary biliary cirrhosis, and ankylosing spondylitis [85–93], with SLE being most commonly associated [85, 94–97]. The onset of autoimmunity can occur before, during, or after the diagnosis of TTP. A study by Roriz et al. [85] found that the presence of anti-dsDNA antibodies and anti-SSA antibodies at TTP diagnosis was significantly associated with later development of autoimmunity. One case series at Texas Children's Hospital describes the development of SLE in seven out of eight patients initially diagnosed with TTP, leading the authors to conclude that TTP may be an initial manifestation of SLE [98]. During an episode of antibody-mediated acquired TTP, ADAMTS13 levels usually fall to less than 5–10% of normal secondary to plasma IgG antibodies that inhibit the normal function of the enzyme; ADAMTS13 levels most often return to normal after recovery from an acquired TTP episode, but the inhibitory antibodies may persist, leading to relapses or refractory disease [2, 46, 47, 99].

Epitope mapping has determined that most acquired TTP patients possess multiple autoantibodies against ADAMTS13 that bind to several different domains [100–103]; the most frequent epitope region is present within the spacer domain of the protease [101, 102, 104–110]. Not all ADAMTS13 autoantibodies neutralize the protease activity of ADAMTS13 but are thought to alter the function by some other means, i.e., by prohibiting ADAMTS13 binding to various receptors or ligands or by accelerating clearance of ADAMTS13 from the circulation [111, 112]. The anti-ADAMTS13 antibodies that do disrupt the cleavage of VWF do not always cause

TTP [100]; additionally, these antibodies have been detected in up to 18% of patients with non-TTP thrombocytopenia [113]. These observations suggest that TTP onset is multifactorial.

Other Etiologies of Acquired TTP

While autoimmunity is the prevailing cause of TTP, the disorder can be triggered by other entities, including sepsis, liver failure, pancreatitis, pregnancy, infections, HIV, cancer, organ transplant, and drugs. ADAMTS13 levels can be decreased in sepsis, disseminated intravascular coagulation (DIC), and liver disease [66, 114–117]. It is postulated that the acute release of cytokines during an episode of pancreatitis can lead to abundant release of ULVWF multimers from endothelial cells, overwhelming the cleavage capacity of ADAMTS13 [118, 119]. It is also hypothesized that ADAMTS13 may be degraded by pancreatic enzymes [118]. TTP patients with pancreatitis often have ADAMTS13 levels below normal, but rarely to less than 10%, and the presence of inhibitory antibodies is rare [118]. TTP in pregnancy is likely secondary to a combination of increased ULVWF multimer output and decreased ADAMTS13 production that occurs in pregnancy [114, 120], as well as ADAMTS13 autoantibody development. Surprisingly, up to 24% of pregnancy-induced TTP may be secondary to previously undiagnosed congenital ADAMTS13 deficiency [121]. Infections are a well-described trigger for initiation or relapse of TTP [122, 123], possibly secondary to the effect of cytokines or other endothelial cell stimulants present during infection that lead to a surge in the release of ULVWF multimers from endothelial cells [124]. HIV infection is thought to cause TTP through direct infection of the endothelial cells and consumption of ADAMTS13; however, severe ADAMTS13 deficiency has not been commonly identified in HIV patients with TTP [125]. TTP can be the first manifestation of cancer or can be secondary to the chemotherapy given as treatment [126]. A host of drugs have been implicated in the development of TTP, including mitomycin C, cyclosporine and other immunosuppresants, quinine, ticlopidine, clopidogrel, and micafungin [127–132]. The pathogenesis of drug-induced TTP is usually secondary to antibody development to ADAMTS13 or to direct endothelial toxicity by the drug [130, 132].

Newer Concepts in the Pathogenesis of TTP: The Alternative Complement Pathway

Over-activation of the alternative complement pathway (AP) is a pathophysiologic mechanism of atypical hemolytic uremic syndrome (aHUS), another thrombotic microangiopathic disorder with clinical features nearly indistinguishable from TTP. Because of the two distinct mechanisms of disease, aHUS and TTP have been considered distinct entities; however, recent in vitro studies have demonstrated a molecular linkage between ULVWF multimers and AP activation, and case reports have documented complement activation in patients with TTP. These findings suggest a possible role for the AP in the pathogenesis of TTP.

The Alternative Complement Pathway (Fig. 9.3)

The complement system is composed of three pathways—the classical, lectin, and alternative pathways—important in innate immunity and responsible for ridding the body of foreign invaders or damaged tissue. The AP is initiated when complement component C3 is cleaved to C3b upon contact with an activating surface. C3b attaches to the surface [133, 134], factor B (FB) then binds to C3b to form C3bB [135, 136], and factor D (FD) cleaves FB in this complex to form C3bBb, which is known as the C3 convertase [137]. The C3 convertase is stabilized by the binding of factor P (FP, properdin) [138–140]. The Bb in the C3 convertase cleaves C3 to generate additional C3b by an amplification loop; as the ratio of C3b to Bb increases, C3bBbC3b (the C5 convertase) forms and cleaves C5 to C5b [137, 141]. C5b then

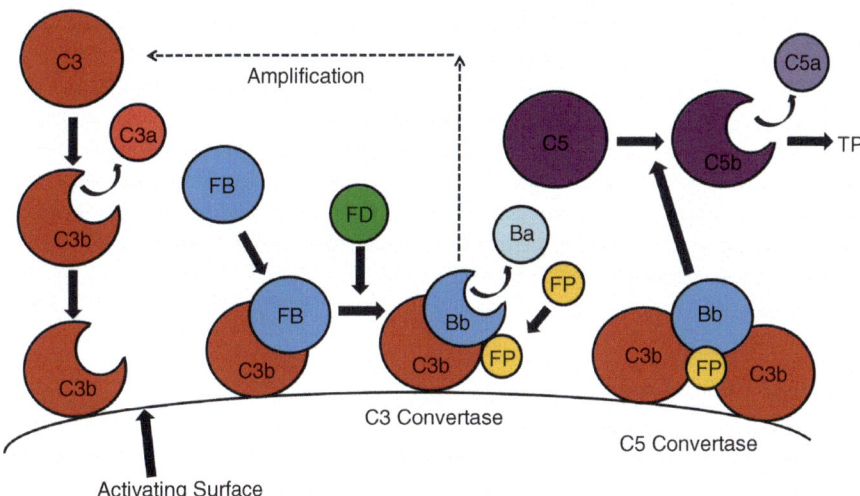

Fig. 9.3 The alternative complement pathway. The AP is initiated when C3b is cleaved from C3 and attaches to an activating surface, releasing a soluble C3a fragment in the process. FB then combines with C3b to form C3bB, and FD cleaves FB in this complex to form C3bBb (C3 convertase), releasing the activation product Ba. The C3 convertase is stabilized by FP. The Bb in C3bBb cleaves C3 to generate additional C3b as part of an amplification loop; as the ratio of C3b to Bb increases, C3bBbC3b (C5 convertase) forms and cleaves C5 to C5b, releasing the C5a fragment. C5b then enters into the terminal complement pathway. *AP:* alternative complement pathway; *FB:* factor B, *FD;* factor D; *FP:* factor P (properdin); *TP:* terminal complement pathway

enters into the terminal complement pathway (TP), where ultimately the membrane attack complex (MAC), capable of inserting into the membranes of foreign invaders, is formed. The AP is regulated by both soluble and cell surface-bound proteins: factor H (FH) and factor I (FI) are soluble inhibitory regulators of the AP, while CD46, CD55, and CD141 are cell surface membrane regulatory proteins [142–149].

AP Activation on ULVWF Strings and the Implications in TTP

In 2013 it was discovered by several groups that AP components bind to ULVWF strings in vitro [150–152]. Experiments performed by Turner et al. [150] demonstrated that ULVWF strings secreted from, and anchored to, HUVECs in culture serve as activating surfaces for the AP. In these experiments, addition of purified proteins to HUVECs was not required because HUVECs, and other endothelial cells, express mRNA for all complement components. They found that C3, FB, FD, FP, and C5 bind to endothelial cell secreted/anchored ULVWF strings in patterns consistent with the assembly of the AP C3 and C5 convertases, resulting in activation of the AP (Fig. 9.4) [150]. Because TTP patients have an abundance of ULVWF multimers secondary to the severe decrease in ADAMTS13, it is conceivable that patients with TTP may also have over-activation of the AP. Further activation of the terminal complement pathway and formation of the MAC in these patients may lead to endothelial injury, and perhaps, microangiopathic hemolytic anemia and schistocyte formation, providing an additional pathophysiologic mechanism for the disease [153]. This pathophysiologic mechanism may explain the conundrum of TTP-like syndromes in patients who have only mild or modest reductions in plasma ADAMTS13 (20–60% of normal): some of these patients may have a heterozygous defect of the *ADAMTS13* gene, resulting in decreased cleavage of ULVWF not sufficient enough to cause the degree of platelet adhesion/aggregation observed in TTP, but adequate enough to cause excessive activation of the AP [153].

Clinical Evidence of AP Activation in TTP

While it is not common practice to evaluate complement parameters in patients with TTP, there is growing evidence that the AP may be over-activated in these patients. In one small series, eight patients with TTP demonstrated evidence of AP activation [154]. A subsequent larger report found that 23 patients with antibody-mediated TTP had evidence of increased activation of all three complement pathways [155]. A larger retrospective study found that 38 patients with acquired TTP had elevations in Bb and C5b-9 (MAC), consistent with AP activation [156]. In a recent study comparing 52 patients with acquired TTP to 30 normal controls, plasma levels of the AP activation product Bb were significantly higher in the TTP patients [157]. There are also case reports of patients with two distinct abnormalities: mutations in,

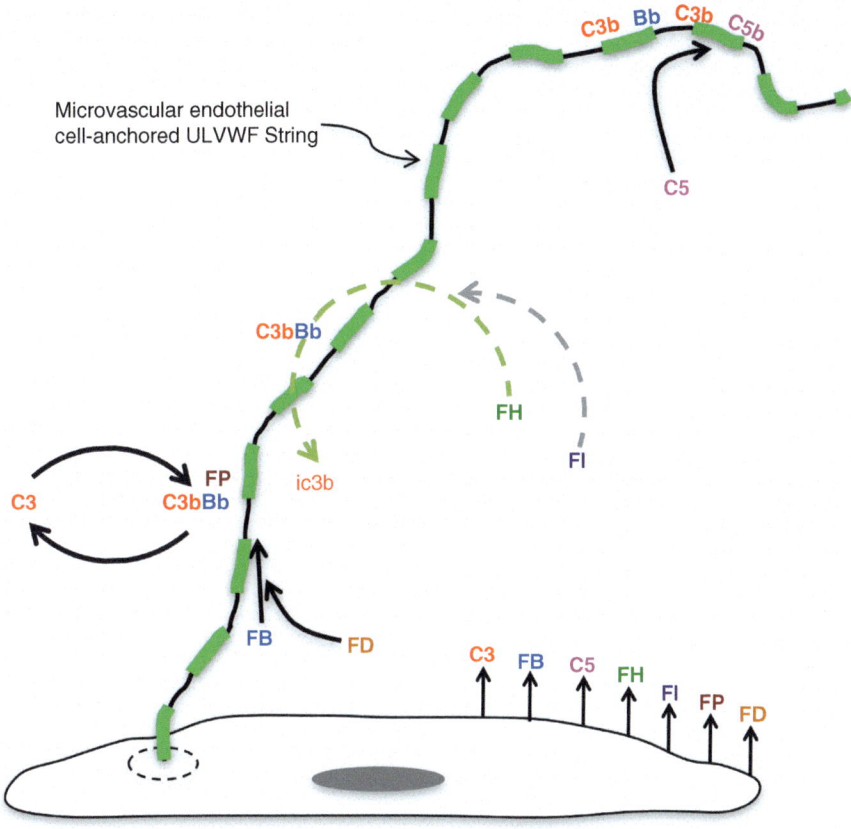

Fig. 9.4 Assembly and activation of the AP on ULVWF multimeric strings secreted by, and anchored to, microvascular endothelial cells. Endothelial cells produce and release AP components and regulators constitutively. Upon stimulation, ULVWF strings are secreted from, and anchor to, microvascular endothelial cells. C3 (as C3b), FB (as Bb), and C5 (as C5b) bind to the anchored ULVWF strings in patterns consistent with the assembly of the C3 and C5 convertases of the AP. FH and FI control AP activation on ULVWF strings by inactivating C3b bound to the strings. *AP:* alternative complement pathway; *FB:* factor B; *ULVWF:* ultra-large von Willebrand factor; *FH:* factor H; *FI:* factor I. Figure provided by Nancy A Turner, used with permission

or autoantibodies to, AP components or regulators with concomitant presence of inhibitory autoantibodies to ADAMTS13 [158, 159]. Evidence for successful therapeutic complement inhibition in TTP is demonstrated by a case report of a patient with ADAMTS13-deficient (<5%) TTP refractory to standard TTP treatment regimens, who was treated with the monoclonal antibody eculizumab [160]. This drug functions by inhibiting cleavage of complement component C5, thereby preventing initiation of the terminal complement pathway and formation of the MAC. While this patient did not have abnormalities in plasma levels of complement components or regulators, he was found to have endothelial deposition of C5b-9 on skin biopsy, prompting use of the anti-complement agent. The patient's platelet count, creatinine, and LDH normalized by day 29, with continued normalization of ADAMTS13 activity by day 54, after eculizumab initiation. These reviews and case reports suggest additional immune-mediated mechanisms for the pathogenesis of TTP, allowing for alternative therapeutic interventions.

Conclusion

In summary, TTP is a devastating disorder characterized by endothelial injury and systemic thrombosis of the microvasculature, ultimately resulting in MAHA, thrombocytopenia, and end-organ failure. The disorder is caused by a severe deficiency of the ADAMTS13 protease, which functions normally to cleave ULVWF multimers attached to microvascular endothelial surfaces. Deficiencies in ADAMTS13 are most commonly secondary to acquired inhibitory autoantibodies to ADAMTS13, although inheritance of *ADAMTS13* gene mutations occurs as well. TTP is generally considered an autoimmune disorder but can also develop secondary to other entities. More recently, evidence has suggested an association between AP activation and TTP pathophysiology, improving the understanding of the pathogenesis of TTP and providing another possible target for therapeutic intervention in immune-mediated TTP.

References

1. Furlan M, Robles R, Lammle B. Partial purification and characterization of a protease from human plasma cleaving von Willebrand factor to fragments produced by in vivo proteolysis. Blood. 1996;87:4223–34.
2. Furlan M, Robles R, Galbusera M, Remuzzi G, Kyrle PA, Brenner B, et al. von Willebrand factor-cleaving protease in thrombotic thrombocytopenic purpura and the hemolytic-uremic syndrome. N Engl J Med. 1998;339:1578–84.
3. Tsai HM. Physiologic cleavage of von Willebrand factor by a plasma protease is dependent on its conformation and requires calcium ion. Blood. 1996;87:4235–44.
4. Jaffe EA, Hoyer LW, Nachman RL. Synthesis of antihemophilic factor antigen by cultured human endothelial cells. J Clin Invest. 1973;52:2757–64.
5. Jaffe EA, Hoyer LW, Nachman RL. Synthesis of von Willebrand factor by cultured human endothelial cells. Proc Natl Acad Sci U S A. 1974;71:1906–9.
6. Nachman R, Levine R, Jaffe EA. Synthesis of factor VIII antigen by cultured guinea pig megakaryocytes. J Clin Invest. 1977;60:914–21.
7. Wagner DD, Olmsted JB, Marder VJ. Immunolocalization of von Willebrand protein in Weibel-Palade bodies of human endothelial cells. J Cell Biol. 1982;95:355–60.
8. Cramer EM, Meyer D, le Menn R, Breton-Gorius J. Eccentric localization of von Willebrand factor in an internal structure of platelet alpha-granule resembling that of Weibel-Palade bodies. Blood. 1985;66:710–3.
9. Bernardo A, Ball C, Nolasco L, Moake JF, Dong JF. Effects of inflammatory cytokines on the release and cleavage of the endothelial cell-derived ultralarge von Willebrand factor multimers under flow. Blood. 2004;104:100–6.

10. Rickles FR, Hoyer LW, Rick ME, Ahr DJ. The effects of epinephrine infusion in patients with von Willebrand's disease. J Clin Invest. 1976;57:1618–25.
11. Harrison RL, McKee PA. Estrogen stimulates von Willebrand factor production by cultured endothelial cells. Blood. 1984;63:657–64.
12. Hamilton KK, Sims PJ. Changes in cytosolic Ca2+ associated with von Willebrand factor release in human endothelial cells exposed to histamine. Study of microcarrier cell monolayers using the fluorescent probe indo-1. J Clin Invest. 1987;79:600–8.
13. Levine JD, Harlan JM, Harker LA, Joseph ML, Counts RB. Thrombin-mediated release of factor VIII antigen from human umbilical vein endothelial cells in culture. Blood. 1982;60: 531–4.
14. Loesberg C, Gonsalves MD, Zandbergen J, Willems C, van Aken WG, Stel HV, et al. The effect of calcium on the secretion of factor VIII-related antigen by cultured human endothelial cells. Biochim Biophys Acta. 1983;763:160–8.
15. Ribes JA, Francis CW, Wagner DD. Fibrin induces release of von Willebrand factor from endothelial cells. J Clin Invest. 1987;79:117–23.
16. Shelton-Inloes BB, Titani K, Sadler JE. cDNA sequences for human von Willebrand factor reveal five types of repeated domains and five possible protein sequence polymorphisms. Biochemistry. 1986;25:3164–71.
17. Shelton-Inloes BB, Broze GJ, Miletich JP, Sadler JE. Evolution of human von Willebrand factor: cDNA sequence polymorphisms, repeated domains, and relationship to von Willebrand antigen II. Biochem Biophys Res Commun. 1987;144:657–65.
18. Verweij CL, Diergaarde PJ, Hart M, Pannekoek H. Full-length von Willebrand factor (vWF) cDNA encodes a highly repetitive protein considerably larger than the mature vWF subunit. EMBO J. 1986;5:1839–47.
19. Cruz MA, Yuan H, Lee JR, Wise RJ, Handin RI. Interaction of the von Willebrand factor (vWF) with collagen localization of the primary collagen-binding site by analysis of recombinant vWF A domain polypeptides. J Biol Chem. 1995;270:19668.
20. Foster PA, Fulcher CA, Marti T, Titani K, Zimmerman TS. A major factor VIII binding domain resides within the amino-terminal 272 amino acid residues of von Willebrand factor. J Biol Chem. 1987;262:8443–6.
21. Jenkins PV, Pasi KJ, Perkins SJ. Molecular modeling of ligand and mutation sites of the type A domains of human von Willebrand factor and their relevance to von Willebrand's disease. Blood. 1998;91:2032–44.
22. Sugimoto M, Mohri H, McClintock RA, Ruggeri ZM. Identification of discontinuous von Willebrand factor sequences involved in complex formation with botrocetin. A model for the regulation of von Willebrand factor binding to platelet glycoprotein Ib. J Biol Chem. 1991;266:18172–8.
23. Zhou YF, Eng ET, Zhu J, Lu C, Walz T, Springer TA. Sequence and structure relationships within von Willebrand factor. Blood. 2012;120:449–58.
24. Ruggeri ZM, Ware J. von Willebrand factor. FASEB J. 1993;7:308–16.
25. Arya M, Anvari B, Romo GM, Cruz MA, Dong JF, LV MI, et al. Ultralarge multimers of von Willebrand factor form spontaneous high-strength bonds with the platelet glycoprotein Ib-IX complex: studies using optical tweezers. Blood. 2002;99:3971–7.
26. Sadler JE. Biochemistry and genetics of von Willebrand factor. Annu Rev Biochem. 1998;67:395–424.
27. Siedlecki CA, Lestini BJ, Kottke-Marchant KK, Eppell SJ, Wilson DL, Marchant RE. Shear-dependent changes in the three-dimensional structure of human von Willebrand factor. Blood. 1996;88:2939–50.
28. Miura S, Li CQ, Cao Z, Wang H, Wardell MR, Sadler JE. Interaction of von Willebrand factor domain A1 with platelet glycoprotein Ibalpha-(1-289). Slow intrinsic binding kinetics mediate rapid platelet adhesion. J Biol Chem. 2000;275:7539–46.
29. Ruggeri ZM. Developing basic and clinical research on von Willebrand factor and von Willebrand disease. Thromb Haemost. 2000;84:147–9.

30. Savage B, Shattil SJ, Ruggeri ZM. Modulation of platelet function through adhesion receptors. A dual role for glycoprotein IIb-IIIa (integrin alpha IIb beta 3) mediated by fibrinogen and glycoprotein Ib-von Willebrand factor. J Biol Chem. 1992;267:11300–6.
31. Brinkhous KM, Sandberg H, Garris JB, Mattsson C, Palm M, Griggs T, et al. Purified human factor VIII procoagulant protein: comparative hemostatic response after infusions into hemophilic and von Willebrand disease dogs. Proc Natl Acad Sci U S A. 1985;82:8752–6.
32. Fay PJ, Coumans JV, Walker FJ. von Willebrand factor mediates protection of factor VIII from activated protein C-catalyzed inactivation. J Biol Chem. 1991;266:2172–7.
33. Koedam JA, Meijers JC, Sixma JJ, Bouma BN. Inactivation of human factor VIII by activated protein C. Cofactor activity of protein S and protective effect of von Willebrand factor. J Clin Invest. 1988;82:1236–43.
34. Koppelman SJ, van Hoeij M, Vink T, Lankhof H, Schiphorst ME, Damas C, et al. Requirements of von Willebrand factor to protect factor VIII from inactivation by activated protein C. Blood. 1996;87:2292–300.
35. Turner NA, Moake JL. Factor VIII is synthesized in human endothelial cells, packaged in Weibel-Palade bodies and secreted bound to ULVWF strings. PLoS One. 2015;10: e0140740.
36. Suzuki M, Murata M, Matsubara Y, Uchida T, Ishihara H, Shibano T, et al. Detection of von Willebrand factor-cleaving protease (ADAMTS-13) in human platelets. Biochem Biophys Res Commun. 2004;313:212–6.
37. Turner N, Nolasco L, Tao Z, Dong JF, Moake J. Human endothelial cells synthesize and release ADAMTS-13. J Thromb Haemost. 2006;4:1396–404.
38. Uemura M, Tatsumi K, Matsumoto M, Fujimoto M, Matsuyama T, Ishikawa M, et al. Localization of ADAMTS13 to the stellate cells of human liver. Blood. 2005;106:922–4.
39. Zhou W, Inada M, Lee TP, Benten D, Lyubsky S, Bouhassira EE, et al. ADAMTS13 is expressed in hepatic stellate cells. Lab Investig. 2005;85:780–8.
40. Crawley JT, de Groot R, Xiang Y, Luken BM, Lane DA. Unraveling the scissile bond: how ADAMTS13 recognizes and cleaves von Willebrand factor. Blood. 2011;118:3212–21.
41. Tsai HM, Sussman II, Nagel RL. Shear stress enhances the proteolysis of von Willebrand factor in normal plasma. Blood. 1994;83:2171–9.
42. Nolasco L, Nolasco J, Feng S, Afshar-Kharghan V, Moake J. Human complement factor H is a reductase for large soluble von Willebrand factor multimers—brief report. Arterioscler Thromb Vasc Biol. 2013;33:2524–8.
43. Turner N, Nolasco L, Moake J. Generation and breakdown of soluble ultralarge von Willebrand factor multimers. Semin Thromb Hemost. 2012;38:38–46.
44. Dong JF, Moake JL, Nolasco L, Bernardo A, Arceneaux W, Shrimpton CN, et al. ADAMTS-13 rapidly cleaves newly secreted ultralarge von Willebrand factor multimers on the endothelial surface under flowing conditions. Blood. 2002;100:4033–9.
45. Levy GG, Nichols WC, Lian EC, Foroud T, JN MC, BM MG, et al. Mutations in a member of the ADAMTS gene family cause thrombotic thrombocytopenic purpura. Nature. 2001;413:488–94.
46. Furlan M, Robles R, Solenthaler M, Lämmle B. Acquired deficiency of von Willebrand factor-cleaving protease in a patient with thrombotic thrombocytopenic purpura. Blood. 1998;91:2839–46.
47. Tsai HM, Lian EC. Antibodies to von Willebrand factor-cleaving protease in acute thrombotic thrombocytopenic purpura. N Engl J Med. 1998;339:1585–94.
48. Furlan M, Robles R, Solenthaler M, Wassmer M, Sandoz P, Lammle B. Deficient activity of von Willebrand factor-cleaving protease in chronic relapsing thrombotic thrombocytopenic purpura. Blood. 1997;89:3097–103.
49. George JN, Nester CM. Syndromes of thrombotic microangiopathy. N Engl J Med. 2014;371:1847–8.
50. Burns ER, Zucker-Franklin D. Pathologic effects of plasma from patients with thrombotic thrombocytopenic purpura on platelets and cultured vascular endothelial cells. Blood. 1982;60:1030–7.

51. Gore I. Disseminated arteriolar and capillary platelet thrombosis; a morphologic study of its histogenesis. Am J Pathol. 1950;26:155–75, incl 4 pl.
52. Wada H, Kaneko T, Ohiwa M, Tanigawa M, Hayashi T, Tamaki S, et al. Increased levels of vascular endothelial cell markers in thrombotic thrombocytopenic purpura. Am J Hematol. 1993;44:101–5.
53. Mori Y, Wada H, Okugawa Y, Tamaki S, Nakasaki T, Watanabe R, et al. Increased plasma thrombomodulin as a vascular endothelial cell marker in patients with thrombotic thrombocytopenic purpura and hemolytic uremic syndrome. Clin Appl Thromb Hemost. 2001;7:5–9.
54. Jimenez JJ, Jy W, Mauro LM, Horstman LL, Ahn YS. Elevated endothelial microparticles in thrombotic thrombocytopenic purpura: findings from brain and renal microvascular cell culture and patients with active disease. Br J Haematol. 2001;112:81–90.
55. Tandon NN, Rock G, Jamieson GA. Anti-CD36 antibodies in thrombotic thrombocytopenic purpura. Br J Haematol. 1994;88:816–25.
56. Praprotnik S, Blank M, Levy Y, Tavor S, Boffa MC, Weksler B, et al. Anti-endothelial cell antibodies from patients with thrombotic thrombocytopenic purpura specifically activate small vessel endothelial cells. Int Immunol. 2001;13:203–10.
57. Koenig DW, Barley-Maloney L, Daniel TO. A western blot assay detects autoantibodies to cryptic endothelial antigens in thrombotic microangiopathies. J Clin Immunol. 1993;13:204–11.
58. Wright JF, Wang H, Hornstein A, Hornstein A, Hogarth M, Mody M, et al. Characterization of platelet glycoproteins and platelet/endothelial cell antibodies in patients with thrombotic thrombocytopenic purpura. Br J Haematol. 1999;107:546–55.
59. Noris M, Ruggenenti P, Todeschini M, Figliuzzi M, Macconi D, Zoja C, et al. Increased nitric oxide formation in recurrent thrombotic microangiopathies: a possible mediator of microvascular injury. Am J Kidney Dis. 1996;27:790–6.
60. Gangemi S, Allegra A, Sciarrone P, Russo S, Cristani M, Gerace D, et al. Effect of therapeutic plasma exchange on plasma levels of oxidative biomarkers in a patient with thrombotic thrombocytopenic purpura. Eur J Haematol. 2015;94:368–73.
61. Mikes B, Sinkovits G, Farkas P, Csuka D, Schlammadinger A, Rázsó K, et al. Elevated plasma neutrophil elastase concentration is associated with disease activity in patients with thrombotic thrombocytopenic purpura. Thromb Res. 2014;133:616–21.
62. Mitra D, Jaffe EA, Weksler B, Hajjar KA, Soderland C, Laurence J. Thrombotic thrombocytopenic purpura and sporadic hemolytic-uremic syndrome plasmas induce apoptosis in restricted lineages of human microvascular endothelial cells. Blood. 1997;89:1224–34.
63. Dang CT, Magid MS, Weksler B, Chadburn A, Laurence J. Enhanced endothelial cell apoptosis in splenic tissues of patients with thrombotic thrombocytopenic purpura. Blood. 1999;93:1264–70.
64. Moake JL, Turner NA, Stathopoulos NA, Nolasco L, Hellums JD. Shear-induced platelet aggregation can be mediated by vWF released from platelets, as well as by exogenous large or unusually large vWF multimers, requires adenosine diphosphate, and is resistant to aspirin. Blood. 1988;71:1366–74.
65. Moake JL, Turner NA, Stathopoulos NA, Nolasco LH, Hellums JD. Involvement of large plasma von Willebrand factor (vWF) multimers and unusually large vWF forms derived from endothelial cells in shear stress-induced platelet aggregation. J Clin Invest. 1986;78:1456–61.
66. Tsai HM. Pathophysiology of thrombotic thrombocytopenic purpura. Int J Hematol. 2010;91:1–19.
67. Asada Y, Sumiyoshi A, Hayashi T, Suzumiya J, Kaketani K. Immunohistochemistry of vascular lesion in thrombotic thrombocytopenic purpura, with special reference to factor VIII related antigen. Thromb Res. 1985;38:469–79.
68. Hosler GA, Cusumano AM, Hutchins GM. Thrombotic thrombocytopenic purpura and hemolytic uremic syndrome are distinct pathologic entities. A review of 56 autopsy cases. Arch Pathol Lab Med. 2003;127:834–9.
69. George JN. Clinical practice. Thrombotic thrombocytopenic purpura. N Engl J Med. 2006;354:1927–35.

70. George JN. How I treat patients with thrombotic thrombocytopenic purpura: 2010. Blood. 2010;116:4060–9.
71. Sadler JE, Moake JL, Miyata T, George JN. Recent advances in thrombotic thrombocytopenic purpura. Hematol Am Soc Hematol Educ Prog. 2004;2004:407–23.
72. Remuzzi G. HUS and TTP: variable expression of a single entity. Kidney Int. 1987;32:292–308.
73. Eknoyan G, Riggs SA. Renal involvement in patients with thrombotic thrombocytopenic purpura. Am J Nephrol. 1986;6:117–31.
74. Vesely SK, George JN, Lammle B, Studt JD, Alberio L, El-Harake MA, et al. ADAMTS13 activity in thrombotic thrombocytopenic purpura-hemolytic uremic syndrome: relation to presenting features and clinical outcomes in a prospective cohort of 142 patients. Blood. 2003;102:60–8.
75. Zafrani L, Mariotte E, Darmon M, Canet E, Merceron S, Boutboul D, et al. Acute renal failure is prevalent in patients with thrombotic thrombocytopenic purpura associated with low plasma ADAMTS13 activity. J Thromb Haemost. 2015;13:380–9.
76. Hawkins BM, Abu-Fadel M, Vesely SK, George JN. Clinical cardiac involvement in thrombotic thrombocytopenic purpura: a systematic review. Transfusion. 2008;48:382–92.
77. Gami AS, Hayman SR, Grande JP, Garovic VD. Incidence and prognosis of acute heart failure in the thrombotic microangiopathies. Am J Med. 2005;118:544–7.
78. Patschan D, Witzke O, Duhrsen U, Erbel R, Philipp T, Herget-Rosenthal S. Acute myocardial infarction in thrombotic microangiopathies—clinical characteristics, risk factors and outcome. Nephrol Dial Transplant. 2006;21:1549–54.
79. Ridolfi RL, Hutchins GM, Bell WR. The heart and cardiac conduction system in thrombotic thrombocytopenic purpura. A clinicopathologic study of 17 autopsied patients. Ann Intern Med. 1979;91:357–63.
80. Podolsky SH, Zembowicz A, Schoen FJ, Benjamin RJ, Sonna LA. Massive myocardial necrosis in thrombotic thrombocytopenic purpura: a case report and review of the literature. Arch Pathol Lab Med. 1999;123:937–40.
81. Wajima T, Johnson EH. Sudden cardiac death from thrombotic thrombocytopenic purpura. Clin Appl Thromb Hemost. 2000;6:108–10.
82. Hughes C, McEwan JR, Longair I, Hughes S, Cohen H, Machin S, et al. Cardiac involvement in acute thrombotic thrombocytopenic purpura: association with troponin T and IgG antibodies to ADAMTS 13. J Thromb Haemost. 2009;7:529–36.
83. Brain MC, Dacie JV, Hourihane DO. Microangiopathic haemolytic anaemia: the possible role of vascular lesions in pathogenesis. Br J Haematol. 1962;8:358–74.
84. Tsai HM. Platelet activation and the formation of the platelet plug: deficiency of ADAMTS13 causes thrombotic thrombocytopenic purpura. Arterioscler Thromb Vasc Biol. 2003;23:388–96.
85. Roriz M, Landais M, Desprez J, Barbet C, Azoulay E, Galicier L, et al. Risk factors for autoimmune diseases development after thrombotic thrombocytopenic purpura. Medicine (Baltimore). 2015;94:e1598.
86. Amoura Z, Costedoat-Chalumeau N, Veyradier A, Wolf M, Ghillani-Dalbin P, Cacoub P, et al. Thrombotic thrombocytopenic purpura with severe ADAMTS-13 deficiency in two patients with primary antiphospholipid syndrome. Arthritis Rheum. 2004;50:3260–4.
87. Trent K, Neustater BR, Lottenberg R. Chronic relapsing thrombotic thrombocytopenic purpura and antiphospholipid antibodies: a report of two cases. Am J Hematol. 1997;54:155–9.
88. Espinosa G, Bucciarelli S, Cervera R, Lozano M, Reverter JC, de la Red G, et al. Thrombotic microangiopathic haemolytic anaemia and antiphospholipid antibodies. Ann Rheum Dis. 2004;63:730–6.
89. Asamiya Y, Moriyama T, Takano M, Iwasaki C, Kimura K, Ando Y, et al. Successful treatment with rituximab in a patient with TTP secondary to severe ANCA-associated vasculitis. Intern Med. 2010;49:1587–91.
90. Yamashita H, Takahashi Y, Kaneko H, Kano T, Mimori A. Thrombotic thrombocytopenic purpura with an autoantibody to ADAMTS13 complicating Sjögren's syndrome: two cases and a literature review. Mod Rheumatol. 2013;23:365–73.

91. Suzuki E, Kanno T, Asano T, Tsutsumi A, Kobayashi H, Watanabe H, et al. Two cases of mixed connective tissue disease complicated with thrombotic thrombocytopenic purpura. Fukushima J Med Sci. 2013;59:49–55.
92. Manadan AM, Harris C, Block JA. Thrombotic thrombocytopenic purpura in the setting of systemic sclerosis. Semin Arthritis Rheum. 2005;34:683–8.
93. Pallot-Prades B, Benvenuto V, Riffat G, Alexandre C. Thrombotic thrombocytopenic purpura and ankylosing spondylarthritis. Apropos of a case. Rev Med Interne. 1993;14:115–6.
94. Jiang H, An X, Li Y, Sun Y, Shen G, Tu Y, et al. Clinical features and prognostic factors of thrombotic thrombocytopenic purpura associated with systemic lupus erythematosus: a literature review of 105 cases from 1999 to 2011. Clin Rheumatol. 2014;33:419–27.
95. Letchumanan P, Ng HJ, Lee LH, Thumboo J. A comparison of thrombotic thrombocytopenic purpura in an inception cohort of patients with and without systemic lupus erythematosus. Rheumatology (Oxford). 2009;48:399–403.
96. Musio F, Bohen EM, Yuan CM, Welch PG. Review of thrombotic thrombocytopenic purpura in the setting of systemic lupus erythematosus. Semin Arthritis Rheum. 1998;28:1–19.
97. Kwok SK, Ju JH, Cho CS, Kim HY, Park SH. Thrombotic thrombocytopenic purpura in systemic lupus erythematosus: risk factors and clinical outcome: a single centre study. Lupus. 2009;18:16–21.
98. Muscal E, Edwards RM, Kearney DL, Hicks JM, Myones BL, Teruya J. Thrombotic microangiopathic hemolytic anemia with reduction of ADAMTS13 activity: initial manifestation of childhood-onset systemic lupus erythematosus. Am J Clin Pathol. 2011;135:406–16.
99. Veyradier A, Obert B, Houllier A, Meyer D, Girma JP. Specific von Willebrand factor-cleaving protease in thrombotic microangiopathies: a study of 111 cases. Blood. 2001;98:1765–72.
100. Grillberger R, Casina VC, Turecek PL, Zheng XL, Rottensteiner H, Scheiflinger F. Anti-ADAMTS13 IgG autoantibodies present in healthy individuals share linear epitopes with those in patients with thrombotic thrombocytopenic purpura.[letter]. Haematologica. 2014;99(4):e58–60.
101. Yamaguchi Y, Moriki T, Igari A, Nakagawa T, Wada H, Matsumoto M, et al. Epitope analysis of autoantibodies to ADAMTS13 in patients with acquired thrombotic thrombocytopenic purpura. Thromb Res. 2011;128:169–73.
102. Klaus C, Plaimauer B, Studt JD, Dorner F, Lämmle B, Mannucci PM, et al. Epitope mapping of ADAMTS13 autoantibodies in acquired thrombotic thrombocytopenic purpura. Blood. 2004;103:4514–9.
103. Zander CB, Cao W, Zheng XL. ADAMTS13 and von Willebrand factor interactions. Curr Opin Hematol. 2015;22:452–9.
104. Pos W, Crawley JT, Fijnheer R, Voorberg J, Lane DA, Luken BM. An autoantibody epitope comprising residues R660, Y661, and Y665 in the ADAMTS13 spacer domain identifies a binding site for the A2 domain of VWF. Blood. 2010;115:1640–9.
105. Pos W, Sorvillo N, Fijnheer R, Feys HB, Kaijen PH, Vidarsson G, et al. Residues Arg568 and Phe592 contribute to an antigenic surface for anti-ADAMTS13 antibodies in the spacer domain. Haematologica. 2011;96:1670–7.
106. Igari A, Nakagawa T, Moriki T, Yamaguchi Y, Matsumoto M, Fujimura Y, et al. Identification of epitopes on ADAMTS13 recognized by a panel of monoclonal antibodies with functional or non-functional effects on catalytic activity. Thromb Res. 2012;130:e79–83.
107. Luken BM, Turenhout EA, Kaijen PH, Greuter MJ, Pos W, van Mourik J, et al. Amino acid regions 572-579 and 657-666 of the spacer domain of ADAMTS13 provide a common antigenic core required for binding of antibodies in patients with acquired TTP. Thromb Haemost. 2006;96:295–301.
108. Pos W, Luken BM, Sorvillo N, Kremer Hovinga JA, Voorberg J. Humoral immune response to ADAMTS13 in acquired thrombotic thrombocytopenic purpura. J Thromb Haemost. 2011;9:1285–91.
109. Schaller M, Vogel M, Kentouche K, Lämmle B, Kremer Hovinga JA. The splenic autoimmune response to ADAMTS13 in thrombotic thrombocytopenic purpura contains recurrent antigen-binding CDR3 motifs. Blood. 2014;124:3469–79.

110. Luken BM, Kaijen PH, Turenhout EA, Kremer Hovinga JA, van Mourik JA, Fijnheer R, et al. Multiple B-cell clones producing antibodies directed to the spacer and disintegrin/thrombospondin type-1 repeat 1 (TSP1) of ADAMTS13 in a patient with acquired thrombotic thrombocytopenic purpura. J Thromb Haemost. 2006;4:2355–64.

111. Scheiflinger F, Knöbl P, Trattner B, Plaimauer B, Mohr G, Dockal M, et al. Nonneutralizing IgM and IgG antibodies to von Willebrand factor-cleaving protease (ADAMTS-13) in a patient with thrombotic thrombocytopenic purpura. Blood. 2003;102:3241–3.

112. Shelat SG, Smith P, Ai J, Zheng XL. Inhibitory autoantibodies against ADAMTS-13 in patients with thrombotic thrombocytopenic purpura bind ADAMTS-13 protease and may accelerate its clearance in vivo. J Thromb Haemost. 2006;4:1707–17.

113. Rieger M, Mannucci PM, Kremer Hovinga JA, Herzog A, Gerstenbauer G, Konetschny C, et al. ADAMTS13 autoantibodies in patients with thrombotic microangiopathies and other immunomediated diseases. Blood. 2005;106:1262–7.

114. Mannucci PM, Canciani MT, Forza I, Lussana F, Lattuada A, Rossi E. Changes in health and disease of the metalloprotease that cleaves von Willebrand factor. Blood. 2001;98:2730–5.

115. Uemura M, Matsuyama T, Ishikawa M, Fujimoto M, Kojima H, Sakurai S, et al. Decreased activity of plasma ADAMTS13 may contribute to the development of liver disturbance and multiorgan failure in patients with alcoholic hepatitis. Alcohol Clin Exp Res. 2005;29:264S–71S.

116. Ono T, Mimuro J, Madoiwa S, Soejima K, Kashiwakura Y, Ishiwata A, et al. Severe secondary deficiency of von Willebrand factor-cleaving protease (ADAMTS13) in patients with sepsis-induced disseminated intravascular coagulation: its correlation with development of renal failure. Blood. 2006;107:528–34.

117. Nguyen TC, Liu A, Liu L, Ball C, Choi H, May WS, et al. Acquired ADAMTS-13 deficiency in pediatric patients with severe sepsis. Haematologica. 2007;92:121–4.

118. McDonald V, Laffan M, Benjamin S, Bevan D, Machin S, Scully MA. Thrombotic thrombocytopenic purpura precipitated by acute pancreatitis: a report of seven cases from a regional UK TTP registry. Br J Haematol. 2009;144:430–3.

119. Ali MA, Shaheen JS, Khan MA. Acute pancreatitis induced thrombotic thrombocytopenic purpura. Indian J Crit Care Med. 2014;18:107–9.

120. Sánchez-Luceros A, Farías CE, Amaral MM, Kempfer AC, Votta R, Marchese C, et al. von Willebrand factor-cleaving protease (ADAMTS13) activity in normal non-pregnant women, pregnant and post-delivery women. Thromb Haemost. 2004;92:1320–6.

121. Moatti-Cohen M, Garrec C, Wolf M, Boisseau P, Galicier L, Azoulay E, et al. Unexpected frequency of Upshaw-Schulman syndrome in pregnancy-onset thrombotic thrombocytopenic purpura. Blood. 2012;119:5888–97.

122. Niv E, Segev A, Ellis MH. Staphylococcus aureus bacteremia as a cause of early relapse of thrombotic thrombocytopenic purpura. Transfusion. 2000;40:1067–70.

123. Creager AJ, Brecher ME, Bandarenko N. Thrombotic thrombocytopenic purpura that is refractory to therapeutic plasma exchange in two patients with occult infection. Transfusion. 1998;38:419–23.

124. Tsai HM. The molecular biology of thrombotic microangiopathy. Kidney Int. 2006;70:16–23.

125. Park YA, Hay SN, Brecher ME. ADAMTS13 activity levels in patients with human immunodeficiency virus-associated thrombotic microangiopathy and profound CD4 deficiency. J Clin Apher. 2009;24:32–6.

126. Pirrotta MT, Bucalossi A. Thrombotic microangiopathy and occult neoplasia. Cardiovasc Hematol Disord Drug Targets. 2010;10:87–93.

127. Tsai HM, Rice L, Sarode R, Chow TW, Moake JL. Antibody inhibitors to von Willebrand factor metalloproteinase and increased binding of von Willebrand factor to platelets in ticlopidine-associated thrombotic thrombocytopenic purpura. Ann Intern Med. 2000;132:794–9.

128. Bennett CL, Connors JM, Carwile JM, Moake JL, Bell WR, Tarantolo SR, et al. Thrombotic thrombocytopenic purpura associated with clopidogrel. N Engl J Med. 2000;342:1773–7.

129. Zakarija A, Kwaan HC, Moake JL, Bandarenko N, Pandey DK, JM MK, et al. Ticlopidine-and clopidogrel-associated thrombotic thrombocytopenic purpura (TTP): review of clinical, laboratory, epidemiological, and pharmacovigilance findings (1989–2008). Kidney Int Suppl. 2009;75:S20–4.
130. Nazzal M, Safi F, Arma F, Nazzal M, Muzaffar M, Assaly R. Micafungin-induced thrombotic thrombocytopenic purpura: a case report and review of the literature. Am J Ther. 2011;18:e258–60.
131. Reese JA, Bougie DW, Curtis BR, Terrell DR, Vesely SK, Aster RH, et al. Drug-induced thrombotic microangiopathy: experience of the Oklahoma Registry and the BloodCenter of Wisconsin. Am J Hematol. 2015;90:406–10.
132. Al-Nouri ZL, Reese JA, Terrell DR, Vesely SK, George JN. Drug-induced thrombotic microangiopathy: a systematic review of published reports. Blood. 2015;125:616–8.
133. Law SK, Levine RP. Interaction between the third complement protein and cell surface macromolecules. Proc Natl Acad Sci U S A. 1977;74:2701–5.
134. Pangburn MK, Ferreira VP, Cortes C. Discrimination between host and pathogens by the complement system. Vaccine. 2008;26(Suppl 8):I15–21.
135. Law SK, Dodds AW. The internal thioester and the covalent binding properties of the complement proteins C3 and C4. Protein Sci. 1997;6:263–74.
136. Schreiber RD, Pangburn MK, Lesavre PH, Müller-Eberhard HJ. Initiation of the alternative pathway of complement: recognition of activators by bound C3b and assembly of the entire pathway from six isolated proteins. PNAS. 1978;75:3948–52.
137. Rawal N, Pangburn M. Formation of high-affinity C5 convertases of the alternative pathway of complement. J Immunol. 2001;166:2635–42.
138. Fearon DT, Austen KF, Ruddy S. Formation of a hemolytically active cellular intermediate by the interaction between properdin factors B and D and the activated third component of complement. J Exp Med. 1973;138:1305–13.
139. Pillemer L, Blum L, Lepow IH, Ross OA, Todd EW, Wardlaw AC. The properdin system and immunity. I. Demonstration and isolation of a new serum protein, properdin, and its role in immune phenomena. Science. 1954;120:279–85.
140. Weiler JM, Daha MR, Austen KF, Fearon DT. Control of the amplification convertase of complement by the plasma protein beta1H. Proc Natl Acad Sci U S A. 1976;73:3268–72.
141. Kinoshita T, Takata Y, Kozono H, Takeda J, Hong KS, Inoue K. C5 convertase of the alternative complement pathway: covalent linkage between two C3b molecules within the trimolecular complex enzyme. J Immunol. 1988;141:3895.
142. Kazatchkine MD, Fearon DT, Austen KF. Human alternative complement pathway: membrane-associated sialic acid regulates the competition between B and beta1 H for cell-bound C3b. J Immunol. 1979;122:75–81.
143. Whaley K, Ruddy S. Modulation of the alternative complement pathways by beta 1 H globulin. J Exp Med. 1976;144:1147–63.
144. Harrison RA, Lachmann PJ. The physiological breakdown of the third component of human complement. Mol Immunol. 1980;17:9–20.
145. Delvaeye M, Noris M, De Vriese A, Esmon CT, Esmon NL, Ferrell G, et al. Thrombomodulin mutations in atypical hemolytic-uremic syndrome. N Engl J Med. 2009;361:345–57.
146. Liszewski MK, Post TW, Atkinson JP. Membrane cofactor protein (MCP or CD46): newest member of the regulators of complement activation gene cluster. Annu Rev Immunol. 1991;9:431–55.
147. Fearon DT. Regulation of the amplification C3 convertase of human complement by an inhibitory protein isolated from human erythrocyte membrane. Proc Natl Acad Sci U S A. 1979;76:5867–71.
148. Fearon DT. Identification of the membrane glycoprotein that is the C3b receptor of the human erythrocyte, polymorphonuclear leukocyte, B lymphocyte, and monocyte. J Exp Med. 1980;152:20–30.

149. Nicholson-Weller A, Burge J, Fearon DT, Weller PF, Austen KF. Isolation of a human erythrocyte membrane glycoprotein with decay-accelerating activity for C3 convertases of the complement system. J Immunol. 1982;129:184–9.
150. Turner NA, Moake J. Assembly and activation of alternative complement components on endothelial cell-anchored ultra-large von Willebrand factor links complement and hemostasis-thrombosis. PLoS One. 2013;8:e59372.
151. Tati R, Kristoffersson AC, Stahl AL, Rebetz J, Wang L, Licht C, et al. Complement activation associated with ADAMTS13 deficiency in human and murine thrombotic microangiopathy. J Immunol. 2013;191:2184–93.
152. Feng S, Liang X, Cruz MA, Vu H, Zhou Z, Pemmaraju N, et al. The interaction between factor H and Von Willebrand factor. PLoS One. 2013;8:e737.
153. Turner N, Sartain S, Moake J. Ultralarge Von Willebrand factor-induced platelet clumping and activation of the alternative complement pathway in thrombotic thrombocytopenic purpura and the hemolytic-uremic syndromes. Hematol Oncol Clin North Am. 2015;29:509–24.
154. Ruiz-Torres MP, Casiraghi F, Galbusera M, Macconi D, Gastoldi S, Todeschini M, et al. Complement activation: the missing link between ADAMTS-13 deficiency and microvascular thrombosis of thrombotic microangiopathies. Thromb Haemost. 2005;93:443–52.
155. Reti M, Farkas P, Csuka D, Razso K, Schlammadinger A, Udvardy ML, et al. Complement activation in thrombotic thrombocytopenic purpura. J Thromb Haemost. 2012;10:791–8.
156. Cataland SR, Holers VM, Geyer S, Yang S, Wu HM. Biomarkers of terminal complement activation confirm the diagnosis of aHUS and differentiate aHUS from TTP. Blood. 2014;123:3733–8.
157. Cao W, Pham HP, Williams LA, McDaniel J. Human neutrophil peptides and complement factor Bb in pathogenesis of acquired thrombotic thrombocytopenic purpura. Haematologica. 2016;101(11):1319–26.
158. Tsai E, Chapin J, Laurence JC, Tsai HM. Use of eculizumab in the treatment of a case of refractory, ADAMTS13-deficient thrombotic thrombocytopenic purpura: additional data and clinical follow-up. Br J Haematol. 2013;162:558–9.
159. Patschan D, Korsten P, Behlau A, Vasko R, Heeg M, Sweiss N, et al. Idiopathic combined, autoantibody-mediated ADAMTS-13/factor H deficiency in thrombotic thrombocytopenic purpura-hemolytic uremic syndrome in a 17-year-old woman: a case report. J Med Case Rep. 2011;5:598.
160. Chapin J, Weksler B, Magro C, Laurence J. Eculizumab in the treatment of refractory idiopathic thrombotic thrombocytopenic purpura.[letter]. Br J Haematol. 2012;157(6):772–4.

Chapter 10
Evaluation and Treatment of Thrombotic Thrombocytopenic Purpura

Satheesh Chonat

Clinical Presentation

The classic pentad of clinical presentation described in TTP includes microangiopathic hemolytic anemia (MAHA), thrombocytopenia, fever, and neurological and renal dysfunction. While MAHA and thrombocytopenia are almost always seen at presentation in TTP, other signs are not always present at the time of diagnosis. Table 10.1 lists some of the presenting clinical features seen in TTP. Most centers now rely on the combination of clinical features (MAHA and low platelets) and severe deficiency of ADAMTS13 activity. Since the laboratory evaluation of ADAMTS13 activity might not be readily available, empiric therapy should be instituted if microangiopathic hemolytic anemia and thrombocytopenia are present without an obvious underlying cause.

Laboratory Diagnosis

Laboratory testing is vital in distinguishing acquired TTP from congenital TTP and other TMA syndromes. Laboratory diagnosis of acquired TTP is typically made using a combination of the measurement of plasma ADAMTS13 activity and detection of anti-ADAMTS13 autoantibodies. Determination of the ADAMTS13 antigen level is infrequently needed. Please also refer to Table 10.2 for additional testing and Fig. 10.1 for a diagnostic algorithm in any suspected patient with TTP.

S. Chonat, MD
Pediatric Hematology, Department of Pediatrics, Emory University School of Medicine and Aflac Cancer and Blood Disorders Center, Children's Healthcare of Atlanta,
Atlanta, GA, USA
e-mail: satheesh.chonat@emory.edu

© Springer International Publishing AG, part of Springer Nature 2018   189
J. M. Despotovic (ed.), *Immune Hematology*,
https://doi.org/10.1007/978-3-319-73269-5_10

Table 10.1 Spectrum of clinical features in TTP

Organ system	Clinical features
Hematological	Microangiopathic hemolytic anemia (schistocytes on peripheral smear), symptoms of anemia, jaundice, thrombocytopenia, and associated bleeding manifestations
Renal	Hematuria, proteinuria, acute kidney injury, hypertension
Neurological	Headache, confusion, visual disturbances, focal neurological signs (aphasia, motor, or sensory abnormalities), coma, stroke, seizure
Cardiac	Chest pain, arrhythmias, myocardial infarction (ST and non-ST elevation), raised serum troponin, congestive heart failure, cardiac arrest, cardiogenic shock
Gastrointestinal	Abdominal pain, nausea, vomiting, diarrhea
Eye	Pain, blurred vision, ocular hemorrhage, retinal vessel occlusion
Miscellaneous/ systemic	Fever, fatigue, arthralgia, myalgia, venous thromboembolism, multiple organ failure, early death

Table 10.2 Suggested laboratory testing

Hematological	ADAMTS13 activity and anti-ADAMTS13 IgG assay
	Complete blood count, peripheral blood smear, reticulocyte count, haptoglobin, free plasma hemoglobin, LDH, bilirubin
	Prothrombin time, activated partial thromboplastin time, fibrinogen
	Blood group, antibody screen, direct antiglobulin test
Renal and metabolic	BUN, creatinine, calcium, thyroid function test
Gastrointestinal	Liver function test
Cardiac	Serum troponin, electrocardiogram, echocardiogram
Infection	HIV, hepatitis, CMV, and EBV serology
Urine, stool	Urine pregnancy testing, urinalysis, urine protein/creatinine ratio, Shiga toxin in stool
Autoimmune testing	Erythrocyte sedimentation rate, antinuclear antibodies, dsDNA, rheumatoid factor, lupus anticoagulant testing panel
Imaging	Cranial imaging (CT or MRI) and other appropriate imaging if malignancy is suspected

In most laboratories, the activity assay is initially performed to measure the ability of the ADAMTS13 enzyme to cleave vWF multimers (patient's plasma added to a mixture containing normal vWF peptide). The split products are then commonly detected either using immunoassay (ELISA) or fluorescence resonance energy transfer (FRET). In the former, a recombinant fusion protein (GST-VWF73-His) is used as a substrate for Y1605-M1606 peptide bond in the vWF. This is cleaved by ADAMTS13 present in the patient's plasma, and the resulting Y1605 residue is recognized by the enzyme-linked mouse monoclonal antibody conjugated to horseradish peroxidase [1]. In the FRET assay, a synthetic 73-amino acid peptide (FRET-VWF730) containing the Y1605-M1606 cleavage site is cleaved by ADAMTS13 enzyme, and the quantitative release of the fluorescence is directly proportional to the concentration of the enzyme activity. This is essentially a simple assay with

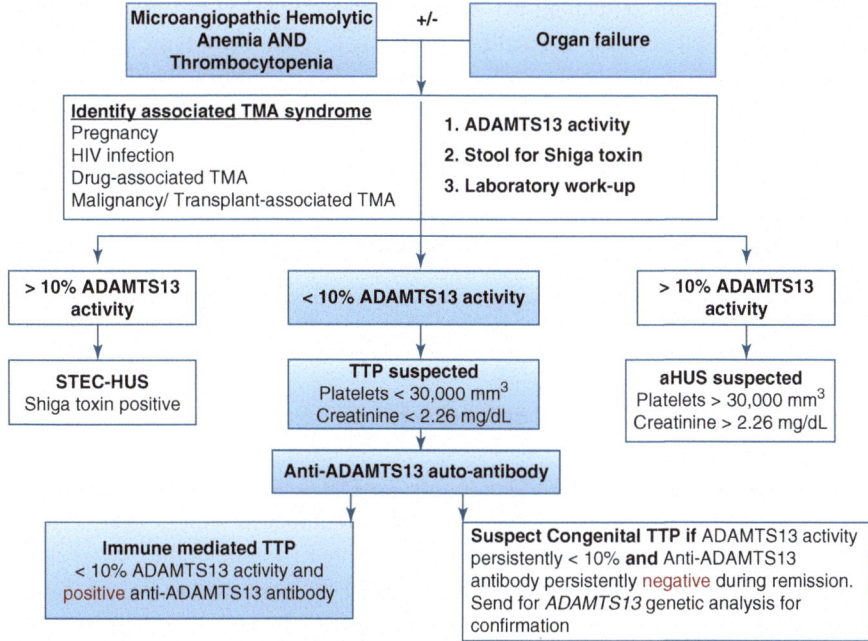

Fig. 10.1 Diagnostic algorithm for TTP

many advantages including being highly reproducible between multiple runs, which take about 4–6 h per run and is able to detect even <5% activity [2].

When there is a severe decrease in the activity of ADAMTS13 to less than 30%, the presence of functional anti-ADAMTS13 autoantibodies is assessed. These antibodies can be detected quantitatively using a Bethesda-like assay (used to detect inhibitors to Factor VIII in Hemophilia patients). This is a mixing study performed by adding patient's plasma (presumably with inhibitory antibodies) to a plasma pool from healthy controls. The result is reported as "inhibitor units," where one inhibitor unit reduces the ADAMTS13 activity in control plasma by 50%. Another method used is enzyme-linked immunosorbent assay (ELISA) to detect these autoantibodies (IgG or rarely IgM) in plasma of patients with deficient ADAMTS13 activity.

The plasma antigen level of ADAMTS13 can be measured using ELISA but is not routinely used for initial testing or considered pertinent in the diagnosis of acquired TTP.

Treating clinicians should be aware of some of the limitations and nuances with these assays. Most centers use local reference laboratories for these tests. Therefore, the results are not immediately available, and initial treatment is instituted prior to the availability of ADAMTS13 activity data. It is also important to recognize that recent red cell transfusion, platelet transfusion, plasma exchange, or plasma infusion can affect the level of the ADAMTS13 activity as well as the level of any inhibitors present. An ADAMTS13 ELISA-based antibody assay is less specific than a functional inhibitor assay. A mild to moderate reduction of ADAMTS13 activity (>10%) with or without the presence of anti-ADAMTS13 antibodies can also be seen in other medical conditions such as atypical hemolytic uremic syndrome (aHUS), systemic lupus erythematosus (SLE), antiphospholipid syndrome, disseminated intravascular coagulation, and sepsis, among others [3]. The dilution of plasma to run some of these tests can further affect the sensitivity of enzyme activity and inhibitor levels. One important limitation of FRET assay is that hemolysis with resulting free hemoglobin and hyperbilirubinemia can interfere with florescence detection leading to falsely lower ADAMTS13 activity. Therefore, these diagnostic tests should ideally be sent to laboratories that analyze them on a regular basis and have the expertise to interpret the results appropriately.

Initial Management of Acquired TTP

Upon suspicion of TTP, one should promptly send laboratory workup as outlined in the previous section. However, given the high likelihood of sudden deterioration and associated complications, a patient with presumed TTP should be treated expeditiously as a medical emergency, without waiting for confirmatory testing. Initial steps should focus on stabilization of a critical patient as well as consideration of transfer to a center with expertise in managing patients with TTP. Plasma exchange (see below) requires a central venous catheter (CVC) to be inserted by experienced critical care or surgical team member under ultrasound guidance in a compressible vein such as the femoral or jugular vein. Transfusion of platelets is generally contraindicated in TTP except in the setting of refractory life-threatening bleeding. These CVCs can be safely inserted by experienced personnel even with a lower platelet count [4], but this risk should be discussed among the treating physicians, as bleeding from the insertion site and pulmonary hemorrhage and retroperitoneal hemorrhage related to plasma exchange in patient with TTP have been reported [5]. Packed red cells can be safely administered to maintain blood volume in patients with TTP. Delays in providing immediate care to patients with TTP can be prevented by consulting a multidisciplinary team from intensive care unit, hematology, nephrology, surgery, and apheresis. Please refer to Table 10.3 for a summary of available treatment modalities and Fig. 10.2 for treatment algorithm.

Plasma Therapy

Plasma therapy includes simple plasma infusion (PI) and plasma exchange (PEX). While the former is preferred in cTTP, ADAMTS13 testing results are usually not available promptly enough to definitively differentiate cTTP from iTTP. Furthermore, delay in obtaining ADAMTS13 activity data often precludes definitive differentiation of TTP from other TMAs as well. Therefore, PEX is often started prior to a definitive diagnosis of TTP is made. PEX is superior to PI for acquired TTP since it

Table 10.3 Treatment modalities

	Replaces ADAMTS13 enzyme	Reduces anti-ADAMTS13 autoantibodies	Immune suppression	Blocks vWF binding to platelet GP1b
Plasma infusion	Yes	–	–	–
Plasma exchange	Yes	Yes	–	–
Steroids	–	–	Yes	–
Rituximab and immune-modulating agents	–	Yes	Yes	–
Splenectomy	–	Yes	–	–
vWF A1 domain therapy (ALX-0081, ALX-0681) and N-acetylcysteine	–	–	–	Yes
Recombinant ADAMTS13	Yes	–	–	–

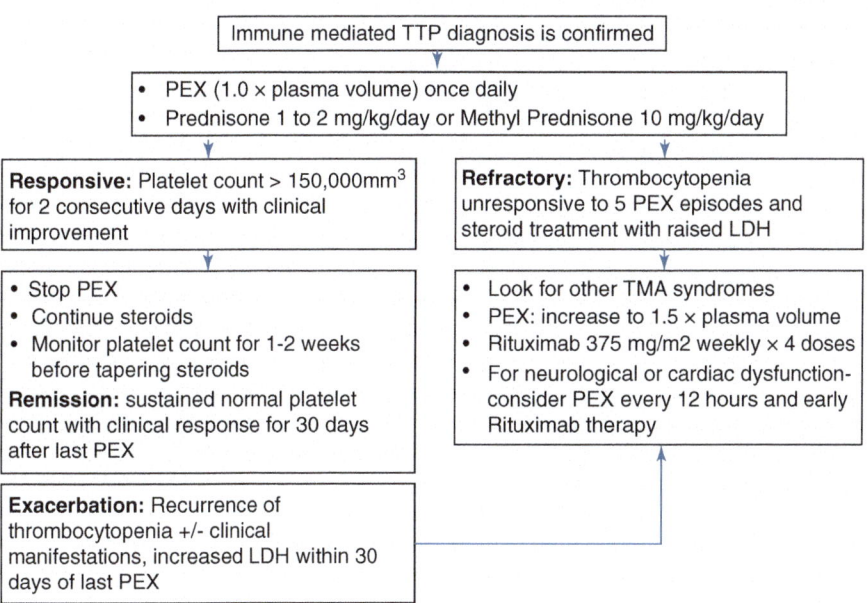

Fig. 10.2 Treatment algorithm for Acute iTTP

replenishes ADAMTS13 and removes anti-ADAMTS13 autoantibodies, as well as ULVWF multimers. Plasma exchange should be initiated as early as possible in any patient with suspected TTP, as delay in starting this therapy is associated with significantly increased mortality and morbidity [6–9]. If delays in initiating PEX are expected, PI should be initiated as a temporizing measure, especially if there is high clinical suspicion for cTTP.

The recommended volume for initial therapy with PEX is 1.0 to 1.5 times the plasma volume [8, 10, 11]. This is typically continued daily until platelet count normalization (150,000/mm^3) is achieved for two consecutive days along with stabilization of hemolysis and organ dysfunction (clinical response). PEX is performed every 12 h in some centers for refractory acquired TTP or TTP with severe symptoms of cardiac or neurological dysfunction. Fresh frozen plasma or solvent-based plasma can be used as the replacement fluid in PEX. Most centers prefer to use centrifugation-based blood component separation over membrane-based system for PEX, as the former is more efficient in plasma removal and treatment time is shorter.

Complications of PEX are usually catheter related (bleeding, infection, thrombosis, pneumothorax, death), plasma related (anaphylaxis, hypotension, arrhythmias, serum sickness, death), or citrate related (hypocalcemia) [12, 13]. While PEX is ongoing, initiation of immune-modulation therapies should be strongly considered. Dosing and timing of these medications during PEX is critical to ensure adequate effect.

Corticosteroids

Among the immune-modulation therapies, initiation of corticosteroids along with PEX therapy is the standard of care for the initial management of acquired TTP. Methylprednisolone at 1 g (or 10 mg/kg/day) should be given intravenously daily for 3 days along with PEX therapy, as oral therapy can be a challenge in critically ill patients. High-dose methylprednisolone (MP) administered intravenously in combination with PEX was shown to achieve remission in 77% of patients compared to 47% of patients using a lower dose [14]. The mechanism of corticosteroid effect is not completely clear but likely involves suppression of antibody production and/or downregulation of the cytokine storm involved in endothelial activation [15]. Concurrent use of steroids with PEX has been shown to reduce the duration of PEX and its related complications [5]. This initial high dose of methylprednisolone is typically transitioned to oral prednisone 1–2 mg/kg/day for the next several weeks [10, 11, 16].

Rituximab

Rituximab is a monoclonal antibody against CD20 and has been used in the management of various hematological malignancies and autoimmune conditions such as immune thrombocytopenic purpura and rheumatoid diseases. This antibody binds to B lymphocytes expressing CD20 and eliminates these B cells through a variety of mechanisms. In a prospective trial involving patients with relapsed/refractory acquired TTP, patients who received rituximab (375 mg/m^2 intravenously weekly for 4 weeks) had a complete hematological and clinical remission within 1–3 weeks of the first dose. This was coupled with fall in IgG antibody levels and rise in ADAMTS13 activity [17].

Since rituximab is removed from the circulation by PEX therapy, doses should be delivered immediately after PEX. The time to B cell depletion is not altered when given in combination with PEX therapy [18]. A prospective open-label French study looked at rituximab clearance by PEX with dosing on days 1, 3, 7, and 14. This regimen resulted in significant B cell depletion lasting for 9 months, with no severe side effects [19]. This frequent dosing schedule can be potentially used in those who are slow to respond with persistence of anti-ADAMTS13 autoantibodies and low ADAMTS13 activity. There have not been any reports of specific safety issues with use of rituximab in acquired TTP. Recovery of B cells has been found to occur between 6 and 15 months following therapy [18, 19].

While there are no robust data from randomized controlled trials, the use of rituximab along with PEX has resulted in reduced duration of PEX and fewer relapses. In a prospective trial of 40 patients who received rituximab in England, only 4 of them relapsed (10%) at a median duration of 27 months. This was significantly better in comparison to their historical controls (57% relapse rate at a median duration of 18 months) [20]. The Oklahoma registry reported on their experience in 16 adults who had received rituximab; only two relapsed at 2.5 and 9.9 years (12.5% relapse rate compared to 42% in controls) [21]. In the above-mentioned open-label French study, of the 19 patients who received rituximab and were available for follow-up, none relapsed within the first year (compared to 9.4% in the control group) [19]. These results and other retrospective case reports that have been nicely compiled in the recent review article [11] encourage the use of rituximab, in conjunction with PEX and steroids, as frontline therapy in adults with acquired TTP [13, 19, 20, 22].

Monitoring After Initial Management of Acquired TTP

With prompt initiation of PEX, the mortality has decreased from over 90% [6, 23] to less than 20% [8, 24]. Once a patient with acquired TTP is in clinical remission (clinical response for over 30 days from cessation of PEX), close monitoring with routine blood counts, LDH and ADAMTS13 activity level for several months, and during acute illnesses and/or pregnancy is essential. It is advisable that the patient is treated and followed up at least for the initial period by a hematologist with experience in managing patients with acquired TTP. It is also important to monitor for any clinical or laboratory signs of connective tissue disorders (such as SLE, Sjögren syndrome, rheumatoid arthritis, etc.), as these patients can present either before, at the time of, or during follow-up for acquired TTP [25]. One systematic review revealed that 19% of children and 11% of adults with SLE had acquired TMA [26]. These patients can either present as connective tissue disease-related TMA with mild to moderate decrease in ADAMTS13 activity or significant decrease in ADAMTS13 activity levels with presence of anti-ADAMTS13 autoantibodies indicative of acquired TTP. For more detailed information, please refer to Chap. 2 on pathophysiology of TTP.

Risk Factors and Prevention of Relapse

Relapse of acquired TTP occurs in about 40% of patients, the majority of which occur in the first year [27]. Some of the important risk factors for such relapse include older age, persistently severely decreased ADAMTS13 activity levels during remission, and organ damage reflected by increased LDH, elevated troponin, and neurological features [28, 29]. Among these, the only biomarker that is predictive of iTTP relapse is a persistently severely low ADAMTS13 activity during clinical remission. Among the Oklahoma TTP registry patients in remission who had severely decreased ADAMTS13 activity (<10%), up to 60% experienced at least one relapse [30]. These and other similar data from the French registry encourages one to consider prophylactic rituximab in patients with severe ADAMTS13 deficiency during remission [31]. While there are no other drugs that have been formally studied to prevent relapsing or recurrent acquired TTP, splenectomy has been shown to significantly decrease relapses [32].

Management of Refractory/Relapsing Acquired TTP

Refractory TTP is defined by lack of clinical response to more than five episodes of PEX (1–1.5 × plasma volume) every 12–24 h and steroid treatment, with persistent thrombocytopenia (<30,000 to 50,000 mm^3) and elevated LDH (>1.5 × ULN). Often clinical response is noted within 10–15 days of starting PEX. Patients who had an initial response and then deteriorated within a short time frame (15 days) are included in this definition of refractory TTP. This is different than "exacerbation" where there is recurrence of thrombocytopenia (<150,000 mm^3) and increased LDH necessitating PEX therapy within 30 days from an initial treatment response. Exacerbation occurring after 30 days to initial response is termed "relapsing" TTP [29].

Currently, there is no consensus in the management of refractory/relapsing TTP. If response to PEX therapy and steroids is suboptimal, intensification of PEX therapy (increase to 1.5 × plasma volume) should be tried and/or be given every 12 h. Rituximab should be promptly administered if not part of the initial management. Immunomodulatory agents outlined below and splenectomy are some of the salvage therapy options, but newer treatment options are being trialed and used with varying frequency [13, 33].

Immunomodulatory Agents

Cyclosporine A

There are reports of cyclosporine A (CSA) being effective in increasing the ADAMTS13 activity and in preventing relapses of acquired TTP [34]. However, a recent prospective randomized clinical trial comparing CSA to corticosteroids as adjunctive therapy to PEX showed no significant difference in the relapse rate between the two groups; however, corticosteroids were superior to CSA in suppressing autoantibody levels and improving the ADAMTS13 activity [35].

Vincristine

Vincristine has had some success in its use for refractory/relapsing acquired TTP patients in spite of its side effect profile, but since the emergence of rituximab, it is seldom used prior to a trial of rituximab and steroids [16, 36].

Cyclophosphamide

Cyclophosphamide is one of the immunomodulatory options in refractory acquired TTP. It has been used as a salvage therapy when PEX, steroids, rituximab, and vincristine have failed. Its use can help with recovery of platelet count and ADAMTS13 activity. Given the associated adverse effects of cyclophosphamide such as bone marrow suppression, infections, and decreased fertility, it is not used in up-front therapy [37].

Mycophenolate Mofetil

This immunosuppressive agent is widely used to prevent acute rejection after solid organ transplants and in various other autoimmune diseases. Experience with its use in acquired TTP is limited to a few case reports in patients with autoimmune and connective tissue disorders and often in conjunction with other immunomodulatory agents such as steroids and rituximab [38].

Bortezomib

Bortezomib, a proteasome inhibitor, has been in use for multiple myeloma and antibody-mediated rejection of transplanted solid organs for some time, among other emerging uses. Bortezomib was initially trialed in a patient with acquired TTP refractory to PEX and immunosuppression, with a depleted B cell compartment but thought to have autoantibodies originating from plasma cells, and resulted in a prompt response. Per report, four doses of bortezomib (1.3 mg/m^2/dose) resulted in recovery of platelet count and neurological function [39]. Since then, multiple case reports regarding its use in refractory acquired TTP have emerged [40], and it is currently considered an adjunct therapy option in relapsed/refractory acquired TTP.

Splenectomy

While splenectomy was in use for the treatment of acquired TTP before PEX came into use as frontline therapy, its role in the era of PEX, steroids, and rituximab is minimal, as it is now generally reserved for a salvage option. A retrospective study which included 33 patients who underwent splenectomy for plasma refractory or recurrent TTP demonstrated a 10-year relapse-free survival of 70% [32]. In another literature review of 74 cases involving 15 studies of refractory TTP, only 8% of patients failed to respond to splenectomy [41]. Similar to immune thrombocytopenia, it has a limited use in patients in whom the autoantibodies are thought to be produced by B cells that have escaped the rituximab treatment.

Newer Agents

N-acetylcysteine

N-acetylcysteine (NAC) has been in use for acetaminophen poisoning and as a mucolytic agent in pulmonary diseases. In the latter, it works by breaking the disulfide bonds in mucoproteins, which lowers the viscosity of mucus. In a similar fashion, NAC has been shown in vitro and in animal models, to reduce the disulfide bond present in the A1 domain of vWF that interacts with platelet glycoprotein 1b. This reduces the size of ULVWF multimers and inhibits platelet adherence and aggregation [42].

Animal data also suggest that NAC is effective in preventing thrombus formation and MAHA when given along with PEX, but not in resolution of already formed thrombi [43], again emphasizing that it can be a useful adjunct with PEX therapy. Its benefit in refractory TTP in conjunction with PEX and steroids has been demonstrated via evidence of platelet count recovery [44, 45]. Easy availability in most emergency departments, low cost, and acceptable safety profile has increased its appeal within the treatment options for TTP. Its potential for up-front therapy along with PEX is being studied in a pilot trial at a dose of 150 mg/kg loading dose over 60 min followed by 150 mg/kg over 17 h (NCT01808521).

Targeted Therapy in TTP

The vWF A1 domain-platelet glycoprotein 1b has been targeted using small molecule technology.

ARC1779 is a small oligonucleotide aptamer that binds to A1 domain of vWF and blocks vWF-dependent platelet function. In a Phase II trial, this aptamer along with PEX also demonstrated benefit as evidenced by increased platelet counts [46].

GBR600 is a humanized anti-vWF monoclonal antibody that has been studied in baboons. This inhibitory antibody given during acute TTP resulted in platelet recovery and was also noted to protect baboons from acquired TTP [47].

ALX-0081 and ALX-0681 are humanized bivalent single-chained nanobodies which bind to the N-terminus of the vWF A1 domain and block the interaction of any sizes of vWF to the platelet glycoprotein Ib. ALX-0081 is an intravenous active drug, while ALX-0681 is given subcutaneously. These two agents were studied in vitro and in preclinical animal models (baboon) and showed efficacy as an adjunct with PEX with no signs of excessive bleeding [48, 49]. Subsequently, a multicenter, single-blind, randomized, placebo-controlled study (TITAN) assessed the use of caplacizumab (ALX-0081) along with PEX in 75 patients (36 received caplacizumab and 39 received placebo). There was a 39% reduction in median time to recovery of platelet count in the caplacizumab group compared to the placebo group. Exacerbation of acquired TTP was also greater in the placebo group (11 patients) compared to caplacizumab group (3 patients). Mild to moderate bleeding-related adverse events were more common in the caplacizumab group compared to the placebo group (54% vs. 38%), but these did not require any intervention. The study group had eight patients relapse within 10 days of withdrawal of the study drug, while the placebo group had none. Seven of those eight patients who relapsed had persistent ADAMTS13 activity of <10%, indicating the continual presence of anti-ADAMTS13 autoantibodies. There were two deaths in the placebo group in patients who were refractory to treatment, and no deaths were reported in the study group [50]. A multinational, double-blind, placebo-controlled Phase III study utilizing caplacizumab (HERCULES) was recently closed after recruiting 145 patients (NCT02553317), with data forthcoming. In addition, investigation regarding the long-term safety and efficacy of caplacizumab (Post-HERCULES) is in progress (NCT02878603).

These agents are very promising for the initial management of acquired TTP. While PEX and immunosuppressive therapy help to remove anti-ADAMTS13 autoantibodies and restore ADAMTS13 activity in the acute phase of disease, the vWF A1 domain inhibitors prevent the microangiopathy which occurs during the acute phase of disease, in addition to preventing subsequent thrombocytopenia, organ ischemia, and morbidity/mortality.

Recombinant ADAMTS13

Recombinant ADAMTS13 (rADAMTS13) was developed as a replacement product for use in cTTP, anticipating potential replacement of chronic plasma infusion therapy. Additionally, a recombinant product may have potential use in the treatment of acquired TTP [51]. This product was initially studied in vitro, where addition of rADAMTS13 to the plasma from two brothers with cTTP resulted in normalization of vWF multimer processing activity [52]. Further in vitro experiments in 36 plasma samples from acquired TTP patients showed that the concentration of rADAMTS13 required for vWF processing activity was in linear relationship to the inhibitor titers of those samples [53].

This effect in iTTP was confirmed in rat models; inhibitor titer-adjusted rADAMTS13 concentrations were given to rats who were treated with goat anti-ADAMTS13 IgG, and reconstitution of ADAMTS13 activity in the plasma of these rats was achieved [54]. Preclinical studies were conducted in ADAMTS13 knockout animal models using a new rADAMTS13 product (BAX930), and platelet counts stabilized with no severe adverse effects. However, formation of anti-ADAMTS13 antibodies was noted. This may not be clinically significant in humans, however, as most cTTP results from compound heterozygous defects [55]. rADAMTS13 is currently being trialed in a Phase I study in patients with cTTP (NCT02216084).

Long-Term Outcomes

A significant number of TTP survivors have varying degrees of neuropsychological deficits affecting their quality of life. These include difficulties with memory, cognition, concentration, and processing of information. The deficits are sometimes subtle and do not appear to improve over time. These changes do not correlate with the neurological symptoms at the presentation of acute acquired TTP [12, 56, 57]. Screening performed on 52 patients within the Oklahoma TTP-HUS registry revealed that 29% report being severely depressed at least once. Eighty-nine percent of these had further psychiatric evaluation and were confirmed to have major depressive disorder. This finding did not correlate with relapses or ADAMTS13 activity levels [58]. Another significant finding among long-term survivors of acquired TTP is the presence of arterial hypertension in up to 40% [59].

Conclusion

There have been considerable advances in the diagnosis and management of acquired TTP in the past decade, resulting in a dramatic decline in morbidity and mortality. Newer adjuvant therapies and up-front rituximab could continue to improve outcomes. A high clinical suspicion, early initiation of plasma exchange, and prompt diagnosis remain critical. Additionally, these patients require ongoing long-term close follow-up for early detection of relapse, diagnosis of comorbid autoimmune disorders, and neuropsychological sequelae. Ongoing research is needed to continue improving the outcome for patients affected with acquired TTP.

References

1. Kato S, Matsumoto M, Matsuyama T, Isonishi A, Hiura H, Fujimura Y. Novel monoclonal antibody-based enzyme immunoassay for determining plasma levels of ADAMTS13 activity. Transfusion. 2006;46(8):1444–52.
2. Kokame K, Nobe Y, Kokubo Y, Okayama A, Miyata T. FRETS-VWF73, a first fluorogenic substrate for ADAMTS13 assay. Br J Haematol. 2005;129(1):93–100.

3. Rieger M. ADAMTS13 autoantibodies in patients with thrombotic microangiopathies and other immunomediated diseases. Blood. 2005;106(4):1262–7.
4. Riviere E, Saint-Léger M, James C, Delmas Y, Clouzeau B, Bui N, et al. Platelet transfusion and catheter insertion for plasma exchange in patients with thrombotic thrombocytopenic purpura and a low platelet count. Transfusion. 2015;55(7):1798–802.
5. Som S, Deford CC, Kaiser ML, Terrell DR, Kremer Hovinga JA, Lämmle B, et al. Decreasing frequency of plasma exchange complications in patients treated for thrombotic thrombocytopenic purpura-hemolytic uremic syndrome, 1996 to 2011 (CME). Transfusion. 2012;52(12):2525–32.
6. Ridolfi RL, Bell WR. Thrombotic thrombocytopenic purpura. Report of 25 cases and review of the literature. Medicine. 1981;60(6):413–28.
7. Pereira A, Mazzara R, Monteagudo J, Sanz C. Thrombotic thrombocytopenic purpura/hemolytic uremic syndrome: a multivariate analysis of factors predicting the response to plasma exchange. Ann Hematal. 1995;70(6):319–23.
8. Rock GA, Shumak KH, Buskard NA, Blanchette VS, Kelton JG, Nair RC, et al. Comparison of plasma exchange with plasma infusion in the treatment of thrombotic thrombocytopenic purpura. Canadian Apheresis Study Group. N Engl J Med. 1991;325(6):393–7.
9. George JN, Gilcher RO, Smith JW, Chandler L, Duvall D, Ellis C. Thrombotic thrombocytopenic purpura-hemolytic uremic syndrome: diagnosis and management. J Clin Apher. 1998;13(3):120–5.
10. Scully M, Hunt BJ, Benjamin S, Liesner R, Rose P, Peyvandi F, et al. Guidelines on the diagnosis and management of thrombotic thrombocytopenic purpura and other thrombotic microangiopathies. Br J Haematol. 2012;158(3):323–35.
11. Joly BS, Coppo P, Veyradier A. Thrombotic thrombocytopenic purpura. Blood. 2017;129(21):2836–46.
12. George JN. How I treat patients with thrombotic thrombocytopenic purpura: 2010. Blood. 2010;116(20):4060–9.
13. Page EE, Hovinga J, Terrell DR, Vesely SK. Thrombotic thrombocytopenic purpura: diagnostic criteria, clinical features, and long-term outcomes from 1995 through 2015. Blood. 2017;1:590–600.
14. The Italian TTP Study Group, Balduini CL, Gugliotta L, Luppi M, Laurenti L, Klersy C, et al. High versus standard dose methylprednisolone in the acute phase of idiopathic thrombotic thrombocytopenic purpura: a randomized study. Ann Hematol. 2009;89(6):591–6.
15. Rojnuckarin P, Watanaboonyongcharoen P, Akkawat B, Intragumtornchai T. The role of pulse dexamethasone in acquired idiopathic thrombotic thrombocytopenic purpura. J Thromb Haemost. 2006;4(5):1148–50.
16. Sayani FA, Abrams CS. How I treat refractory thrombotic thrombocytopenic purpura. Blood. 2015;125(25):3860–7.
17. Scully M, Cohen H, Cavenagh J, Benjamin S, Starke R, Killick S, et al. Remission in acute refractory and relapsing thrombotic thrombocytopenic purpura following rituximab is associated with a reduction in IgG antibodies to ADAMTS-13. Br J Haematol. 2007;136(3):451–61.
18. Mcdonald V, Manns K, Mackie IJ, Machin SJ, Scully MA. Rituximab pharmacokinetics during the management of acute idiopathic thrombotic thrombocytopenic purpura. J Thromb Haemost. 2010;8(6):1201–8.
19. Froissart A, Buffet M, Veyradier A, Poullin P, Provôt F, Malot S, et al. Efficacy and safety of first-line rituximab in severe, acquired thrombotic thrombocytopenic purpura with a suboptimal response to plasma exchange. Experience of the French thrombotic microangiopathies reference center. Crit Care Med. 2012;40(1):104–11.
20. Scully M, Mcdonald V, Cavenagh J, Hunt BJ, Longair I, Cohen H, et al. A phase 2 study of the safety and efficacy of rituximab with plasma exchange in acute acquired thrombotic thrombocytopenic purpura. Blood. 2011;118(7):1746–53.
21. Page EE, Kremer Hovinga JA, Terrell DR, Vesely SK, George JN. Rituximab reduces risk for relapse in patients with thrombotic thrombocytopenic purpura. Blood. 2016;127(24):3092–4.
22. Westwood JP, Webster H, McGuckin S, Mcdonald V, Machin SJ, Scully M. Rituximab for thrombotic thrombocytopenic purpura: benefit of early administration during acute episodes and use of prophylaxis to prevent relapse. J Thromb Haemost. 2013;11(3):481–90.

23. Amorosi EL, Ultmann JE. Thrombotic thrombocytopenic purpura: report of 16 cases and review of the literature. Medicine. 1966;45:139–59.
24. Bell WR, Braine HG, Ness PM, Kickler TS. Improved survival in thrombotic thrombocytopenic purpura-hemolytic uremic syndrome. Clinical experience in 108 patients. N Engl J Med. 1991;325(6):398–403.
25. Roriz M, Landais M, Desprez J, Barbet C, Azoulay E, Galicier L, et al. Risk factors for autoimmune diseases development after thrombotic thrombocytopenic purpura. Medicine. 2015;94(42):e1598–8.
26. Reese JA, Muthurajah DS, Hovinga JAK, Vesely SK, Terrell DR, George JN. Children and adults with thrombotic thrombocytopenic purpura associated with severe, acquired Adamts13 deficiency: comparison of incidence, demographic and clinical features. Pediatr Blood Cancer. 2013;60(10):1676–82.
27. Hovinga J, Vesely SK, Terrell DR, Lämmle B. Survival and relapse in patients with thrombotic thrombocytopenic purpura. Blood. 2010;115(8):1500–11.
28. Jin M, Casper TC, Cataland SR, Kennedy MS, Lin S, Li YJ, et al. Relationship between ADAMTS13 activity in clinical remission and the risk of TTP relapse. Br J Haematol. 2008;141(5):651–8.
29. Scully M, Cataland S, Coppo P, de la Rubia J, Friedman KD, Kremer Hovinga J, et al. Consensus on the standardization of terminology in thrombotic thrombocytopenic purpura and related thrombotic microangiopathies. J Thromb Haemost. 2016;15(2):312–22.
30. Page EE, Hovinga J, Terrell DR, Vesely SK. Clinical importance of ADAMTS13 activity during remission in patients with acquired thrombotic thrombocytopenic purpura. Blood. 2016;128(17):2175–8.
31. Hie M, Gay J, Galicier L, Provot F, Presne C, Poullin P, et al. Preemptive rituximab infusions after remission efficiently prevent relapses in acquired thrombotic thrombocytopenic purpura. Blood. 2014;124(2):204–10.
32. Kappers-Klunne MC, Wijermans P, Fijnheer R, Croockewit AJ, Holt B, Wolf JTM, et al. Splenectomy for the treatment of thrombotic thrombocytopenic purpura. Br J Haematol. 2005;130(5):768–76.
33. Coppo P. French Reference Center for Thrombotic Microangiopathies. Treatment of autoimmune thrombotic thrombocytopenic purpura in the more severe forms. Transfus Apher Sci. 2017;56(1):52–6.
34. Cataland SR, Holers VM, Geyer S, Yang S, Wu HM. Biomarkers of the alternative pathway and terminal complement activity at presentation confirms the clinical diagnosis of aHUS and differentiates aHUS from TTP. Blood. 2014;23(24):3733–8.
35. Cataland S, Yang S, Masias Castanon C, McGookey M, Wu H, Geyer S, et al. A prospective, randomized study of cyclosporine or corticosteroids as an adjunct to plasma exchange for the treatment of thrombotic thrombocytopenic purpura. Blood. 2016;128(22):133.
36. Ziman A, Mitri M, Klapper E, Pepkowitz SH, Goldfinger D. Combination vincristine and plasma exchange as initial therapy in patients with thrombotic thrombocytopenic purpura: one institution's experience and review of the literature. Transfusion. 2005;45(1):41–9.
37. Beloncle F, Buffet M, Coindre J-P, Munoz-Bongrand N, Malot S, Pène F, et al. Splenectomy and/or cyclophosphamide as salvage therapies in thrombotic thrombocytopenic purpura: the French TMA reference center experience. Transfusion. 2012;52(11):2436–44.
38. Ahmad HN, Thomas-Dewing RR, Hunt BJ. Mycophenolate mofetil in a case of relapsed, refractory thrombotic thrombocytopenic purpura. Eur J Haematol. 2007;78(5):449–52.
39. Shortt J, Oh DH, Opat SS. ADAMTS13 antibody depletion by bortezomib in thrombotic thrombocytopenic purpura. N Engl J Med. 2013;368(1):90–2.
40. Eskazan AE. Bortezomib therapy in patients with relapsed/refractory acquired thrombotic thrombocytopenic purpura. Ann Hematol. 2016;95(11):1–6.
41. Dubois L, Gray DK. Case series: splenectomy: does it still play a role in the management of thrombotic thrombocytopenic purpura? Can J Surg. 2010;53(5):349–55.

42. Chen J, Reheman A, Gushiken FC, Nolasco L, Fu X, Moake JL, et al. N-acetylcysteine reduces the size and activity of von Willebrand factor in human plasma and mice. J Clin Invest. 2011;121(2):593–603.
43. Tersteeg C, Roodt J, Van Rensburg WJ, Dekimpe C, Vandeputte N, Pareyn I, et al. N-acetylcysteine in preclinical mouse and baboon models of thrombotic thrombocytopenic purpura. Blood. 2017;129(8):1030–8.
44. Cabanillas G, Popescu-Martinez A. N-Acetylcysteine for relapsing thrombotic thrombocytopenic purpura: more evidence of a promising drug. Am J Ther. 2016;23(5):e1277–9.
45. Rottenstreich A, Hochberg-Klein S, Rund D, Kalish Y. The role of N-acetylcysteine in the treatment of thrombotic thrombocytopenic purpura. J Thromb Thrombolysis. 2015;41(4):678–83.
46. Cataland SR, Peyvandi F, Mannucci PM. Initial experience from a double-blind, placebo-controlled, clinical outcome study of ARC1779 in patients with thrombotic thrombocytopenic purpura. Am J Hamatol. 2012;87(4):430–2.
47. Feys HB, Roodt J, Vandeputte N, Pareyn I, Mottl H, Hou S, et al. Inhibition of von Willebrand factor-platelet glycoprotein Ib interaction prevents and reverses symptoms of acute acquired thrombotic thrombocytopenic purpura in baboons. Blood. 2012;120(17):3611–4.
48. Ulrichts H, Silence K, Schoolmeester A, de Jaegere P, Rossenu S, Roodt J, et al. Antithrombotic drug candidate ALX-0081 shows superior preclinical efficacy and safety compared with currently marketed antiplatelet drugs. Blood. 2011;118(3):757–65.
49. Callewaert F, Roodt J, Ulrichts H, Stohr T, van Rensburg WJ, Lamprecht S, et al. Evaluation of efficacy and safety of the anti-VWF Nanobody ALX-0681 in a preclinical baboon model of acquired thrombotic thrombocytopenic purpura. Blood. 2012;120(17):3603–10.
50. Peyvandi F, Scully M, Kremer Hovinga JA, Cataland S, Knöbl P, Wu H, et al. Caplacizumab for acquired thrombotic thrombocytopenic purpura. N Engl J Med. 2016;374(6):511–22.
51. Plaimauer B. Cloning, expression, and functional characterization of the von Willebrand factor-cleaving protease (ADAMTS13). Blood. 2002;100(10):3626–32.
52. Antoine G, Zimmermann K, Plaimauer B. ADAMTS13 gene defects in two brothers with constitutional thrombotic thrombocytopenic purpura and normalization of von Willebrand factor-cleaving. Br J Haematol. 2003;120(5):821–4.
53. Plaimauer B, Kremer hovinga JA, Juno C, Wolfsegger MJ, Skalicky S, Schmidt M, et al. Recombinant ADAMTS13 normalizes von Willebrand factor-cleaving activity in plasma of acquired TTP patients by overriding inhibitory antibodies. J Thromb Haemost. 2011;9(5):936–44.
54. Plaimauer B, Schiviz A, Kaufmann S, Höllriegl W, Rottensteiner H, Scheiflinger F. Neutralization of inhibitory antibodies and restoration of therapeutic ADAMTS-13 activity levels in inhibitor-treated rats by the use of defined doses of recombinant ADAMTS-13. J Thrombosis Haemostasis. 2015;13(11):2053–62.
55. Kopić A, Benamara K, Piskernik C, Plaimauer B, Horling F, Höbarth G, et al. Preclinical assessment of a new recombinant ADAMTS-13 drug product (BAX930) for the treatment of thrombotic thrombocytopenic purpura. J Thromb Haemost. 2016;14(7):1410–9.
56. Lewis QF, Lanneau MS, Mathias SD, Terrell DR, Vesely SK, George JN. Long-term deficits in health-related quality of life after recovery from thrombotic thrombocytopenic purpura. Transfusion. 2009;49(1):118–24.
57. Kennedy AS, Lewis QF, Scott JG, Kremer Hovinga JA, Lämmle B, Terrell DR, et al. Cognitive deficits after recovery from thrombotic thrombocytopenic purpura. Transfusion. 2009;49(6):1092–101.
58. Han B, Page EE, Stewart LM, Deford CC, Scott JG, Schwartz LH, et al. Depression and cognitive impairment following recovery from thrombotic thrombocytopenic purpura. Am J Hematol. 2015;90(8):709–14.
59. Deford CC, Reese JA, Schwartz LH, Perdue JJ, Kremer hovinga JA, Lämmle B, et al. Multiple major morbidities and increased mortality during long-term follow-up after recovery from thrombotic thrombocytopenic purpura. Blood. 2013;122(12):2023–9.

Part IV
Autoimmune Neutropenia (AIN)

Chapter 11
Background and Pathophysiology of Autoimmune Neutropenia

Jacquelyn M. Powers

Overview of Neutropenia

Neutropenia is defined as a decrease in the absolute neutrophil count (ANC) in the peripheral blood. The normal ANC range is dependent on an individual's racial and ethnic background and age. For Caucasian children 1 year of age and older, neutropenia is defined as an ANC less than 1500 cell/μL. For infants less than 1 year, 1000 cell/μL is considered the lower limit of normal. Most Caucasian and Asian populations have ANCs in the range of 1500–7000 cell/μL [1]. In persons of African descent, approximately 5% have ANCs less than 1500 cell/μL, which is associated with the Duffy negative blood group and sometimes referred to as "ethnic pseudoneutropenia." Clinically significant or severe neutropenia is considered when the ANC is under 500 cell/μL [2].

Neutropenia, as with other decreased hematopoietic cell lines, can be considered in terms of decreased production, margination from the circulating pool, or increased utilization and/or destruction. Classification can also be made based on the etiology. For neutropenia, broad underlying categories include infectious, drug-related, malignancy, congenital, or autoimmune. Transient neutropenia, enduring less than 3 months, may occur frequently in association with acute viral infections. Autoimmune neutropenia is considered a chronic condition lasting a minimum of 3 months. The primary focus of this chapter will be primary autoimmune neutropenia.

Autoimmune neutropenia and chronic benign neutropenia of infancy and childhood are often described together due to the challenges in distinguishing the two conditions. Many children diagnosed with chronic idiopathic neutropenia are now thought to be secondary to autoimmunity against neutrophils as well. These

J. M. Powers, MD, MS
Pediatric Hematology/Oncology, Baylor College of Medicine, Texas Children's Cancer and
Hematology Center, Houston, TX, USA
e-mail: jacquelyn.powers@bcm.edu

© Springer International Publishing AG, part of Springer Nature 2018   207
J. M. Despotovic (ed.), *Immune Hematology*,
https://doi.org/10.1007/978-3-319-73269-5_11

conditions share characteristics of a benign overall course and a good clinical outcome for most affected patients. In contrast to congenital neutropenia related to decreased or absent bone marrow production, patients with increased destruction of neutrophils, as in autoimmune neutropenia, have much lower rates of infection and morbidity and rarely develop severe infections. An appropriate rise in neutrophil count during an acute infection is supportive of the diagnosis. Relatively benign and common childhood infections such as upper respiratory infections, acute otitis media, or skin infections may be present, and in cases of severe neutropenia, mouth sores may occur [3].

Epidemiology of Autoimmune Neutropenia

Autoimmune neutropenia is the most common chronic neutropenia of childhood [4]. Its historically cited prevalence was 1 in 100,000 children per year [5, 6]. However, analysis of data from the Italian Neutropenia Registry estimated an incidence as high as 1 out of 6300 live births [6]. The neutropenia is often detected during an acute febrile illness, which persists upon follow-up testing after resolution of the infection. However, up to 30% of cases are identified incidentally outside the context of an acute infection [7]. Given that most children experience a benign course and may never have a complete blood count assessed, the true incidence is likely underreported.

Autoimmune neutropenia typically presents within the first 2 years of life [7]. There is no clear difference in prevalence based on gender. A Japanese cohort of 18 patients found the average age of onset between 7 and 8 (+/− 3) months of age [8]. Data from the Italian Neutropenia Registry on 157 patients also found that the majority experienced the disease within the first year of life (median age of onset 8–9 months), though the diagnosis was often not confirmed until 3–4 months from the time of onset [4, 6]. All patients presented before the age of 5, with 82% presenting before 18 months of age. Three children presented within the first month of life after having alloimmune neutropenia ruled out. The condition spontaneously resolves in the majority of children (>95%) by age 5, with remission occurring within 18–24 months from the time of diagnosis [8, 9]. Children beyond 5 years of age with chronic autoimmune neutropenia are more likely to be secondary to other immune or autoimmune conditions [1].

Six percent of patients within the Italian Registry had an elevated immunoglobulin (Ig) G at the time of diagnosis, and IgA deficiency was found in 3% [6]. Two-thirds of patients who recovered had a sudden resolution with no subsequent neutropenia. One-third had a transient, intermittent neutropenia phase lasting up to 2 years prior to complete resolution. A favorable outcome (earlier recovery) was associated with early age at onset and a lack of monocytosis at diagnosis. However, remission can occur in patients even after prolonged time courses and beyond the age of 5 [6].

Pathophysiology of Immune Neutropenia

Neonatal Immune Neutropenia

Immune neutropenia in the neonatal period can be alloimmune or autoimmune. The former occurs from alloimmunization against fetal neutrophil-specific antigens that are not present on maternal white blood cells [9]. The neutropenia can be severe and result in life-threatening infections to the newborn including omphalitis, cellulitis, or sepsis. While the immune destruction typically remits within 6 weeks, neutropenia may persist for up to 6 months. Neonates can also develop autoimmune neutropenia from maternal antineutrophil IgG autoantibodies that cross the placenta in a mother affected with autoimmune neutropenia. Though rare, this form of neutropenia may also result in severe infections in the newborn.

Primary Autoimmune Neutropenia

Outside the neonatal period, many, but not all children with presumptive autoimmune neutropenia have autoantibodies directed against neutrophil surface antigens. The resulting neutropenia is due to peripheral destruction of antibody-coated neutrophils, and phagocytosis of neutrophils in the spleens of autoimmune neutropenia patients has been observed [10]. The precise mechanism for autoantibody production is unknown. Potentially, antibodies to foreign antigens such as viruses cross-react with self-antigens [11]. No specific viral antigens have been associated with the development of autoimmune neutropenia, including one study of 240 affected infants and children, which found no significant association with parvovirus B19 infection [3]. In a healthy functioning immune system, this cross-reactivity is self-limited.

The relatively longer duration of autoimmune neutropenia (typically 18 months) may be due to the lack of full suppressor T-cell function development during the first years of life, which could allow autoantibody production as a consequence of a "surveillance escape event" [12]. The Italian Neutropenia Registry demonstrated that 13% of children had been born premature, which would support this notion of an immature suppressor system playing a role in the pathophysiology [6]. The eventual remission from autoimmune neutropenia would then relate to the maturation of suppressor T-cell function. A similar but alternative mechanism in secondary autoimmune neutropenia would be the loss of suppression of a clone of cells that are able to react with self-antigens due to immune dysregulation, rather than an immature immune system.

In 2015, 11 human neutrophil antigens (HNAs) had been described [7]. HNA-1 is the most immunogenic glycoprotein, located on the immunoglobulin membrane receptor FcγRIIIb (CD16), which is only expressed by neutrophils [2, 7]. The most commonly involved alleles are HNA-1a, HNA-1b, and HNA-1c, with the first two being the principal antigens implicated in autoimmune neutropenia of infancy [1]. Additional antigens include HNA-2a (glycoprotein 58–64, CD177), HNA-3a and 3b (choline transporter-like protein 2), HNA-4a and HNA-4bw (CD11b), and HNA5a and HNA-5bw (CD11a) [7]. The antibodies directed against the neutrophil cell surface membrane have no relationship with antineutrophil cytoplasmic antibodies (ANCA).

Bruin et al. found that early in the disease course of autoimmune neutropenia, pan-FcγRIIIb antibodies were detected in most patients [4]. Later, HNA-1a- and HNA-1b-specific antibodies developed in those with primary autoimmune neutropenia. Sera from patients with secondary autoimmune neutropenia, however, demonstrated persistent pan-FcγRIIIb antibodies [11]. The disappearance of antibody over time precedes eventual ANC recovery, but no specific predictors of time to recovery have been identified [4]. This group hypothesized that at the onset of primary autoimmune neutropenia, nonselective antibody production exists initially followed by selection toward antibodies with a higher affinity over time, similar to autoantibodies produced in celiac disease and systemic lupus erythematosus. Or, at the onset of disease, there may be a loss of tolerance in which naïve, autoreactive B cells receive inappropriate costimulatory signals. This phenomenon is sometimes referred to as bystander activation and occurs in the setting of posttransfusion purpura, in which B cells receive inappropriate costimulatory signals from memory alloreactive T cells [4].

HNA phenotype varies across racial and ethnic groups. On average, 4% of individuals express HNA-1a, HNA-1b, and HNA-1c [7]. Less than 2% are HNA-1a-1b-1c null. Within the United States, HNA-1a is expressed in approximately 37% of Caucasians, 31% of African Americans, 53% of persons of Hispanic/Latino ethnicity, and 55% of Native Americans [7]. HNA-1b is found in 63% of Caucasians, 69% of African Americans, 47% of persons of Hispanic/Latino ethnicity, and 45% of Native Americans. Due to this variability, the specific autoantibodies and expression level are dependent not only on the phase of the disease but also on an individuals' racial and ethnic background [11]. The labile nature of granulocytes makes it difficult to detect autoantibodies in persons with presumptive autoimmune neutropenia. However, antineutrophil antibodies can be detected in many patients when combining both agglutination and immunofluorescence assays, though repeat testing is often necessary (see Chapter 12 on Evaluation and Management of Autoimmune Neutropenia) [10].

More than half of patients with autoimmune neutropenia present with severe neutropenia. Leukopenia may be present, but in up to half of cases, the total white blood cell count is normal; monocytosis may also be present [6]. Most bone marrow examinations performed in patients with primary autoimmune neutropenia have normal to increased cellularity with an increased myeloid to erythroid ratio and without a relative decrease in mature granulocyte precursors [6, 13]. In one series of 240 patients with confirmed autoimmune neutropenia in whom 133 evaluable bone marrow examinations were performed, only 3% had hypocellular marrow [3]. In such cases, antibodies are thought to bind to granulocyte precursors in the marrow, in addition to binding the mature neutrophils found in the peripheral blood. This antibody-mediated destruction for segmented neutrophils and base forms may mimic maturation arrest in the myelocyte and metamyelocyte stage [3].

Secondary Autoimmune Neutropenia

As with children with other immune-mediated cytopenias, such as immune thrombocytopenia purpura or autoimmune hemolytic anemia, patients with chronic autoimmune neutropenia persisting beyond age 5 years are more likely to have a secondary form related to other chronic disease or immune-mediated processes [9]. Secondary autoimmune neutropenia can present at any age and has a variable clinical course. In older children and adolescents, there is a higher frequency in females, increased association with other autoimmune disorders, and less likelihood of a spontaneous remission [7]. As mentioned previously, autoantibody formation differs from that of primary autoimmune neutropenia in that affinity maturation to specific HNAs does not occur. Alternatively, regulation of self-recognition is too disturbed to correct the loss of tolerance, which leads to antibodies with pan-FcγRIIIb specificity [4]. Thus, patients who develop autoimmune neutropenia beyond a very young age have disease persistent for more than 3 years or who develop additional cell lineage abnormalities should be assessed for secondary forms [12].

References

1. Newburger PE, Dale DC. Evaluation and management of patients with isolated neutropenia. Semin Hematol. 2013;50(3):198–206.
2. Newburger PE. Autoimmune and other acquired neutropenias. Hematol Am Soc Hematol Educ Prog. 2016;2016(1):38–42.
3. Bux J, Behrens G, Jaeger G, Welte K. Diagnosis and clinical course of autoimmune neutropenia in infancy: analysis of 240 cases. Blood. 1998;91(1):181–6.
4. Bruin M, Dassen A, Pajkrt D, Buddelmeyer L, Kuijpers T, de Haas M. Primary autoimmune neutropenia in children: a study of neutrophil antibodies and clinical course. Vox Sang. 2005;88(1):52–9.
5. Lyall EG, Lucas GF, Eden OB. Autoimmune neutropenia of infancy. J Clin Pathol. 1992;45(5):431–4.
6. Farruggia P, Fioredda F, Puccio G, Porretti L, Lanza T, Ramenghi U, et al. Autoimmune neutropenia of infancy: data from the Italian neutropenia registry. Am J Hematol. 2015;90(12): E221–2.
7. Farruggia P, Dufour C. Diagnosis and management of primary autoimmune neutropenia in children: insights for clinicians. Ther Adv Hematol. 2015;6(1):15–24.
8. Taniuchi S, Masuda M, Hasui M, Tsuji S, Takahashi H, Kobayashi Y. Differential diagnosis and clinical course of autoimmune neutropenia in infancy: comparison with congenital neutropenia. Acta Paediatr. 2002;91(11):1179–82.
9. Teachey DT, Lambert MP. Diagnosis and management of autoimmune cytopenias in childhood. Pediatr Clin N Am. 2013;60(6):1489–511.

10. Dinauer MC, Newburger PE. The phagocyte system and disorders of granulopoiesis and granulocyte function. In: Orkin SH, Nathan DG, Ginsburg D, Look AT, Fisher DE, Lux SE, editors. Nathan and Oski's Hematology of infancy and childhood. 7th ed. Philadelphia, PA: Saunders Elsevier; 2009. p. 1145–9.
11. Bruin MC, von dem Borne AE, Tamminga RY, Kleijer M, Buddelmeijer L, de Haas M. Neutrophil antibody specificity in different types of childhood autoimmune neutropenia. Blood. 1999;94(5):1797–802.
12. Dufour C, Miano M, Fioredda F. Old and new faces of neutropenia in children. Haematologica. 2016;101(7):789–91.
13. Bussel JB, Abboud MR. Autoimmune neutropenia of childhood. Crit Rev Oncol Hematol. 1987;7(1):37–51.

Chapter 12
Evaluation and Management of Autoimmune Neutropenia

Alicia K. Chang

Evaluation and Workup

When a child presents with neutropenia, the most pressing emphasis remains on ascertaining his or her risk for infection and addressing that risk. Defining the underlying pathology, however, plays a significant role in estimating infection risk in childhood neutropenia. A thorough medical history, physical examination, and family history can often narrow the differential diagnoses in a child presenting with neutropenia. Further laboratory investigation and bone marrow evaluation are usually not indicated for a child whose history strongly suggests AIN [1]. Antineutrophil antibodies in the peripheral blood can help to diagnose AIN; however, this test is limited by low sensitivity, as will be discussed in detail in the following section. Onset and age of presentation, history of prior infections, drug exposures and maternal history can be helpful. A careful physical exam documenting growth retardation, dysmorphic features, organomegaly, or lab data documenting other cytopenias or organ dysfunction can also be useful in delineating etiologies of neutropenia.

Autoimmune neutropenia is most common in the first 2 years of life and usually presents in an otherwise well child [1]. Physical exam is often non-specific in children with AIN, with possible findings of aphthous stomatitis or mild infections of otitis media or upper respiratory infections [2, 3], but generally no severe infections despite typically severe peripheral neutropenia. Occasionally, these children can present with a preceding viral illness, although interestingly, a case report of 240 infants with AIN failed to find a correlation with parvovirus infection and AIN [3].

A. K. Chang, MD
Section of Hematology-Oncology, Department of Pediatrics,
Baylor College of Medicine, Texas Children's Hospital, Houston, TX, USA
e-mail: akchang@txch.org

© Springer International Publishing AG, part of Springer Nature 2018   213
J. M. Despotovic (ed.), *Immune Hematology*,
https://doi.org/10.1007/978-3-319-73269-5_12

In contrast, congenital causes of neutropenia may present with recurrent fevers and infections at an early age [1], as well as a strong family history of infections and/or neutropenia. An investigation into the underlying cause of neutropenia is important, as this may predict clinical severity and guide both medical intervention and anticipatory guidance for families.

Secondary causes of AIN are more common in older children and adults [1]. A non-exhaustive list of secondary causes include connective tissue and autoimmune systemic diseases, medications, and malignancy [2]. The cause of neutropenia in secondary forms is often multifactorial; antineutrophil antibodies, other mechanisms of neutrophil peripheral destruction, and decreased granulopoiesis from the bone marrow may all contribute to the neutropenia seen in these secondary forms [4]. Splenomegaly and other concerning physical findings along with additional cytopenias should prompt bone marrow examination for underlying malignancy or myelodysplasia [5].

Both Felty syndrome (classically comprised of rheumatoid arthritis, splenomegaly, and neutropenia) and systemic lupus erythematosus (SLE) have been the systemic autoimmune diseases most commonly associated with neutropenia in the adult population [4]. Neutropenia in the setting of SLE has been well described, with a 47% incidence of neutropenia in patients with SLE reported in one prospective study [6]. This may be due to a similarity between a neutrophil surface antigen and Ro/SSA in SLE patients who have anti-Ro/SSA antibodies [2]. Interestingly, anti-neutrophil antibodies have been detected in patients with SLE with or without the presence of neutropenia [7].

Neutropenia seen in Felty syndrome may be caused by both immune complexes and antineutrophil antibodies adherent to neutrophil antigens [4] and by inflammatory cytokines (TNF-alpha, interferon-gamma) that may stall neutrophil bone marrow production [2, 4]. Secondary AIN in the setting of Felty syndrome can also be caused by large granular lymphocytic (LGL) leukemia, a clonal malignancy of CD8+ T cells [2]. Typically, anti-neutrophil antibody testing, which will be discussed in the following sections, has less clinical utility given its low sensitivity and specificity [5].

Differential Diagnosis of Isolated Childhood Neutropenia

Cyclic Neutropenia

Cyclic neutropenia is a rare, autosomal dominant disorder caused by mutations in the neutrophil elastase gene (*ELANE*). Mutations in this enzyme are thought to accelerate myeloid cell death; however, the exact cyclic mechanism of neutropenia has yet to be completely elucidated [1]. These patients often initially present with severe neutropenia in the setting of mouth sores and bacterial infection. Bone marrow evaluation shows periods of normal tri-lineage hematopoiesis and times of myelocyte maturational arrest in predictable intervals. These "cycles" often occur in 21-day intervals and consist of a 3–5-day period of severe neutropenia with a rapid recovery to neutrophil counts greater than 1.5×10^9/L [1, 8]. Often at ANC nadir, patients suffer from stomatitis, abscesses, and severe infections [1]. Because of the cyclical nature, diagnosis can be elusive and requires serial blood counts three times a week for 6 weeks documenting regularly the occurring periods of neutropenia [1, 8].

Severe Congenital Neutropenia (SCN)

SCN, also known as Kostmann syndrome, is a rare, heterogeneous group of diseases often associated with severe neutropenia and life-threatening infections early in life [9]. The severe neutropenia is constant, and patients develop deep tissue infections, pneumonias, and overwhelming sepsis [1]. Genetic mutations, such as *ELANE* and *HAX1* mutations, have been described in patients with SCN [1]. These patients may have accompanying dysmorphic features and metabolic derangements [1, 9, 10]. Bone marrow typically shows a maturational arrest at the promyelocyte phase [9]. Twenty to thirty percent of these patients are at risk for developing myelodysplastic syndrome and leukemias [1, 11]. Other bone marrow failure syndromes should also be considered for a patient with significant infections, chronic neutropenia, or other supportive clinical and/or laboratory findings.

Neutropenia Secondary to Drug Administration and Nutrient Deficiencies

The causative drugs are beyond the scope of this review; however, antiepileptic and antibiotic medications are most frequently described in cases of non-chemotherapy drug-induced agranulocytosis. The exact mechanism of neutropenia is debatable, but the findings of antineutrophil antibodies in some patients suggest a possible immune-mediated process [12]. Onset after exposure can be variable, and it may take between 1 week and 1 month for counts to normalize after removal of the offending agent. Vitamin B12, folate, or copper deficiencies have also been implicated as causes for neutropenia, and this resolves once these nutrient stores have been replenished [9].

AIN Associated With Other Autoimmune Diseases

Evans syndrome (the presence of two or more immune cytopenias, most classically autoimmune hemolytic anemia and ITP) and autoimmune thrombocytopenia are the most common autoimmune entities associated with neutropenia in the pediatric population, but can also be seen in SLE and other autoimmune disorders [9]. Typically, children with secondary autoimmune disease tend to be older and female.

Because it may be difficult to distinguish at initial presentation, one study suggests the characterization of antineutrophil antibodies may help discriminate between primary and secondary AIN [13], as HNA-1a- and HNA-1b-specific antibodies were found in patients with primary AIN compared to pan-FcγRIIIb specificity in secondary AIN [13].

Diagnosis

The history and physical exam findings are the most important aspects of the initial evaluation of a child with neutropenia. If a detailed review of the child's personal and family history are non-revealing, the physical exam is normal, and the suspected cause is autoimmune neutropenia; limited laboratory evaluation is recommended. A complete blood count and review of the peripheral blood smear to document neutropenia and to rule out other cytopenias or morphological abnormalities suggestive of other disorders should be done in all cases. Anti-neutrophil antibody testing can be performed, although as previously mentioned the sensitivity and specificity for AIN are low. Further testing should be considered for patients with history of more significant infections, growth or development abnormalities, or other atypical features. Bone marrow evaluation is not indicated for classic AIN but can be helpful if a production defect is suspected.

Neutrophil Antibody Detection Methods

Boxer and colleagues in 1975 first detected circulating antineutrophil antibodies that caused accelerated reticuloendothelial system-induced neutrophil destruction in three out of five hospitalized patients [4, 14]. This was corroborated by Hadley and colleagues in 1986, who published detection of increased anti-granulocyte opsonic activity in more than half of their patients with neutropenia, suggesting a possible immune basis [15]. Earlier animal studies had already demonstrated infusion of antineutrophil antibodies could lead to neutropenia by similar mechanisms of opsonization and enhanced phagocytosis [16]. However, case studies of patients with AIN have reported variable levels of circulating antineutrophil antibodies in patients strongly suspected of AIN, possibly due to circulating titers lower than the detectable limit. Moreover, a lack of relationship between the levels of circulating autoantibodies and the severity of neutropenia has also been observed in patients strongly suspected of AIN [4].

The diagnosis of AIN remains clinical, as accurate detection of antineutrophil antibodies is challenging, and the sensitivity and specificity is low. The International Granulocyte Serology Workshops have sought to establish a standardized method of detecting antineutrophil antibodies as accurate diagnostic tools to identify antineutrophil antibodies are needed for other disease entities such as febrile transfusion reactions, immune neutropenias after stem cell transplant, and transfusion-related acute lung injury (TRALI) as well [17]. Their second international workshop recommended that at least two methods, the indirect granulocyte agglutination test (GAT) and the granulocyte immunofluorescence test (GIFT), be used to detect anti-neutrophil antibodies [18]. However, each of these tests has its own limitations. It has been recognized that the GAT test can lead to false positives since neutrophils can agglutinate spontaneously [4, 19]; however, it has the capability to detect aggregated antibodies, such as anti-HNA-3a [20]. The direct GIFT test detects neutrophil autoantibodies using fluoresceinated human anti-immunoglobulin antibodies, whereas the indirect GIFT exposes patient serum to control neutrophils and detects autoantibodies using fluoresceinated anti-immunoglobulin antiserum [4]. The monoclonal antibody-specific immobilization of granulocyte antigen (MAIGA) assay can overcome some of these false positives, since specific monoclonal antibodies bind neutrophil antigens bound to human antibodies; however, this assay is not routinely available [4, 19], and as of yet, cannot detect anti-HNA-3a antibodies, which are most commonly implicated in fatal TRALI reactions [20]. Recently, a flow cytometric white blood cell immunofluorescence test (Flow-WIFT) has been developed to aid in the precision of this diagnosis. A recent study found this test to detect more granulocyte reactive antibodies than the GIFT, suggesting it may play a role as a screening tool in the future [20].

Human Neutrophil Alloantigens

Lalezari and Bernard in 1966 were the first to describe antineutrophil antibodies found in two infants with alloimmune neutropenia. Since then, 11 antigens have been characterized on five human proteins on the granulocyte membrane [9]. These five proteins make up the human neutrophil antigen (HNA) systems, and their revised nomenclature established in 1998 by an International Society of Blood Transfusion (ISBT) group [21] is the main classification system used today. The grouping is based on the unique surface glycoprotein location of each antigen, and polymorphisms of each antigen are labeled alphabetically and in sequential order of discovery [21, 22].

HNA-1

The most well-described component of the HNA system is HNA-1, comprised of three polymorphisms HNA-1a, HNA-1b, and HNA-1c (formerly known as NA1, NA2, and SH antigens, respectively). Approximately 35% of neutrophil autoantibodies are specific for HNA-1a and HNA-1b in patients with primary AIN of infancy [3, 9, 22]. All are located on the human neutrophil Fc gamma receptor IIIb (FcγRIIIb), a highly glycosylated protein only expressed on the surface of neutrophils and encoded by the *FCGR3B* gene located on the long arm of chromosome 1 [21, 22]. FcγRIIIb protein consists of 184 amino acids and is bound to the neutrophil membrane via a 16-amino acid peptide [23]. This protein functions to enhance both clearance of immune complexes and phagocytosis of opsonized pathogens [23].

FcγRIIIb contains two IgG-like domains, one of which has a high affinity for ligand binding and the other whose function remains unclear [22, 23]. Each antigenic polymorphism, characterized by three alleles, alters the FcγIIIb function [22]. Clinically, HNA-1a individuals have higher affinity for IgG1 and IgG3, lending to increased phagocytosis of opsonized antigens. HNA-1b individuals haves a lower affinity for phagocytosis of opsonized bacteria; thus they are more likely to develop periodontal diseases [23].

The polymorphisms have different ethnic predilections, with HNA-1a seen mainly in native American, Chinese, and Japanese populations; and HNA-1b expressed largely in Caucasian and African populations [22]. Few individuals do not express FCγRIIIb on their neutrophil membranes due to a *FCGR3B* gene deficiency and are called the HNA-1 null phenotype [22, 23]. Pregnant women with this gene defect have risk of forming specific alloantibodies which subsequently cause alloimmune neutropenia in their infants, while they themselves do not suffer from autoimmune diseases [21, 23]. Moreover, FCγRIIIb has been implicated as the target for antibodies in drug-induced immune neutropenia as well [22, 23].

HNA-2

HNA-2 was first described by Lalezari's group in 1971 and is also exclusively found on neutrophils [21]. HNA-2 has been found to be expressed on the neutrophils of 97% of Caucasians and approximately 90% of Japanese individuals [22]. HNA-2 is found on CD177 and located on chromosome 19. HNA-2 positive individuals express two neutrophil populations: one which expresses CD177 and another lacking CD177 caused by a lack of gene transcription [23]. CD177 is involved in the adhesion and migration of neutrophils into tissues by binding platelet endothelial cell adhesion molecule-1 (PECAM-1) [21, 23]. Clinically, antibodies directed against HNA-2 and HNA-3a have been detected in patients with transfusion-related acute lung injury (TRALI) [23].

HNA-3

HNA-3 is found on choline transporter-like protein 2 (CTL2), and unlike HNA-1 and HNA-2, it lacks specificity for neutrophils. It can be found in the inner ear, B- and T-lymphocytes, and platelets [23]. CTL2 is encoded by *SLC44A2* located on chromosome 19; and CTL2 antibodies induce autoimmune hearing loss.

Additionally, HNA-3a antibodies have been reported in severe TRALI cases and febrile transfusion reactions [23].

HNA-4a and HNA-5a

HNA-4a and HNA-5a are polymorphisms caused by single-point mutations in the CD11a and CD11b subunits of the leukocyte adhesion molecules (B2 integrins) found on neutrophils, monocytes, and natural killer cells (Bux 2002). HNA-4a is found on the CD11b/αM subunit of αMβ2-integrin. CD11b is encoded by the ITGAM gene locus on chromosome 16 and functions as a transmembrane protein. The αMβ2-integrin is involved in cell transmigration, phagocytosis, and oxidative burst [23]. It is unclear if the polymorphism affects these functions [23]. Two types of HNA-4a allo-antibodies exist—one is asymptomatic and the other has been reported in neonatal alloimmune neutropenia. HNA-5a is located on a leukocyte-specific adhesion mole-cule CD11a, and antibodies may also act to inhibit leukocyte interactions [23].

Treatment

Typically, primary AIN in children is self-limiting, and severe infection is exceed-ingly rare due to preservation of the bone marrow storage pool of mature neutro-phils. There is no clear consensus on the approach to fever workup in a child with classic AIN. Numerous treatment modalities, such as corticosteroids, intravenous immunoglobulin, and granulocyte-colony stimulating factor (G-CSF), have been trialled and reported in the literature, but only G-CSF was found to be effective at raising the neutrophil count [2]. Rituximab, an anti-CD20 monoclonal antibody, was used to treat six patients with AIN in one case report, with little efficacy [24].

Recombinant human granulocyte-colony stimulating factor (G-CSF) stimulates granulopoiesis and demargination of neutrophils from tissue and decreases neutro-phil apoptosis [2]. It is generally effective in raising neutrophil counts to greater than 1×10^9/L and preventing infections [1]. In patients with cyclic neutropenia or severe congenital neutropenia, fatal bacterial infections have been documented [1], and treatment with G-CSF is therefore recommended in these conditions [1].

In 2011, the Neutropenia Committee of the Marrow Failure Syndrome Group of the Associazione Italiana di Emato-Oncologia Pediatrica (AIEOP) assembled a group of international experts to make recommendations on AIN treatment in the setting of acute infection or surgery and timing of follow-up. G-CSF dosing was based on underlying disease state and target ANC range was set as $>1.0 \times 10^9$/L and $\leq 5.0 \times 10^9$/L. For rare cases of infection in AIN, a starting dose of 1–2 μg/kg/day for 1 week was suggested, with allowance to increase by 1–2 μg/kg/day every 5–7 days if ANC remained $<1.0 \times 10^9$/L [25]. In general, patients with AIN show a quick and robust response to G-CSF due to adequate marrow stores, and G-CSF therapy (especially high doses) may lead to significant bone pain [5]. If treatment is clinically indicated in AIN, the experts recommended monthly follow-up to document neutropenia resolution. If neutropenia persists, repeat testing for indirect autoantibodies against neutrophils is recommended. Of note, this same body of experts does not recommend routine use of prophylactic antibiotics for patients with AIN [25].

Use of prophylactic antibiotics such as cotrimoxazole is generally not indicated for classic AIN and is usually reserved for patients with recurrent moderate infections typical of other disorders. In the same retrospective study of 240 cases of infants with primary AIN discussed previously, 90% of cases were associated with benign infections that resolved with systemic antibiotics despite severe peripheral neutropenia [3]. Eighty-nine percent of these patients received prophylaxis with cotrimoxazole, and prophylaxis was started only after recurrent infection events. Fioredda et al. reported an infection incidence of 40% in their patients with AIN, with the most common being skin and soft tissue infections [26].

Conclusions

Autoimmune neutropenia is caused by autoantibodies against neutrophil membrane proteins, leading to enhanced peripheral clearance. Though the degree of neutropenia can be peripheral neutropenia may be severe, the bone marrow storage pool and response to bacterial challenge is generally normal. The clinical course of AIN is usually benign and the majority will resolve within 1–3 years. The diagnosis remains clinical, as neutrophil autoantibodies remain difficult to detect with current methods, even in the setting of optimal testing utilization which combines agglutination and immunofluorescence assays. The characterization of neutrophil surface antigens continues to progress and will provide further insight into the pathophysiology of immune neutropenia. Routine treatment with prophylactic antibiotics and/or G-CSF is generally not indicated and may be used for rare patients with recurrent infections or other clinical indications on an individualized but infrequent basis.

References

1. Dale DC. How I manage children with neutropenia. Br J Haematol. 2017;178(3):351–63.
2. Afzal W, Owlia MB, Hasni S. Autoimmune neutropenia updates: etiology, pathology and treatment. South Med J. 2017;110(4):300–7.
3. Bux J, Behrens G, Jaeger G, Welte K. Diagnosis and clinical course of autoimmune neutropenia in infancy: analysis of 240 cases. Blood. 1998;91:181–6.
4. Capsoni F, Sarzi-Puttini P, Zanella A. Primary and secondary autoimmune neutropenia. Arthritis Res Ther. 2005;7(50):208–14.
5. Newburger PE. Autoimmune and other acquired neutropenias. Hematol Am Soc Hematol Educ Prog. 2016;2016(1):38–42.
6. Nossent JC, Swaak AJ. Prevalence and significance of haematological abnormalities in patients with systemic lupus erythematosus. Q J Med. 1991;80:605–12.

7. Starkebaum G, Arend WP. Neutrophil-binding immunoglobulin G in systemic lupus erythematosus. J Clin Invest. 1979;64:902–12.
8. Dale DC, Welte K. Cyclic and chronic neutropenia. Cancer Treat Res. 2011;157:97–108.
9. Farrugia P, Dufour C. Diagnosis and management of primary autoimmune neutropenia in children: insights for clinicians. Ther Adv Hematol. 2015;6(1):15–24.
10. Stroncek D. Granulocyte gene polymorphisms and mutations: effects on immune response and neutrophil proliferation. Vox Sang. 2004;87(Suppl 2):101–4.
11. Rosenberg PS, Zeidler C, Bolyard AA, Alter BP, Bonilla MA, Boxer LA, et al. Stable long-term risk of leukemia in patients with severe congenital neutropenia maintained on G-CSF therapy. Br J Haematol. 2010;150:196–9.
12. Andres E, Zimmer J, Affenberger S. Idiosyncratic drug-induced agranulocytosis: update of an old disorder. Eur J Intern Med. 2006;17:529–35.
13. Bruin MCA, Borne AE, Tamminga RY, Kleijer M, Buddelmeijer L, de Haas M. Neutrophil antibody specificity in different types of childhood autoimmune neutropenia. Blood. 1999;94(5):1797–802.
14. Boxer LA, Greenberg MS, Boxer GJ, Stossel TP. Autoimmune neutropenia. N Engl J Med. 1975;293:748–53.
15. Hadley AG, Holburn AM, Bunch C, Chapel H. Anti-granulocyte opsonic activity and autoimmune neutropenia. Br J Haematol. 1986;63(3):581–9.
16. Simpson DM, Ross R. Effects of heterologous anti-neutrophil serum in guinea pigs. Hematologic and ultrastructural observations. Am J Pathol. 1971;65:79–102.
17. Bux J. Molecular Nature of Antigens implicated in immune neutropenias. International Journal Hematology. 2002;76 Suppl 1:399–403.
18. Bux J, Chapman J. Report on the second international granulocyte serology workshop. Transfusion. 1997;37(9):997–83.
19. Farrugia P. Immune neutropenias of infancy and childhood. World J Pediatr. 2016;12(2):142–8.
20. Heinzl MW, Schonbacker M, Dauber E, Panzer S, Mayr WR, Körmöczi GF. Detection of granulocyte-reactive antibodies: a comparison of different methods. Vox Sang. 2015;108:287–93.
21. Moritz E, Norcia A, Cardone J, Kuwano ST, Chiba AK, Yamamoto M, et al. Human neutrophil alloantigens systems. An Acad Bras Cienc. 2009;81(3):559–69.
22. Bux J. Human neutrophil alloantigens. Vox Sang. 2008;94:277–85.
23. Muschter S, Berthold T, Greinacher A. Developments in the definition and clinical impact of human neutrophil antigens. Curr Opin Hematol. 2011;18:452–60.
24. Dungerwalla M, Marsh JC, Tooze JA, Lucas G, Ouwehand W, Pettengell R, et al. Lack of clinical efficacy of rituximab in the treatment of autoimmune neutropenia and pure red cell aplasia: implications for their pathophysiology. Ann Hematol. 2007;86(3):191–7.
25. Fioredda F, Calvillo M, Bananomi S, Coliva T, Tucci F, Farruggia P, et al. Congenital and acquired neutropenias consensus guidelines on therapy and follow-up in childhood from the neutropenia committee of the marrow failure syndrome group of the AIEOP. Am J Hematol. 2012;87(2):238–43.
26. Fioredda F, Calvillo M, Burlando O, Riccardi F, Caviglia I, Tucci F, et al. Infectious complications in children with severe congenital autoimmune or idiopathic neutropenia: a retrospective study from the Italian neutropenia registry. Pediatr Infect Dis J. 2013;32(4):410–2.

Index

The manufacturer's authorised representative in the EU is Springer
Nature Customer Service Centre GmbH, Europaplatz 3, 69115 Heidelberg,
Germany. If you have any concerns regarding our products, please
contact ProductSafety@springernature.com

Printed and bound by CPI Group (UK) Ltd, Croydon, CR0 4YY

29/04/2026

02099451-0005